Modern Food, Moral Food

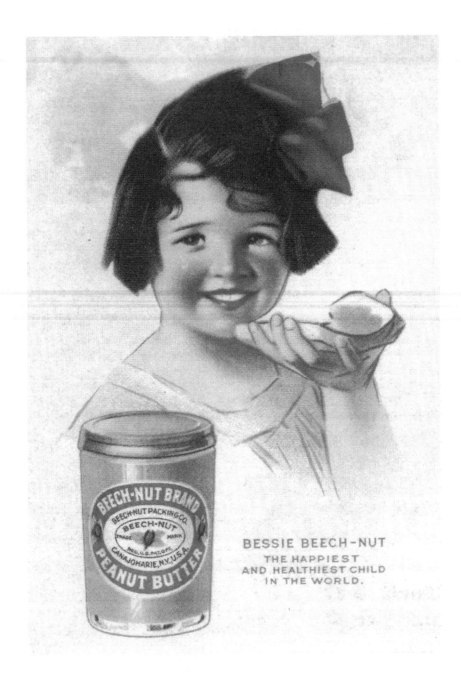

BESSIE BEECH-NUT
THE HAPPIEST
AND HEALTHIEST CHILD
IN THE WORLD.

MODERN FOOD, MORAL FOOD

Self-Control, Science, and the

Rise of Modern American Eating in the

Early Twentieth Century

Helen Zoe Veit

The University of North Carolina Press
Chapel Hill

This book was published with the assistance of the
Anniversary Fund of the University of North Carolina Press.

Library of Congress Cataloging-in-Publication Data
Veit, Helen Zoe, author.
Modern food, moral food : self-control, science, and the rise of modern
American eating in the early twentieth century / Helen Zoe Veit.
p. ; cm.
Includes bibliographical references and index.
ISBN 978-1-4696-0770-2 (cloth : alk. paper)
ISBN 978-1-4696-2647-5 (pbk.   )
I. Title. [DNLM: 1. Diet—history—United States. 2. Body Image—United States.
3. Food—history—United States. 4. Food Habits—psychology—United States.
5. History, 20th Century—United States. 6. Nutritional Requirements—
United States. 7. Social Conditions—history—United States. QT 11 AA1]
362.1—dc23
2012049092

Portions of this work appeared previously in somewhat different
form in Helen Zoe Veit, "'So Few Fat Ones Grow Old': Diet, Health, and
Virtue in the Golden Age of Rising Life Expectancy," *Endeavour* 35, no. 2–3
(June–September 2011): 91–98 (reprinted with permission from Elsevier); and
Helen Zoe Veit, "'We Were a Soft People': American Asceticism and World War I
Food Conservation," *Food, Culture and Society: An International Journal of
Multidisciplinary Research* 10, no. 2 (Summer 2007): 167–90
(reprinted with permission from Berg Publishers).

CONTENTS

ILLUSTRATIONS

ACKNOWLEDGMENTS

This book is immeasurably better than it could have been because of the guidance I got as a graduate student. I had extraordinary support at Yale, especially from Glenda Gilmore. As a scholar, a writer, and a teacher, she is a model and an inspiration. She was a source of voluminous feedback and frank advice, as well as a constant source of encouragement. I learned over time that if I had a question or a problem, she would usually have an answer of some sort back to me within hours. It's hard to overemphasize what a difference it made during some very solitary stretches of research and writing to know that she was available, if I needed her, to nudge me in the right direction. Dan Kevles supported this project from the very beginning, even before I fully realized that what I had on my hands was a book topic. He has been a rock for me, both when I was in graduate school and as a professor myself, and there was more than one time when a kind word from him gave me an injection of confidence just when I needed it most. He has been extraordinarily generous with his time and his thoughts, and I am grateful to count him as a friend. Jay Winter was indispensable, always pushing my ideas and encouraging me to think more broadly about my topic. His advice and constructive criticism made the project much stronger than it would have been otherwise. Seth Fein's enthusiasm, warmth, and boundless intellectual energy were also a great boon to this project. His high standards of academic excellence would have been daunting if not for his seemingly limitless willingness to work with me until I met them. It was also wonderful to have David Blight's support; he brought many new insights to the project, often encouraging me to trace what I had thought of as strictly twentieth-century phenomena back to their nineteenth-century roots.

I am also extremely grateful for the help of other friends and mentors from my time as a graduate student at Yale. Thank you to Jean-Christophe Agnew, Ted Bromund, Bruno Cabanes, Michael Denning, Laura Englestein, John Faragher, Paul Freedman, Joanne Freeman, Beverly Gage, Valerie Hansen, Paul Kennedy, Bettyann Kevles, Ben Kiernan, Sue Lederer, John Merriman, Kevin Repp, Jim Scott, Tim Snyder, and Chuck Walton. And thank you to the many staff members in Yale's history department who helped to make my time there happier and more productive, including Caryn Carson, Wanda Figueroa-Amaro, Carolyn Fitzgerald, Liza Joyner, Marcy Kaufman, Dana Lee, Barbara McKay, and the late Florence Thomas.

This book is much stronger than it ever would have been as a result of the extensive advice—sometimes tough to take, but usually right—that I received as part of a writing group in graduate school. My sincere thanks and affection to Adam Arenson, Gretchen Heefner, Theresa Runstedtler, Jenifer Van Vleck, and Erin Wood. Jen, in particular, has been a source of unparalleled support throughout. She worked in archives and libraries with me in three states and two continents, she read more of the manuscript than any other friend, and she always provided insightful and far-reaching comments. I am deeply grateful for her thoughts, encouragement, and friendship. Thanks also to Charles Lansing, Lindsay O'Neill, Johanna Ransmeier, and Emily Setina, friends who worked alongside me day in and day out during months of writing, and who transformed what could have been a miserable stretch into one that was fun as well as productive.

I'm exceptionally thankful for the wonderful support I got from friends throughout my time at graduate school. Thank you to Kathleen Belew, Daniel Brueckenhaus, Gerry Cadava, Kate Cambor, Sarah Cameron, Haydon Cherry, Rachel Chrastil, Amanda Ciafone, Sahr Conway-Lanz, Caitlin Crowell, Helen Curry, Nandini Deo, Catherine Dunlop, Marco Duranti, Katie Scharf Dykes, Joe Fronczak, Dan Gilbert, Blake Gilpin, Alison Greene, Julia Guarneri, Gisela Guerenstein, Robert Goree, Faith Hillis, Khurram Hussain, Tammy Ingram, Julia Irwin, Michael Jo, Scott Kleeb, Andy Knight, Eden Knudsen, Adriane Lentz-Smith, Grace Leslie, Ken Loiselle, Jake Lundberg, Rebecca McKenna Lundberg, Catherine McNeur, Mike Morgan, Aaron O'Connell, Todd Olszewski, Julie May Pepinsky, Tom Pepinsky, Isaac Reed, Laura Robson, Dana Schaffer, Sam Schaffer, Camilla Schofield, Gene Tempest, George Trumbull, Farzin Vejdani, Jason Ward, Wendy Warren, Julie Weise, and Molly Worthen. I'm also very grateful for the support I've received from other friends throughout the long process of researching and writing this book, including Paige Baldwin Ando, Ben Bagocius, Caroline Cameron, Duncan Cameron, Bonnie Crocker, Naomi Davidson, Amanda Gilvin, Rebecca Kent, Jenny Kozik, Deborah Benson Krishnan, Hill Krishnan, Molly Maclaren, Siiri Morley, Matt Mozian, Sharon Mozian, Rebecca Patkus, Emily Robichaud, Cori Scalzo, Jennie Stevenson, and Rebekah Stevenson.

As a professor at Michigan State, I have been part of a network of colleagues and friends who have given generously of time, energy, and advice.

Thank you most sincerely to Nwando Achebe, Katherine Alaimo, Peter Alegi, David Bailey, Peter Beattie, Rich Bellon, Stuart Braiman, Liam Brockey, Kendra Cheruvelil, Pero Dagbovie, Chris Daniels, Barry Decoster, Denise Demetriou, Emine Evered, Cori Fata-Hartley, Laura Fair, Kirsten Fermaglisch, Lisa Fine, Sean Forner, Chris Ganchoff, Naomi Daysog Ganchoff, Teena Gerhardt, Karrin Hanshew, LaShawn Harris, Jackie Hawthorne, Walter Hawthorne, Matt Hedden, Molly Hicks, Christina Kelly, Peter Knupfer, Brie Weaver Largent, Mark Largent, Leslie Moch, Bob Montgomery, Georgina Montgomery, Noemi Morales Sanchez, Cheryl Murphy, Edward Murphy, Christine Neejer, Michael Nelson, Matt Pauly, Rob Pennock, Chris Root, Ani Sarkissian, Kurt Scholler, Ethan Segal, Suman Seth, Sayuri Shimizu, Lewis Siegelbaum, Mónica Leal da Silva, Elizabeth Simmons, Susan Sleeper-Smith, Ben Smith, Mindy Smith, Michael Stamm, Ronen Steinberg, Gordon Stewart, Steve Stowe, Tom Summerhill, Emily Tabuteau, Chantal Tetrault, Sam Thomas, Sean Valles, Heather Varco, Mark Waddell, Naoko Wake, Abby Waller, John Waller, David Wheat, and Erica Windler. I also benefited greatly from the support of Alicia Gardner-Aben, Debra Greer, Kelli Kolasa, and Peggy Medler.

Conversations with scholars outside of Yale and Michigan State also helped to shape the book. I am especially grateful to Peter Atkins, Warren Belasco, Amy Bentley, Brooke Blower, Aaron Bobrow-Strain, Catherine Carstairs, Nancy Cott, Nick Cullather, Deborah Fitzgerald, Susanne Freidberg, Kristin Hoganson, Rachel Laudan, Kelly Sisson Lessens, James McWilliams, Christopher Otter, Kathy Peiss, Gabriella Petrick, Jeffrey Pilcher, David R. Ringrose, Laura Shapiro, Christina Simmons, Robert Mark Spaulding, Ian Tyrrell, and Tom Westerman.

I am very grateful for the generous support I received for the research and writing of this book. The Woodrow Wilson Foundation and the Andrew W. Mellon Foundation provided valuable support early in graduate school. Jim Scott and the Program in Agrarian Studies at Yale helped support my work in the U.S. National Archives, and the Smith Richardson Foundation, the Coca-Cola World Fund, and the Yale Center for International and Area Studies provided generous support for multiple domestic and international research trips. I could not have researched this book without their support.

I spent a happy and productive summer at Cornell University as the Dean's Fellow in the History of Home Economics and Human Nutrition. In addition to having a long period of time to work in Cornell's many excellent collections, the warmth and friendliness of everyone I met there made the experience a dear one to me. I would particularly like to thank the faculty in the College of Human Ecology and in the Department of History, especially Joan Jacobs Brumberg, Jan Jennings, Carol Kammen, S. Kay Obendorf, Margaret Rossiter, and Jeffery Sobal. And I am very grateful to Gret Atkin, whose kindness and competence made the experience a comfortable and easy one.

Thank you to Patricia Hand and other members of the fellowship committee at the Herbert Hoover Presidential Library, which supported my work there. I would also like to thank Paul and Ellen Gignilliat, whose fellowship helped enormously in my last year of graduate school. The Humanities and Arts Research Program Fellowship, through Michigan State, provided a much-needed semester release from teaching during which I finished this book.

The expertise and hard work of many archivists and librarians contributed to this project. I would like to thank the staff members at the National Archives in College Park, Maryland, where I spent many productive months. Thanks especially to Gene Morris, who helped me navigate the finding aids and ordered box after box of Food Administration records from cold storage in Missouri. Thank you, also, to Pamela Anderson at the Kansas City branch of the National Archives for her great help acquiring images from the collection. At Cornell, thank you to my friends at the Division of Rare and Manuscript Collections at Kroch Library, especially Elaine Engst, Heather Furnas, Eileen Keating, and Sarah Keen. At Cornell's Mann Library, thank you to Mary Ochs, and especially to Ashley Miller, who became a friend and who went out of her way to suggest several extremely useful sources. At the Herbert Hoover Presidential Library, I am very grateful to Spencer Howard and the other archivists and librarians there; I have never worked in a friendlier archive. Thank you as well to the very helpful staff at the U.S. Library of Congress, particularly to Margaret Kieckhefer. I am also very grateful to the archivists at the Schlesinger Library at Harvard University and at the Hoover Institution for War, Revolution, and Peace at Stanford University, who helped make my time in those collections extraordinarily smooth and productive. I would also like to thank the staffs at the French National Library, the French National Archives, the French departmental archives of the Somme, the Aisne, and the Marne, and the Spanish National Library. Last, but very far from least, I am enormously grateful to Peter Berg at Michigan State's Special Collections. Peter welcomed me into the exceptional culinary collection there from my first day on campus, and his extraordinary interest, knowledge, and generosity have been an unrivaled support to my research ever since.

I owe a debt of gratitude to many good people at the University of North Carolina Press, especially Chuck Grench, Mary Carley Caviness, and Sara Jo Cohen. A sincere thank you, also, to Sian Hunter.

I am enduringly grateful to the excellent professors I had as an undergraduate at Kenyon College. A sincere thank you to the historians Jeffrey Bowman, Reed Browning, Clifton Crais, Ellen Furlough, Will Scott, and Wendy Singer. In the English department, I am extremely grateful to have worked with Amy Blumenthal, Deborah Laycock, Perry Lentz, Sergei Lobanov-Rostovksy, Ellen Mankoff, and Kim McMullen. Lastly, I am deeply grateful to Peter Rutkoff, with whom I had the excellent good luck to take a history class my first semester in college. I doubt that I would have been a history major if not for that class, and I certainly can't imagine that I would have gone on to pursue a Ph.D. in history if not for him. His passion for American culture and history is contagious, and my highest goal as a teacher is to be the kind of teacher that he was, and still is, to me.

I would like to thank my family. I am deeply grateful for the love and support I get from Euphrosyne Bloom, Bill Keith, Claire Keith, Martin Keith, Minna Liret, Vicki Oeljen, Larry Roesler, Steve Roesler, Marlys Svendsen, and Shea Whittaker. And I would not be the person I am without the unwavering love and encouragement of my parents, Anita and Richard Veit, and my sister, Katherine Whittaker. Thank you for everything.

Finally, Charles. You have been a steadfast supporter and friend throughout this project, and you've seen me, and it, through good days and bad. I am profoundly grateful to be able to spend my life with you. I dedicate this book to you, to Clara, and to Gretchen.

Modern Food, Moral Food

VICTORY OVER OURSELVES

American Food in the Era of the Great War

Now is the hour of our testing.
Let us make it the hour of our victory—victory over ourselves.
—United States Food Administration slogan, 1918

In the 1890s, when a poor African American sharecropper in Mississippi ate a plate of beans, greens, gravy, and corn bread, her dinner seemed a world removed from a Gilded Age restaurant meal of steak, asparagus, béarnaise sauce, and white rolls. Just two decades later, however, by the 1910s, chemical analyses of these foods would reveal disconcerting similarities in their nutritive content. In fact, the poor southern meal—lower in fat and higher in vitamins—would increasingly look like the healthier of the two.[1] By breaking food down into units like vitamins, calories, proteins, and carbohydrates, nutritionists by the 1910s were able to argue convincingly that foods that had long seemed completely different could in fact be nutritionally equivalent. In so doing, they exposed striking similarities in foods from different classes and cultures and regions. It seems commonsensical in hindsight, but at the time this way of thinking about food was revolutionary.

Nutrition science sparked the modernization of American diets, but it was really only the beginning: the ways Americans bought, produced, ate, and thought about their food and their bodies all changed dramatically. And the most radical changes happened during the first two decades of the twentieth century, an extraordinarily short period of time. During these years, modern food science, Progressive impulses, and U.S. involvement in

World War I all came together to fundamentally change American thinking on food. The war was particularly crucial. Immediately after entering the war in 1917, the government created a powerful wartime agency called the United States Food Administration, which aimed to ship food supplies to western European allies and neutrals, where supplies in some places ran desperately low. For almost two years, the war provided a laboratory on the American home front in which the state managed food on a national scale, making food and its management patriotic projects and extending the state's reach into the home, onto dinner plates, and into kitchen cabinets. The Food Administration and the voluntary conservation campaigns that surrounded it marked the high point of a revolution in the ways Americans at all levels of society understood food.

The way we think about food now has its origins in this moment. Today, popular interest in food has never been higher, and Americans are newly vocal about the diverse pleasures of cooking, eating, and thinking about food, as well as the dire results of not thinking about it enough. Movies, magazines, websites, and television shows focusing on food have gained a firm place in mainstream media, while middle-class "foodies" unembarrassedly describe cooking and eating as central to their lives. Grocery stores offering a dizzying array of products, almost unimaginable a generation earlier, have flourished around the country. Meanwhile, driven by concerns ranging from food safety to food quality to environmental degradation to exploitative labor practices, Americans in growing numbers have become invested in knowing where their food comes from and how it is produced. As a result, interest in home food production has seen an unprecedented revival, from home baking, home canning, home brewing, and home cheese making to vegetable gardening to domestic livestock husbandry. At the same time, participation in farm shares and farmers' markets has grown rapidly, while demand for organic and local products in even conventional supermarkets has boomed. Commitment to local, seasonal, and sustainable eating has been fueled by a new genre of books and documentary films that decry the production methods of industrial food systems. Americans' food choices are regularly pointed to as vital factors in public health, social justice, national security, climate change, and even geopolitics. On a scale unrivaled since the Progressive Era, food choices have again become moral choices.

To understand food now, it is crucial to understand the origins of modern eating. In the first decades of the twentieth century, Americans were also living through a time when food had taken on urgent new importance. In the long term, many believed, national strength depended on a stable and abundant food supply, and public health depended upon a population that was literate in nutrition science. Rationalizing food production, distribution, and consumption promised to make U.S. society wealthier and more efficient, with stronger and more productive citizens. To many Americans, indeed, a comprehensive overhaul of U.S. food offered answers to a host of social questions, including physical health, wage strife, women's roles, racial fitness, Americanization, international welfare, and world peace. European food shortages during World War I clarified that world power in the new century would hinge on the ability to marshal and coordinate food resources, both within and without national borders. Whether the goal was global power or individual health, some said there was simply "no question more important" than food.[2]

None of this would have happened in the same way if it had not happened in the Progressive Era. Progressives were first and foremost confident problem solvers, people who identified social problems and set about systematically trying to solve them, whether in groups or as individuals, through private or state initiatives.[3] Classic Progressive methodology relied upon expert authority to generate solutions to social problems and upon bureaucracies to carry out those solutions. An extraordinarily broad array of Americans worked to reform food in the early twentieth century, and not all of them would have described themselves as "Progressives." In fact, most of them probably would not have known exactly what that term meant. But Progressive Era confidence in expertise, social-scientific knowledge, centralized administration, and the possibility of positive social change itself profoundly influenced the many diverse attempts to change American eating during these years.[4]

A major reason that ambitious food reform seemed possible in the first place was that so much about food had recently changed. Food practices in the United States had never been static, but major changes in previous decades had unfastened a whole generation of Americans from habitual ways of dealing with and thinking about food. Since the late nineteenth century, Americans had witnessed the rise of industrialized food production and distribution, a revolution in nutrition science, the institutionalization of home economics within U.S. public schools and universities, the shrinking presence of servants in middle-class homes, repeated attempts by reformers to Americanize the diets of immigrants and improve the diets of the poor, the beginnings of both commercial and domestic refrigeration, and a dramatic spike in food prices. Throughout the late nineteenth and early twentieth centuries it was becoming more normal to eat food that wasn't produced at home, whether it came from a restaurant or a can.[5] By the mid-1910s, the food crisis afflicting western Europe—and the notion that "famine" had struck even "the white race," as one U.S. food administrator put it—made clear that global systems were pitifully vulnerable to disruptions when left to the vagaries of weather and war.[6] High food prices at home and food shortages abroad confirmed the moral mandate to rethink the rules by which Americans ate.

More to the purpose, in fact, they confirmed the mandate to *create* rules for eating where there had seemingly been none before. The great theme of Progressive food reform was the urgent need to make everything about food more rational, and given the stakes, reformers imbued their quest for rational food with a profound sense of morality. Indeed, for many Americans in the Progressive Era the concepts of rationality and morality were virtually inseparable. That was their point. When it came to food, it was especially important to think about it rationally because it was so beguilingly easy to think about it irrationally. Emotions, traditions, and the pleasures of eating were powerful forces pushing Americans to make poor food choices. Eating the wrong things would make Americans less productive—malnourished or even "overweight," a recently coined term for a growing problem.[7] And eating the wrong things in time of war meant that U.S. allies and U.S. soldiers themselves might go hungry.

Downplaying the pleasure of eating—and even renouncing pleasure altogether in some cases—seemed to make it easier to make rational food choices. Doing so, of course, demanded enormous self-discipline, and a growing number of Americans expressed the idea that self-discipline around food was a moral virtue. And it was a virtue not only in its own right but also because it bespoke a general ability to forego immediate gratification and to control animal impulses in the interest of what people knew, intellectually, to be good and right. During a war that the U.S. government styled as an epic contest between democracy and autocracy, Americans described the internal self-control of individuals in a democracy as vastly superior to a dictatorship's external demands. Indeed, they said with growing confidence that individual self-control was the very foundation of a healthy, productive, and democratic society. Thus an astonishingly broad group of Americans in this era held up ascetic self-control as a virtue and as the enlightened pathway to mature citizenship. The Food Administration's "victory over ourselves" slogan emphasized the moral imperative of self-control around food. At the same time, of course, the slogan also acknowledged how difficult such self-control really was.

THE FOOD CRISIS OF WORLD WAR I POLITICIZED FOOD, and the book's first chapter describes how that politicization heralded a new attitude toward eating for a new century. As food administrators worked to send high-calorie, highly transportable commodities like beef, pork, white flour, butter, and sugar to war-torn Europe, they called upon Americans to voluntarily eat less of those foods, daily staples for many, in the name of a greater good. The administration's head, a young Herbert Hoover, had the power to impose a nationwide food rationing system, but instead he relied almost completely on voluntarism and propaganda, and a great many Americans ultimately welcomed the opportunities voluntary food conservation offered to exercise self-discipline. The sensual pleasures of eating went out of fashion in wartime America amid claims from both the government and from ordinary people that overeating and waste threatened moral life. In contrast, Americans who deprioritized pleasure when deciding what to eat supposedly demonstrated the depth of their self-control and, thus, their intellectual and political maturity. In Progressive debates about both food and democracy, self-control became the defining feature of those white American adults, male or female, who were worthy of full political participation.

Food administrators claimed much of their cultural authority from the recent revolution in nutrition science, and chapter 2 explores this revolution and the accompanying attempts to establish a pragmatic logic for the kinds of foods Americans ate. As food reformers in the early twentieth century worked to rationalize American diets, hoping to get people to spend both their money and their physical energy more efficiently, they codified a food philosophy that would define the era: rational decision-making based on science trumped pleasure and tradition every time when it came to eating. The wartime food conservation campaign helped popularize nutrition science, and its popularity was speeded, not slowed, by the moralism embedded in it.[8] In their quest to rationalize food, reformers promoted a variety of what they described as rational foods, ranging from cheap sources of protein and calcium, like peanut butter and cottage cheese, to foods previously considered waste products, like brains and intestines, to unfamiliar animal products, including even the meat of cats and dogs. The extremity of some reformers' dietary suggestions reveal the obsession with use value and efficiency that continued to underpin U.S. diets throughout the twentieth century, as well as what would ultimately prove to be the limits of rational eating.

Besides increasingly thinking about their food choices in terms of nutrition science, Americans also more and more considered the effects of their food choices on the world. The United States was becoming an ascendant world power during the Great War, in part because recipients of American "aid" paid for it by going into deep debt, cementing the U.S. position as postwar creditor to the empires of Europe. Chapter 3 explores how food conservation in the name of international aid was the most direct and meaningful way that ordinary Americans experienced their country's rise to power. International food aid captured Americans' imaginations, and it did so because administrators compellingly connected individuals' food choices to the welfare of people in other countries and to their own country's evolving international role. They also encouraged all Americans to see themselves as both citizens and benefactors of a hungry world. As a result, a much wider cast of characters was involved in this foreign aid project than historians have usually acknowledged, including housewives, children, poor laborers, immigrants, and African Americans—people who believed the U.S. government when it told them they could be heroic participants in international aid every time they stood up to cook or sat down to eat.

Despite its immediate relevance, however, the longest-lasting forum through which Americans considered the political and social implications of their food choices was not international food aid. Instead, it was the seemingly mundane realm of home economics. A young discipline that was expanding rapidly by the 1910s, home economics was central to Progressivism. Chapter 4 examines how home economists throughout the early twentieth century described housework as a scientific occupation with immediate value for state and society, and modern American women as the expert administrators of family diet and health. This persuasive redefinition of what it meant to be a housewife helped change attitudes as the availability of domestic servants dwindled and as middle-class women who had previously employed servants began to accept full-time housework as a personal duty, and even, to some extent, as a privilege. Women in the Progressive Era self-consciously linked their push for political rights to the politicization of cooking and other domestic work, and gender identities were transformed in tandem with social and political changes. In fact, in the context of debates over woman suffrage and the food conservation campaign itself, some women claimed that their own specialized knowledge of food production and domestic management gave them unique political insights. Home economics, together with the wartime food conservation campaign, popularized the belief that housework was public service in the private home, a labor of love *and* a form of political labor that was best performed by educated wives and mothers rather than by servants.

Meanwhile, the ersatz science of eugenics was also repositioning itself in response to changing popular beliefs about food's effects on the body. As nutritionists demonstrated that poor diets hindered both physical and mental development, Americans increasingly expressed the idea that biological parentage was only part of what went into creating healthy, productive adults. If diet could affect individual health and intelligence, it seemed obvious that the dietary habits of a race could steer its course. Chapter 5 looks at food's relationship to the powerful racial discourse of the day, as the nutrition revolution drove even die-hard eugenicists to consider the effects of diet and other environmental factors upon so-called racial development. A new discipline called "euthenics" emerged in this era to tackle the effects of environment on race, complicating eugenicists' claims that breeding was the engine of racial development. Even while maintaining a lively interest in the genetic aspects of race, both white and black euthenists argued that sanitation, exercise, and especially diet also drove racial change. In the context of changing beliefs about the limits and malleability of biological race, food in the Progressive Era became a crucible for debates about racial progress.

The final two chapters trace food changes of the Progressive Era into the 1920s and 1930s. Taking a broad view of race—precisely because that was how people then viewed it—chapter 6 looks to immigrant cuisines, Americanization efforts, and the uneasy incorporation of foreign foods into mainstream American diets throughout the first four decades of the twentieth century. Americanization efforts crested around the time of the Great War, as native-born reformers sought to convince first- and second-generation immigrants to take up nominally "American" habits, including food habits. Yet counterintuitively, at this same time more and more native-born Americans were in fact eagerly sampling what they considered foreign foods, spurred in part by wartime food conservation suggestions to try "foreign" recipes that stretched meat and wheat. Thus in the very midst of Americanization efforts, a number of immigrant dishes actually entered mainstream U.S. cookbooks and diets, especially mixed foods like pasta dishes, stews, and casseroles. The fact that these dishes became utterly commonplace in the decades that followed only points to the depth of this culinary transformation: in the early years of the twentieth century, some Americans had found these foods to be truly disgusting, a disgust sharpened by the conviction that eating gloppy foreign foods had racial consequences. In the end, Americanization efforts had the most drastic effect on the recipes themselves, and blander versions of what had seemed like threateningly exotic recipes emerged as components of a broader U.S. diet that was only strengthened by its limited diversity.

Finally, chapter 7 points to the idealization of thinness as the single most enduring expression of Progressive beliefs in the moral value of asceticism. During the 1910s, Americans made increasingly bold associations between moral righteousness, physical self-discipline, and the unattractiveness of body fat, and these associations directly contributed to the explosion of the thin ideal for both sexes—and especially for women—in the 1920s, 1930s, and beyond. While moderate amounts of excess fat had long seemed like an admirable indication of prosperity, by the late 1910s Americans in large numbers began instead to condemn excess weight as the physical evidence of gluttony and as lack of self-control made manifest. In the midst of international food shortages, Americans described fat as the visible evidence of moral weakness, and that basic idea not only survived the war but thrived in the decades that followed. The idealization of thinness that came to dominate twentieth-century conceptions of beauty grew alongside and gained strength from Progressive ideals of asceticism, moral legibility, and righteous self-discipline.

The modernization of food in the early twentieth century drew upon and contributed to Progressive beliefs about order and self-control, and these beliefs had lasting social, political, and cultural repercussions. Throughout this era, reformers aggressively touted the benefits of making American food more efficient. Far from a peripheral pursuit, they claimed, the quest for rational food could strengthen the economy, enhance public health and racial fitness, clarify women's roles, speed immigrants' assimilation, and elevate America's place in the world. Yet beneath the boosterism, reformers continually acknowledged the profound difficulty of actually extricating food from its messy cultural contexts. Eating rationally meant more than disseminating information about nutrition science, more than getting American consumers to allocate their food budgets more wisely, and more even than submitting agriculture or food processing to industrial methods. On its most basic level, rational food really did call for "victory over ourselves," a series of battles that people would have to wage and re-wage every day against inclination, against habit, and even against the drive for pleasure. Eating rationally, in other words, demanded what proved to be an unsustainable victory over some of peoples' most fundamental instincts and powerful desires.

TO TELL THE STORY OF FOOD'S MODERNIZATION, this book immerses the reader in the complex and sometimes strange world of the American

Progressive Era, letting the voices of real people articulate their own changing beliefs about food. Many of those voices come from an extraordinary source base that no historian had thoroughly explored before: the more than 380,000 letters that Americans wrote to the Food Administration in the late 1910s, housed in the U.S. National Archives' Food Administration collection. These letters provide a truly exceptional window into what ordinary people were thinking about food and eating at a time when food habits were undergoing revolutionary changes. People who wrote to the government were a self-selecting group by definition, but the letters nevertheless reveal that in terms of class, race, age, gender, and geographical location, an astounding diversity of Americans sought to communicate with their government about food. Many wrote either to praise or to denounce federal food policies. Just as often, however, letter writers veered into rich and unpredictable territory. People talked about their food preferences, justifying their likes and dislikes and providing recipes and kitchen tips. Sometimes they inventoried their pantry shelves or listed the kinds of foods growing in their gardens. Occasionally they described their efforts to gain or to lose weight. And over and over they detailed their beliefs about how eating habits could lead alternatively to moral uprightness or to moral corruption. Not only do the letters provide an unparalleled snapshot of Americans' attitudes about food in this historical moment, but the very fact that they exist in such scope and at such a scale underlines the point that food was a passionate issue. I spent months immersed in these letters, and by the end of my time in the National Archives it was obvious that they contained far more valuable material than could ever fit within the reach of a single project. These letters remain a valuable source base that other historians will wish to explore in the future.[9]

Another great boon to this project was the fact that food administrators engaged press-clipping services from 1917 to 1919 in order to gauge public sentiment across the country. During these years, press-clipping employees combed U.S. newspapers ranging from the immense to the miniscule, cutting out and cataloging any article or blurb that mentioned food, cooking, gardening, diets, or, of course, the wartime food conservation campaign itself. The fruits of their labors are also held in the National Archives' Food Administration collection. Thus with great dispatch I was able to browse food-related articles, editorials, letters, cartoons, and recipes from hundreds of newspapers, including many from towns so small it is difficult to find them on a map.[10]

Besides the National Archives, the manuscript draws from research performed at more than a dozen other archives in the United States and

Europe. Among the collections in which I worked are the archives at Cornell University on cookery, extension work, and home economics; the archives of the Hoover Institution at Stanford University; the holdings of the Hoover Presidential Library in West Branch, Iowa; the Schlesinger Library at Harvard University; and the extensive culinary collections at Michigan State University. I also made use of European archives: the French National Archives and National Library, archives in northern France from places that were rich agricultural regions before the war and scenes of some of the bloodiest fighting during the war, and the National Library of Spain.

Historical study of food forces us to confront some of our most basic human beliefs about what is normal, what is right, what is disgusting, and what is natural. Because food can seem like an intimately familiar—even a transhistorical—topic, putting food in historical context underlines the fragility of any casual assumptions about the beliefs and motivations of people in the past. I have written this book around the extraordinary primary sources I found, based on the belief that the thoughts of ordinary people are never more immediate or more revealing than when expressed in their own words. When quoting primary sources, I have attempted to remain as true as possible to the voices and intentions of the writers. Even in the 1910s, the writing of many Americans, especially those with little formal education, did not conform to uniform rules of spelling or grammar. In most cases, therefore, I have used people's words verbatim, without inserting "[sic]" to draw attention to technical errors in spelling or phrasing. Whenever I thought there might be confusion, I have clarified in the endnotes that this was the author's original spelling or grammatical structure rather than a transcription error of mine. Occasionally, quotes contained what was clearly a typo, such as one instance of "teh" in a text whose writer otherwise wrote "the." When I believed that an author would have corrected a minor mistake had she or he noticed it, I have made the correction in the quote and included the author's original words in the endnote. In all cases, I have indicated any changes in the notes.

1

NATIONAL WILLPOWER

American Asceticism and Self-Government

If men have not self-control, they are not capable
of that great thing which we call democratic government.
—Woodrow Wilson, November 1917

In January 1918, 300 of the richest women in New York City asked the government to tell them what to eat. The United States had entered the Great War nine months earlier, and food was one of the most immediate ways that American civilians experienced it. European food shortages were front-page news, and in the minds of many, the outcome of the war and the fate of the country depended on Americans' success in feeding their allies and their soldiers. The government had already launched an elaborate voluntary food conservation program orchestrated by a nationwide network of volunteers, but these wealthy New York women did not *want* their participation to be voluntary. They wanted orders. And so the Food Administration printed special ration cards just for them, setting strict weekly limits on the red meat, butter, wheat flour, and sugar they and their families could eat, although permitting unlimited amounts of milk, vegetables, nonwheat cereals, fish, and poultry.[1] After seeing their ration cards, some of the women called the program a "stiff one," but they added that the government could not ask too much of them if their sacrifices would help win the war.[2]

On one level, it was playacting. These "rations" were utterly unenforced, and compliance with them remained as voluntary as food conservation had always been. If some of those wealthy families chose to feast on pork loin and cake every night, no one was the wiser, and maybe some of them did. But on another level, the sense of obligation conferred by the idea of "rations" was clearly critical to these women. Voluntary food conservation gave them a freedom of choice they did not want; they did not want the burden of *having* to choose to go without pork and cake and all the other foods they liked, night after night. They simply wanted to be "told definitely what to eat," to be able to act morally without a moral dilemma.[3] And it soon became obvious that they were not the only ones who longed for stricter rules and less autonomy when it came to saving food. Within a week, a group of wealthy white women in New Orleans announced that they were adopting the same rationing plan.[4] By the end of another week, society women in Washington, D.C.—including the wives of senators, congressmen, and cabinet members—pledged to submit to rations, too.[5] By springtime, requests for rations were pouring into the Food Administration from across the country, especially from wealthy homes, and newspapers printed the ration plan so that anyone could follow it.[6]

When the United States entered World War I in April 1917, food supplies seemed vitally important to victory. As crop yields fell in Europe and regular distribution lines failed, each side sought to induce capitulation through military and civilian hunger, turning the war into a contest of endurance on and off the battlefield. By 1917, food scarcity had become a central factor in the military strategy of both sides. One of the first steps that President Woodrow Wilson took after American entry into the war was to create the United States Food Administration, a powerful, temporary wartime agency that combined extensive volunteer networks with unprecedented federal power in order to export as much food as possible to western European allies and neutrals. To head the Food Administration, Wilson named Herbert Hoover, a mining engineer turned public servant who had led relief efforts to feed Belgian and French civilians since the beginning of the European war.

Pressed for shipping space, the Food Administration's goal was to send nutrients to Europe in their most concentrated form. By the nutrition standards of the day, this meant prioritizing the export of beef, pork, white flour, butter, and sugar, all of which were packed with desirable calories and kept well during the transatlantic voyage. As a result, the U.S. government actively discouraged its citizens from eating those same foods, dietary staples for many Americans. Officially, the Food Administration did not encourage Americans to eat less, just to eat differently: to eat substitutes like chicken and fish and cornmeal rather than commodities needed for export. The administration's official line, which appeared on

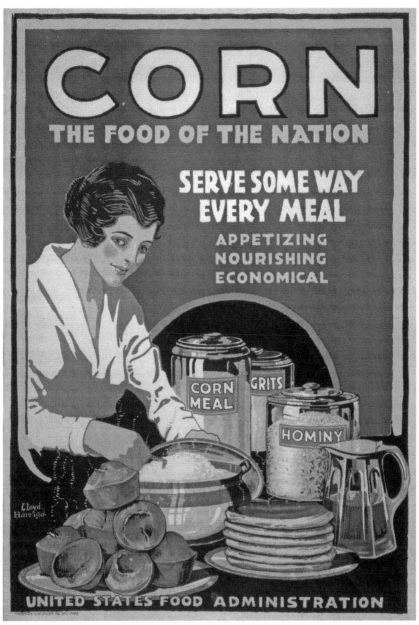

Lloyd Harrison, "Corn: The Food of the Nation," 1918. This Food Administration propaganda poster advertised some of the many uses of corn, one of the most prominent of the substitute foods administrators promoted. Harrison-Landauer Inc., Baltimore, Prints and Photographs Division, Library of Congress, Washington, D.C.

placards, membership cards, posters, and in instructional guidelines for volunteer canvassers, was that Americans "should eat plenty, wisely and without waste."[7]

But despite the official position that there was no need for Americans to reduce their overall consumption, individuals within and without the administration clearly saw the food conservation campaign as an opportunity to champion the moral value of austerity, and they drew parallels between righteous physical self-control and individuals' capacity for political self-control. Large numbers of Americans participated in the voluntary food conservation campaign to some extent, and the most enthusiastic participants often did so because they welcomed the chance to exercise ascetic self-control and to demonstrate their mastery over their own bodies. Throughout the war, administrators and other Americans adopted a rich vocabulary of sacrifice in which austerity and self-discipline figured *both* as the virtues fuelling voluntary food conservation *and* as casts of mind sympathetic to the possibility of righteous mandatory rationing, should it become necessary. Amid Progressive Era disputes over the nature of government and the meaning of democracy, some Americans during World War I came to make striking associations between self-control, a distrust of the pleasures of food, and views of the war as a morally and politically purifying experience.

THE MOST RADICAL BILL EVER ENACTED BY CONGRESS

The Food Administration's motto, "Food Will Win the War," was more than empty rhetoric. German troops had occupied Belgium and parts of northeastern France since the start of the European war in 1914, severing regular distribution networks and stifling production in what had been France's richest agricultural region. Millions of European farmers left their fields for the trenches, while drought and cold weather further depleted crop yields across Europe. The populations of Germany and Britain had come to rely heavily on imported food in previous decades, and both nations took aim at this shared weakness. Both the Allied naval blockade of Germany and the German U-boat campaign aimed to deprive civilians in other countries of food.[8] Western Europeans were not starving, but in some places wartime food shipments were the only bulwark against hunger.[9]

Americans had been hearing about food's importance to the war since 1914, when a young American engineer named Herbert Hoover became head of the Commission for Relief in Belgium.[10] The commission was a philanthropic, ostensibly neutral organization that fed millions of Belgian and French civilians during the war, using contributions from individuals and aid from allied and neutral governments. The German occupation had stifled French agricultural production and severed regular food distribution networks, and it had cut off Belgium from the imports it relied upon for upwards of 80 percent of its cereals.[11] Under Hoover's leadership, the commission was a voluntary and famously efficient organization that had enormous success in provisioning people who otherwise would have faced bleak shortages. By 1917, the commission was feeding nine million people a day, including most of the population of Belgium and occupied northern France.[12] A midwestern orphan and a self-made man, Hoover had forsaken his lucrative engineering work to head wartime food relief efforts, and he made an appealing subject of news stories about the heady potential of a "simon-pure American" abroad.[13] Hoover's coordination of food aid on an international scale was unprecedented, and it earned him a global reputation as the face of U.S. benevolence.[14]

By the time the United States entered the war in 1917, Hoover was the obvious choice to lead a formal American aid program, despite his total absence of nutritional expertise. Even as he awaited congressional approval throughout the first four months of the war, Hoover launched the still unofficial Food Administration and rolled out an extensive food conservation campaign to change the ways Americans ate. In order to export surplus food to Europe, American food administrators needed it in hand in the first place, ready for shipment in their warehouses by the New York ports. But surplus food was hard to come by. In the immediate prewar years, production levels of major American crops had only just exceeded domestic consumption. Securing surplus food required not only getting farmers to produce more beef, pork, wheat, sugar, and butter, but also, somehow, getting American consumers to eat less of them. For food conservation to work, a critical mass of people had to change their eating habits, at least temporarily. Administrators asked Americans to eat one meatless—meaning no red meat—and one wheatless meal each day, and to observe a completely meatless day on Tuesday, a porkless day on Saturday, and a wheatless day on Monday. Wartime pamphlets, posters, and cookbooks instructed Americans how to cook and eat what were to many people unfamiliar wartime substitutes like oatmeal, peanut butter, skim milk, cottage cheese, and pasta.[15]

As they worked to convince Americans to change their eating habits, administrators had to confront the very live issue of soaring food prices.[16] Between William McKinley's inauguration in 1897 and Woodrow Wilson's reelection in 1916, the cost of living in the United States had risen by almost a third.[17] Wages had risen, too, but not in pace with inflation. In early 1917, food prices that already seemed astronomical soared further still, with the price of some commodities nearly doubling, a catastrophic development for poor families who already spent more than 40 percent of their incomes on food.[18] In February and March, food riots erupted in major American cities, including New York, Boston, Baltimore, Philadelphia, Saint Louis, and Chicago.[19] Disgusted at food prices, one woman lambasted supposed American abundance while so many were suffering from chronic hunger: "But poor is the people/ Whose women must cry, / 'We work, but we starve—/ Give us food or we die!' "[20] A few weeks later, when Russian food riots sparked the revolution that toppled the tsar, they seemed like an ominous—or hopeful—herald of American events. During the spring and summer of 1917, thousands of Americans from across the country wrote to the still unofficial Food Administration to complain about prices. Sallie Bardette, a mother of thirteen in West Virginia, spoke for many when she asked "why the food bill cant be pased in a way by witch we may Have a Bite to eat in speaking distance of wages."[21]

The "food bill" to which Bardette referred was the Lever Food and Fuel Control Bill, and it was on the minds of lots of people during the summer of 1917. The Food Administration's official status—and the funding and power that would go with it—awaited the bill's passage, but it stalled in the Senate for five weeks that summer.[22] Legislators intended the bill to define and expand the government's capabilities to dampen food prices while increasing wartime food exports, and it faced fierce opposition from people who objected to its broad expansion of federal power. Especially as it concerned alcohol, food requisitioning, price fixing, and rationing, the Lever Bill generated genuine anxiety, and people called it "despotic," "antagonistic" to democracy, and "the most radical [bill] ever enacted by congress."[23]

The Lever Act *was* radical, in fact. When it finally passed Congress in August 1917, it granted audacious power to the federal government, appropriating more than $150 million for the Food Administration and granting administrators unprecedented ability to intervene in the market. One of the most controversial parts of the act was its authorization of the government to requisition any food or fuel deemed necessary from civilians.[24] In the winter of 1918, the Food Administration routinely received letters from Americans loyally providing an inventory of their pantries, because they had heard a rumor that the Food Administration wanted a "census" of all food in individual homes in advance of requisitioning personal supplies.[25] And when volunteer canvassers went door to door to gather signatures during Food Administration membership drives, they regularly encountered people scared that if they provided their names and addresses the government would come back and confiscate their canned goods and garden produce.[26] Although administrators never did requisition food from civilians and they were convinced that German propaganda was the source of the rumors, it is little wonder that such stories seemed credible given the broad powers the Lever Act granted the government to requisition food.[27]

The Lever Act was controversial in other ways, too. It handed temperance advocates a major victory by making it illegal to use food products to make hard liquor. Even more remarkably, the act also gave the president the power to prohibit the manufacture and importation of *all* alcoholic beverages, including beer and wine, if he later judged it to be necessary.[28] The act also made it illegal for anyone to hoard more than a month's worth of food or fuel or to destroy food or fuel for the purpose of raising the price.[29] The general punishment for anyone found guilty of violating part of the act was a maximum fine of $5,000, the equivalent of about $60,000 today, or two years in jail, or both.[30] It gave the government the power to take over any factory or mine related to food or fuel needs, and it authorized it to buy and sell select foods, including wheat, and to fix the price of any commodity considered necessary to the war effort.[31] Finally, most radically and most controversially of all, the act allowed the government to institute a national system of food rationing.[32]

In other words, the Lever Act made the Food Administration a wartime agency with extraordinary power to regulate the distribution, prices, and consumption of food in the United States. Yet despite the extensive powers granted his administration, Hoover consciously and publicly declined to use many of them.[33] Administrators never seized food or fuel from civilians, for instance. And although the bill allowed administrators to set food prices, they pegged only a wholesale price for wheat, otherwise shunning formal price fixing. Instead, they regulated wholesale distribution and asked newspapers to publish monthly lists of "normal" prices to tip off consumers to price-gouging retailers.[34]

Even more pointedly, as head of an administration that had the power to impose a nationwide rationing system, Hoover publicly embraced voluntarism. A fierce debate over the dangers and merits of rationing raged for the duration of the war, but the Food Administration's official stance remained that voluntary food conservation was greatly superior to compulsory rationing. The strongest power the administration ever exercised over consumers was the "fifty-fifty rule," which stipulated that consumers could purchase unlimited amounts of wheat flour as long as they bought an equal amount of some other grain at the same time, like corn, barley, or rye flour. Otherwise, the war ended without the government ever directly controlling what Americans bought or ate.[35]

The ethos of voluntarism permeated the administration as a whole. Hoover himself was a volunteer; he had accepted the job of Food Administrator on the condition that he receive no salary and that, apart from a clerical staff, unpaid volunteers do all the work.[36] The administration was still big by contemporary standards, but its paid staff of 3,000 people was small compared with the 800,000 volunteers mobilized in networks across the country.[37] Hoover also insisted that his title was "Food Administrator," not "Food Controller" or "Food Dictator," as critics and admirers alike sometimes called him.[38] Voluntarism was a savvy choice, and Hoover knew that the stance would make the gathering of power at the federal level more acceptable to his detractors.

BE YOUR OWN POLICEMAN

To a remarkable degree, voluntary food conservation took hold in the United States during the Great War. Consumption levels of the foods that administrators urged Americans to eat only sparingly, like wheat, beef, pork, and sugar, all decreased, although not by much.[39] Meanwhile, Americans ate more—much more, in some cases—of those foods administrators pushed as substitutes for commodities needed in Europe. In 1917 and 1918, compared with the average from the six years before the war, consumption of rye, barley, and buckwheat increased by 120 percent. Margarine consumption rose by 115 percent. Consumption of nuts increased by 90 percent and rice by almost 80 percent. Legume consumption increased more than 50 percent and potato consumption almost 30 percent. Corn consumption rose by about 20 percent.[40] Due in part to reduced consumption, though mainly to increased production, the United States almost tripled its wheat exports during the war, and it more than quintupled red meat exports.[41]

Why did voluntarism work at all? Certainly, many Americans remained unwilling to modify their diets in the slightest. The Food Administration received tens of thousands of letters critical of its policies, and taking factors like literacy levels, proficiency in English, fear of the government, and plain lack of interest into account, most people who did not like the Food Administration clearly did not write a letter telling them so. Yet the administration also received hundreds of thousands of enthusiastic letters, and more than fourteen million Americans—mainly women, at whom most propaganda was aimed—"joined" the Food Administration by signing membership cards pledging themselves and their families to comply with food conservation measures. After signing the nonbinding pledge, the volunteers received a colored placard to hang in their kitchen proclaiming, "Member of United States Food Administration." By the Food Administration's reckoning, about 70 percent of American families joined the Food Administration during the war.[42]

In part, voluntarism worked because of social pressure and informal surveillance networks. The Food Administration's meatless and wheatless days were a clever strategy, since setting aside specific days for group abstinence both fostered an esprit de corps and made possible the casual surveillance of friends and neighbors, whose purchase and consumption of meat and wheat on the wrong days would be more conspicuous. Some surveillance was more systematic. Howard Heinz, the young condiment magnate and Pennsylvania's state food administrator, organized a "state food police" composed of volunteer undercover snoops who worked with county food administrators to identify noncompliant individuals and to fine any businesses that violated rules.[43] For instance, the Food Administration had stipulated that restaurants could give a maximum of two ounces of bread to patrons at each meal, and when a woman carrying a small set of scales entered restaurants in Pittsburgh in early 1918 and proceeded to weigh the dinner rolls, she panicked local restaurant owners.[44] One small-town Ohio newspaper informed all women residents that if they were loyal patriots, then they should act as "policewomen" and turn in anyone who was not saving food.[45]

Mainly, though, Americans heard advice to "Be Your Own Policeman," and some were clearly eager to do so.[46] Indeed, those people who responded enthusiastically to the voluntary food conservation campaign often did so precisely because they welcomed the opportunities it provided to exercise austerity and self-discipline. To many, overeating, luxury, greed, and waste had all gained too strong a sway over national eating habits, and the country's naturally abundant food resources themselves posed a threat to upright living.[47] The governor of North Carolina called prewar America "a saturnalia of extravagance," while Harvey Wiley, the architect of the Pure Food Act of 1906, described it as "a riot of high living and high eating."[48] Since the Civil War, many lamented, extravagant living had led to physical and spiritual laxity. Because of the plentiful availability of land and good jobs, one woman claimed, Yankee thrift had wilted and in its place had flourished a slipshod and undisciplined "come-easy-go-easy spirit." In light of wartime food needs, she hoped other women would become "so aggressively thrifty that their wasteful neighbors may call them stingy."[49] The war would teach more self-restraint than Americans had known in generations, others predicted, and they would emerge from it all the happier for having learned to subdue their appetites.[50]

According to such thinking, Americans were wasteful in one sense because they were careless about food, buying too much and letting it rot, taking more than they needed onto their plates and then scraping the excess into the garbage.[51] But even more disturbing, Americans also wasted food simply by eating too much.[52] Indeed, Americans' average calorie consumption easily outpaced that of other nations according to a range of calorie-based studies, themselves relatively recent phenomena.[53] Only applied to food energy two decades earlier, by the late 1910s calories had become a powerful tool for nutritionists and bureaucrats alike.[54] According to those who derided American profligacy, however, the number of absolute calories Americans ate mattered less than the fact that Americans ate greedily and childishly. Anytime they could "get their hands on food," one Alabama journalist observed, "Americans stuff and gorge."[55] Americans ate a "scandalous" amount of candy, another journalist declared, which only further stimulated their "gluttony."[56] And when it came to gluttony, no moral equivocation was possible, because it was a biblical sin.

Another form of gluttony was excessive drinking, and there was a long-standing association in America between eating too much and drinking too much. At the turn of the century, for example, one magazine advice columnist had repeated a common warning to mothers not to feed their children too much or to make the food too delicious lest the unnatural cravings it stoked lead to "the habit of intemperate drinking."[57] The anti-alcohol movement was at the height of its power during the Great War, and the food conservation campaign borrowed freely from temperance themes and tactics, especially in its central equation of physical self-control with moral righteousness. The Food Administration's pledge card campaign—in which volunteers went door to door asking Americans to sign pledges committing themselves to go without foods on certain days—was seemingly modeled directly on the pledges temperance advocates had used for decades. Indeed, prohibitionists and food conservationists were aware that their campaigns had kindred spirits, and they amplified the similarities between immoral overeating and immoral overdrinking during the war. For instance, one food administrator who was also a zealous prohibitionist insinuated that excessive sugar consumption, like excessive drink, testified to "low moral resistance."[58] Temperance supporters emphasized that when drinking men poured their wages into the saloon, their children could go hungry as a result, and members of the Woman's Christian Temperance Union made the point by exhibiting huge piles of groceries purchased with the same amount of money it cost to buy two beers a day for a year.[59] Teetotalers were not the only ones to bend food conservation rhetoric to their own purposes, however. For a short time the Greenhut Company ran ads for "Hoover Rye, America's Conservation Whisky" highlighting the fact that it contained no wheat, although the company pulled the ads after the Food Administration wrote them an admonishing letter.[60]

In fact, prohibitionists—seemingly natural allies in the battle against decadent American food habits—initially fought against food conservation efforts. While the Lever Bill was being debated during the summer of 1917, letters poured into the Food Administration protesting any talk of wheat or sugar conservation as long as alcohol manufacture remained legal. Letter writers pointed out that the grain, sugar, and hops used by American brewers and distillers each year contained enough calories to feed seven million people, which happened to be precisely the population of Belgium.[61] When administrators calculated that if every U.S. housewife saved a slice of bread every day for a year they would collectively save seven million bushels of wheat, temperance advocates retorted that that was still only a fifteenth of the wheat used in U.S. beer and liquor production.[62] The Lever Act did outlaw the production of hard alcohol when it was signed into law in August 1917, but Woodrow Wilson did not use the power it granted him to halt beer and wine manufacture, and it outraged temperance supporters that "alcoholic German-American traitors" could continue to waste good grain by making it into alcohol.[63]

Likewise, when Hoover asked American clergymen to support food conservation, he provoked a storm of angry replies about alcohol. A typical response was that of a Presbyterian minister in Idaho who wrote back, "No sir, I have no heart to beg the people to save in minute ways when President Wilson comes out as a champion of the millions of bushels of waste—and worse, going into the making of beer."[64] Wives and mothers demanded, "*Why oh why* should we deprive our children, our hard-working husbands, fathers and sons of food they need and should have when hundreds of bushels of grain are used daily in the manufacture of intoxicating liquor?"[65] But food administrators snapped back, "Who would refuse a slice of bread to a starving child because some other child's father drinks?"[66] Brewers' output in 1917 decreased about 12 percent from the prewar average, and then in early 1918 it fell more than 27 percent from its level in early 1917.[67] Although efforts to include a full prohibition clause in the Lever Bill had not succeeded, wartime food conservation measures directly contributed to growing national sentiment that the use of grain in alcohol production—however Americans might feel about alcohol otherwise—was a luxury the country could not afford. Although it did not go into effect until January 1920, the Eighteenth Amendment, prohibiting the manufacture and sale of intoxicating liquors, was passed in the Senate in December 1917.[68]

Temperance advocates were not the only Progressives to hope that wartime privations would save a nation falling into moral decrepitude. Wealthy city dwellers, with their supposed penchants for multicourse meals, imported foods, high teas, and after-theater suppers, came under special scrutiny in the attacks on waste and excess. Hoover, himself a wealthy man who was quietly making plans to build a lavish twenty-one-room house in Palo Alto at the time, blasted the idle rich for not sharing the food-saving burden.[69] He cautioned that the urban upper class had to do away with extravagant entertainments before the Food Administration could ask the "frugal housewife of the American farm and village" to do any more scrimping.[70] In a *Los Angeles Times* article called "Sumptuous Waste," a journalist described the "gluttony" of the patrons of fancy hotels and resorts, who pretended to practice food conservation while smearing butter on everything and cramming all the bread and meat they could into their "jaded stomachs."[71] Another woman heaped scorn on those "gorging rich wasters" who were now "puffed up like poisoned pups with patriotism because they eat cornbread made with eggs and milk, and fruit with great pitchers of cream," foods many Americans could not afford in the first place.[72]

The choice to live more ascetically was a luxury, and the notion of righteous food conservation struck those with nothing to save as a cruel joke. One of the bitterest objections to food conservation measures was their incompatibility with the economic realities facing poor Americans. Although by the late 1910s Americans on the whole "probably err[ed] on the side of abundance rather than scarcity," as one home economist put it, there were many—especially those living in big cities and in Appalachia and the Deep South—whose diets were already damagingly inadequate.[73] For some people, further economizing on food meant starvation. Like civilians in the most ravaged parts of Belgium and northern France, the poorest Americans had scanty access to milk, fruits and vegetables, or decent meat, and diseases caused by malnutrition, like pellagra and rickets, were epidemic in parts of the country.[74] According to the Chicago postmaster, in

1917 the children in that city who wrote to Santa Claus asked for food more than for any other item.[75] In New York, meanwhile, a caseworker on the East Side recorded stories of desperately poor Jewish families subsisting almost entirely on bread and coffee, with watery noodle soups for dinner and only occasional scraps of meat. One mother she interviewed went to the market three times a day because otherwise her hungry children cried for any food remaining in the house.[76]

Keeping a steady supply of wheat in the United States was as important as maintaining it in France, food administrators believed, because in either place a shortage might "impair morale," as the food administrator and physiologist Alonzo Taylor mildly put it. After the American food riots in early 1917, administrators remained wary of the possibility of more—and more violent—urban unrest.[77] From Michigan, a man named Gust Stohlberg mockingly addressed Hoover as "your highnes" and threatened that 85 percent of the population would not "patiently starve to death" while the rest of the nation "is roling themselves in all concivable luxury."[78] Some people suspected government officials themselves of careless extravagance. One Tennessee woman charged that one need look no farther than Washington, D.C., and the social lives of the leaders who lived there to find a "very striking demonstration of the sin of gourmandizing."[79] Likewise, when Hoover's wife, Lou Henry Hoover, attended a meeting in New York City, one woman stood up to warn her angrily, "There has got to be some coordination between the alleged patriotic saving of the rich and the condition of the poor," or else "we'll have a fine old honest-to-God Bolsheviki here."[80]

Even among Americans who were not destitute, many were pressed up close enough to the "very rock bottom of economy" to resent any implication that they had wasteful habits to correct.[81] Hoover wanted even the poorest Americans to join the Food Administration, but a glaring problem in the administration's public relations was that many of the foods it blithely suggested as wartime substitutes—like eggs, cheese, and various kinds of fowl and fish—cost more than many workers could afford.[82] A southern farmer's daughter wrote to Hoover that their meals were *always* wheatless, meatless, and butterless by necessity, and if he did not believe her he should "come down south and visit a while and get sighted."[83] The voluntary rations adopted by those wealthy women in New York, New Orleans, and elsewhere attracted contempt, especially the clause that they could eat as much as they desired of commodities not needed for export to Europe. "Rationing?" the author of one Georgia editorial smirked. "Lots of us would like to be 'rationed' very frequently with chicken and rice, corn bread, hominy and milk, 'as much as we could desire.' Isn't it the truth!"[84] After reading a few Food Administration circulars on food economy, one Pittsburgh railroad worker wrote furiously, "Economize! If I could follow your directions and give my family what you direct I would consider myself a millionaire."[85]

One Food Administration strategy to diffuse anger over high food prices was to evoke a supposedly common legacy of Civil War privations. Hoover was well aware that parts of the country had suffered prolonged food shortages in living memory, and he tried to use the experience as a selling point for the administration's suggested wheatless diet: "Our population has lived before this on corn. For three years the Southern States lived and put up a good fight with no wheat."[86] One syndicated editorial appeared across the Midwest challenging anyone who dared to grouse about meatless and wheatless days to live off a Civil War diet for a while.[87] Although Miss Ida Beale in Cherrydale, Virginia, pledged cheerfully enough to raise her own "Potators, Cabbage, Turnips, Kale Spinnage," and, with a nod to hungry Belgium, "'*Brussells*' Sprouts," she added that she knew better than any Washington administrator what war and food shortage meant, because she was "old enough to remember the great privation of the South in 1861 and 1865."[88] Food administrators also specifically enlisted—and received—the support of Confederate organizations.[89] The United States entered World War I shortly after the fiftieth anniversary of the ending of the Civil War, and food administrators played on popular celebrations of reconciliation between North and South as they reminded Americans of their supposedly shared historical experience with food shortages.[90]

Indeed, food conservationists exploited antimodern impulses and nostalgia for simpler times in general.[91] In the modern world, they claimed, "temptations to indulgence are on every street-corner and at every family table," whereas in "pioneer days circumstances were the stern teachers of wisdom."[92] Hoover wrote a special message to Americans telling them to "go back" to a simpler way of living, one he implied that they had recently abandoned: "Go back to the simple life, / Be contented with simple food, / Simple pleasures, simple clothes. / Work hard, pray hard, play hard."[93] Hoover's "Simple Life" message appeared in newspapers around the country as well as in all manner of Food Administration literature, and it became the theme of editorials, lectures, and college courses. Warren Harding, then an Ohio senator, said the country would not need formal food conservation at all if everyone would eat like colonial Americans, and an Illinois woman suggested that churches hold colonial-themed conservation suppers where they could serve baked beans, brown bread, creamed codfish, and pickles, along with baked apples and pumpkin pie.[94] Another writer argued that even if twentieth-century Americans could not be expected to truly live like colonial people, they could still try to be as content as their forebears with "simple food" and "wholesome pleasures."[95]

THIS COUNTRY HAS TO SAVE TO SAVE ITSELF

Substitution, not reduced consumption, was the ostensible centerpiece of the food conservation campaign, and Hoover said frequently that no one was asking Americans to starve themselves.[96] Yet in spite of the policies condoning ample consumption of substitute foods, talk of eating *less* riddled food conservation material.[97] A large banner hanging in Grand Central Station during the war proclaimed, "Eat less, look better, feel better, help win the war."[98] The food administrator Ray Wilbur, who was also an esteemed physician, calculated that Americans ate as much as 40 percent more food than their bodies should have.[99] Similarly, Hoover wrote in the *Journal of Public Health* that if the food conservation campaign managed to reduce the amount of food Americans ate, it would greatly improve public health.[100]

The idea that eating less might be healthful was relatively new to most Americans. For decades, public nutritional concern had focused primarily on the problem of undernourishment, a concept long virtually identical with that of malnourishment. Indeed, those concepts were so synonymous that the English language could not readily distinguish between being thin and being poorly nourished until the 1910s: the term "undernourished" was only coined in 1910 and "malnourished" in 1911.[101] It was only during that decade that dramatic advances in nutritional understanding made clear that even someone who appeared to be sleekly well fed might turn out to be suffering from unseen vitamin deficiencies. Meanwhile, a greater general availability of food, advances in transportation, and increasingly sedentary habits were all making excess weight a more common problem. Public interest in food fads and fasting manias had crested a decade or two before the war, but their popularity had also stimulated a growing belief that eating less could be healthful.[102] In 1918, the food faddist extraordinaire Horace Fletcher wrote U.S. food administrators from Europe—where his own failing health embarrassingly belied his pretensions to nutritional expertise—to assure them that fat was totally expendable in the diets of anyone with a warm bed and only light work.[103] The classic home economics textbook of the era, Henry Sherman's *Chemistry of Food and Nutrition*, likewise advocated strict limits on calorie and fat consumption.[104]

Beyond physical health, Progressives increasingly highlighted that moral health could also result from abstention and self-discipline around food. The Food Administration had "awakened the conscience of the American people," one administrator insisted, not just because Americans were sending food to hungry friends abroad but because giving up desired foods was a moral act in itself.[105] Another top administrator told Americans to renounce "tastes and desires" themselves: taste was duplicitous and it could mislead all but the most vigilant into spending too much and eating the wrong things.[106] A blurb in a Tulsa newspaper pointed to the American palate as the "real traitor in every community," while cookbook authors deemed it the housewife's duty to buy food based on its nutrient content and not on family preferences.[107] While particularly important for curbing the whims of fussy children, eating what you were told to eat was a moral practice for adults as well.[108] If people found it unpleasant to eat unfamiliar substitutes, they should just *"keep trying,"* another cookbook writer counseled sternly.[109] Some people did. For example, a Providence woman reported proudly that she forced herself to eat fish on every meatless day, even though she loathed it.[110] When a young Ohio girl reported that she choked down oatmeal without sugar or cream, the editor of the local newspaper praised her sacrifice, adding that "the fact that it was a little disagreeable simply adds to the merit of it."[111] By these lights, individual sacrifice was a moral act in its own right, beyond and in some ways separate from its potential contribution to the war effort.

From Mississippi, likewise, a man named Edward Arps mailed a copy of his homemade treatise on food saving to the Food Administration, in which he argued that Americans could feed millions abroad if they would only accept God's message "to let go of false and vicious eating habits." He provided a handful of sample menus composed of berries, nuts, and milk, and he warned his readers that if the meals "leave an empty feeling stomach, a knawing or craving stomach, just remember that you have a diseased stomach and you dont cure it by filling it up with hot biscuits, cornbread and molasses."[112] According to Food Administration rules, of course, cornbread and molasses *were* ideal substitute foods, since they took the place of wheat and sugar, but for Arps as for many others, the details of Food Administration directions were less important than the structure that wartime food conservation provided to advance food crusades of their own.

Indeed, beyond the immediate obligations to send food to Europe, many believed that food conservation's "greater purpose" was an explicitly religious one.[113] As the historian Robert Crunden has argued, Progressive impulses were often spurred by intense religiosity and by a specifically Protestant brand of social evangelicalism.[114] In the context of saving food, construed as both a patriotic and a humanitarian act, many Americans connected their willingness to sacrifice to their religious convictions. "Oh, heed the appeal of the government to the people that ought to stop gourmandizing," the popular evangelical preacher Billy Sunday urged.[115] In fact, food saving vocabulary was often openly evangelical in tone. Administrators "preached" the "gospel of Food Conservation," especially the "gospel of the clean plate," an expression of Hoover's that became a household phrase.[116] Journalists encouraged Americans to save food with "a truly religious fervor," declaring all instances of food waste to be "sins."[117] Hoover, raised as a Quaker, hoped food conservation might also divert Americans from their peacetime materialism to focus on life's "higher purposes."[118] If Americans followed the food conservation program, according to one Kansas editorial, the country "will emerge from this war nobler, less selfish, [and] nearer to God as a nation."[119]

Food administrators also actively enlisted the involvement of the clergy. Several times during the war, Hoover sent a circular letter to preachers, rabbis, and priests around the country asking for general support and that they devote certain services to food conservation sermons, and thousands wrote back enthusiastically.[120] The Methodist-Episcopalians were one of many denominations to pass a special resolution at their national conference to cooperate with food conservation because the campaign appealed "directly to the spirit of self denial and sacrifice."[121] Seventh-Day Adventists, long-term proponents of health and dietary reforms, were especially active.[122] The Food Administration created a commission to work with Jewish organizations and to carry out food conservation propaganda in Jewish communities, and its leaders said that cooperation with the Food Administration meant "the carrying out of a high moral duty, a Jewish duty, an American duty and a duty owed to all humanity."[123] One condescending fable in a state food administration publication told of how the war converted "Papa and Mamma Rosenbloom"—grocers and former Socialists—into patriotic synagogue-goers who now "wouldn't sell you flour without substitutes for a million in cash."[124]

Federal food administrators also believed that black churches were the most effective way to reach African Americans who were not "too stiff or too limber" to be influenced at all.[125] When the head of the Negro press division drew up a list of African American men in each state who could help organize food conservation among African Americans, every single one was a minister.[126] Likewise, when food administrators invited "representative colored people" to attend a conference on African American food conservation, those representatives were overwhelmingly clergymen.[127] Even in supposedly secular pamphlets aimed at black Americans, food administers made explicitly religious appeals, arguing that food conservation was "a sacred service" offered "to Him who rules the world," and that conserving food meant "serving God."[128] Hoover wrote a letter to black ministers, asking for their help with food conservation, and many responded wholeheartedly.[129] Despite such enthusiasm, however, food administrators did not even include "negro churches" under their regular list of participating churches, but rather under "Work among the Negros."[130]

In spite of the abundance of U.S. foods like corn that were not needed for export, Americans from a variety of religions called for the federal government to establish a "national fast day," modeled on religious fasts and undertaken both as spiritual atonement and to save the rest of the world from hunger.[131] Senator Reed Smoot of Utah, the first Mormon to serve in the U.S. Senate, proposed that Americans follow the Mormon example of observing a monthly fast day, and then donate the money they would have spent on food to relief organizations.[132] While senators with farming constituencies objected to the idea and no official fast day was ever set, others went even further and called for mandatory weekly fasts, an extreme but by no means unprecedented suggestion since communal and national fast days—often infused with religiosity—had taken place periodically since the early days of colonial New England.[133] Meanwhile, articles appeared in newspapers across the country in advance of Lent in 1918 suggesting that it was a good time for everyone, whatever their religion, "to give up extravagant habits of eating and to practice self-control in eating."[134] In his pastoral letter before Lent, James Cardinal Gibbons told all Catholics that they should observe the meatless Tuesdays and porkless Saturdays asked by the Food Administrations in addition to abstaining from meat on Wednesdays and Fridays.[135] In fact, some Catholics wanted priests to ask their congregations to go entirely without meat during Lent, "thereby doing themselves good spiritually and physically," as well as helping to win the war.[136]

To many, Hoover's genius lay in his willingness to harness this religious energy to food conservation and to encourage the idea that "this country has to save to save itself."[137] Food administrators not only drew upon a range of preexisting associations between self-denial and spiritual righteousness, but they worked hard to strengthen those connections. Americans had been "in grave danger of making our bodily wants supreme," according to an article in one of the Food Administration's religious bulletins, but food conservation was teaching Americans that physical pleasures were "subject to higher regulations."[138] The author did not specify whether the higher regulations were those of the Food Administration or those of God.

WE WANT SELFISH PIGS TO SUFFER ALSO

Food conservation was voluntary, which meant that in theory people could eat all the beef, butter, and sugar they wanted and remain within their legal rights. Individuals could only be punished for hoarding or for violating the fifty-fifty rule. As they worked to inculcate a spirit of voluntarism, food administrators began to shape a narrative that went something like this: while over-rationed Germany languished and its demoralized home front began to collapse, the United States was succeeding in feeding its soldiers and allies precisely because it *inspired* Americans to sacrifice instead of forcing them to do so. According to this reasoning, the means of the war were inseparable from its ends: voluntarism trumped compulsion, and democracy trumped autocracy.[139] Of course, the equation of voluntary food conservation with democracy and rationing with autocracy was patently flawed. It was a lopsided comparison—sloppy, really—with its bizarre inference that the only factor differentiating blockaded, war-weary Germany from the crop-rich United States was the imposition or absence of government rations. And it ignored the fact that all the other major Allied governments had imposed strict rations by the end of the war. Despite its flaws, however, prescriptive versions of the formula circulated throughout the war, and administrators celebrated voluntary food conservation as proof that Americans, as citizens of a democracy, could govern themselves physically as well as politically.

Yet if the choice between voluntarism and rationing was a "Test of American Democracy," many others saw this test in a whole different light, and they believed that only nonvoluntary government rations could ensure true democratic equality.[140] Then as now, "democracy" had a range of uses and connotations, but those who clamored for stricter food control often shared an understanding of democracy as the equal obligation of citizens before the state. According to them, "democracy" meant *equality of burden*, and rationing was inherently more democratic because it prevented one group (the patriotic) from bearing the double burden of compensating for another (the shirkers).[141] In a typical comment, one California woman said that compulsory rations seemed "more democratic" since they meant "all should share alike," rather "than that the conscientious should save and the careless waste."[142] Encompassed in this understanding of democracy was an easy assumption that since many people would not naturally deny themselves anything, it was appropriate and just for the state to compel them to sacrifice.

Indeed, the fact that some Americans were eager to sacrifice and to submit to government authority themselves does not contradict arguments that coercion and vigilantism characterized the Great War home front, as put forth by the historian Christopher Capozzola.[143] Far from contradictory, in fact, these impulses were closely related. Americans held diverse views about the war, and those who believed that the war represented an urgent call to arms often said that coercing others to support it—by legal mandate or even by physical violence—was not only acceptable but desirable. Ardent food conservationists routinely expressed a desire to compel others to comply and to see shirkers pay, and people wrote to Hoover all the time expressing the hope that the government would punish neighbors or acquaintances who were ignoring conservation guidelines.[144] One Montana man, for instance, ended up serving almost three years in jail under sedition laws after he was reported for calling food conservation "a joke."[145] Some feared that in the absence of strong laws German Americans would "buy and eat and hoard all the wheat they possibly can."[146] At least one man, suspected of being German, was beaten until he signed the "voluntary" food pledge.[147]

There were varying and specific motivations behind pleas for compulsory rationing. Some people worried that as the rich splurged on delicacies the patriotic poor would suffer real deprivation. Others worried that the poor were squanderers and easily confused, or that servants would never go out of their way to conserve food without government rationing.[148] At a confidential meeting on the "food needs of the poor" held in New York City, home economists working with the Food Administration concluded, "People want orders—not advice."[149] Still others who advocated mandatory rations argued that compulsion inspired cheerful willingness, whereas voluntarism got largely apathetic results.[150] And some people, like Marie Broomfield in Rhode Island, said plainly that "we want selfish pigs to suffer also."[151]

Furthermore, many white Americans endorsed rationing because they believed that poor African Americans and immigrants were otherwise incapable of sustained self-denial. For these people, physical self-control was a central part of white adulthood and the inability to control bodily desires was a defining part of nonwhiteness. After the Armistice, for example, when the Food Administration announced an end to wheat substitutes, the author of one Maryland news article expressed the "joyous" news not in his own voice but in the mocking caricature of an African American: "'Glory be! The good old befo' de' wa' bread am back.'"[152] Reverend Gertrude Coe in Connecticut wrote to Hoover, "You are putting us on 'our honor' and alas, many of us are not yet advanced sufficiently to throw aside self."[153] In such arguments for rations, the evolutionary language about "advancing" toward a state of controlled selflessness was no accident. Nor was it purely to flatter people into saving when one food administrator said that self-control around food was proof of "high intelligence."[154] If people were intelligent and disciplined enough, they could control their appetites, and to the many people steeped in the era's racist evolutionary thinking, intelligence and discipline were advanced traits that only white people really possessed.[155] Self-discipline and the dutiful, even easy, eschewal of pleasure were supposedly distinguishing traits of whiteness, while wholehearted joy in the pleasures of food was a characteristic that whites ascribed to nonwhites.

According to this reasoning, self-control was a central pillar of what it meant to be a white adult, whether a man or a woman, capable of physical self-discipline and political self-government, deserving of full political participation. For the racially fit, self-discipline and voluntary food conservation were supposedly easy, and anyone who had trouble with the minimal sacrifices food conservation demanded was soft and suspect. Nostalgia for rugged colonial American eating sometimes intersected with these racially charged arguments. According to some, white Americans from pioneer stock should have inherited an appreciation of simple food and an ability to withstand deprivations. Pioneers had known "wheatless days in greater number than Mr. Hoover has requested," and anyone "of pioneer ancestry" who complained of the light food conservation rules was a "soft citizen and a poor patriot."[156] The food administrator Ray Wilbur, whose own grandfather was from Connecticut, said that the "clean plate of our New England ancestors must again be the symbol of American thrift."[157] Wilbur well knew that many of his listeners did not literally have New England ancestors, but his rhetoric implied that frugal eating and shopping were ways to claim a place in the symbolic lineage of white New England thrift.

Whatever they might have said publicly, food administrators were increasingly receptive to such calls for mandatory rations. Despite Hoover's vocal defense of voluntarism and his later strident opposition to Franklin

Roosevelt's rationing system in World War II, the fact that the United States never instituted rations during World War I had more to do with the short duration of the war after American involvement than with steadfast ideological conviction. Out of the public eye, administrators seriously contemplated the possibility of imposing rations starting in the fall of 1917.[158] By the summer of 1918, the administration had commissioned a secret report on the British rationing system in order to consider the application of a similar system to the United States.[159] The underlying willingness to impose rations, should Americans not conserve food voluntarily, worked in tandem with the food control message. "If we are going to be selfish," the food administrator Ray Wilbur typically said in one of his speeches, "[w]e will have to say the Prussian system is right—make them do it."[160]

HOOVER'S GOIN' TO GET YOU

To express a willingness to impose rations while simultaneously equating voluntarism with democracy required considerable rhetorical finesse, and no one's rhetoric so successfully balanced these contradictory ideas as that of Ray Lyman Wilbur. An eminent physician and an old college friend of Hoover's as well as the president of their alma mater, Stanford University, Ray Wilbur was a man of staggering energy and self-confidence.[161] During the war, he was also one of the most powerful figures in the Food Administration, the director of its Home Conservation division.[162] Of the administration's leaders, it was Ray Wilbur, towering and gaunt, with flat, wet lips and a fish-eyed stare, who emerged as the most zealous advocate of self-denial as a tenet of food conservation. Wilbur was a fervent Congregationalist and a famously dynamic public speaker, and he toured the country for four months during the war, giving thunderous, sermonlike orations in twenty states.[163] "We were a soft people," he informed his audiences in an imperative past tense, but wartime food conservation was transforming the United States from a spoiled land of plenty into a hard and righteous nation, capable of taking a leading place in the postwar world.[164] Wilbur dismissed complaints about food conservation as mewling weakness and said that Americans needed to toughen up to the realities of war.[165]

Ray Wilbur was the preeminent spokesman for popular asceticism, but others shared his suspicions about the moral fiber of anyone lukewarm about food conservation. "A Little Talk to the Food Hoarder," published in the *Oklahoma City News*, for example, described a woman who complained that the government's food regulations veered toward autocracy. In the author's opinion, the woman's questioning of the Food Administration's rhetoric about democracy and her hesitation to follow orders voluntarily proved her "[i]ncapable of self-government." The government, as a result, would have to make her food choices for her. In suggesting the government had already gone too far, she effectively forced it to go further still, "to tell her definitely just what she has to do." It was her skepticism itself that exposed her as "the kind of woman who makes government regulations necessary," the kind who needed "A Little Talk[ing]" to.[166] According to this logic, to question government regulations—about food or anything else related to the war—was to legitimate them. Similarly, in descriptions of special courses they designed for women students at universities, food administrators made clear that administration policy was to use voluntary cooperation "as much as possible," but to use compulsion "on those individuals or organizations that refuse to cooperate."[167] This remarkable statement was more of a threat than a description of practice, but administrators took pains to encourage the notion that people who failed to volunteer would be forced to cooperate anyway. The United States had "to harden," Wilbur said to the National Security League, and it could best do so by becoming stronger and more efficient: a nation lean not because it was small, but because it was muscular.[168] In Herbert Hoover's hands, Ray Wilbur believed, autocratic power would be a force for good.[169]

During the war, a veritable cult of personality emerged around Herbert Hoover, a figure almost inseparable from the concept of food conservation in the public imagination.[170] Most people who wrote to the Food Administration addressed Hoover directly, and many assumed he would respond personally. So many people sent Hoover samples of homemade conservation foods that one headline quipped that the "Food Administrator Would Welcome Visit from Mice."[171] Other people wrote Hoover asking for advice on personal problems or for loans to help with money troubles, clearly under the impression that he was as expansively kindhearted as he was powerful.[172] Magazines encouraged readers to "Hooverize" and to "Save and Serve with Hoover," and poems and ditties appeared on both sides of the Atlantic with titles like "Hooveritis" or "Hoover's Goin' to Get You," celebrating the Food Administration as Hoover's personal achievement: "Who kept the Belgians' black bread buttered? / Who fed the world when millions muttered? / . . . Hoover—that's all!"[173] One woman kept a framed picture of Hoover on the dining room table to inspire the family to eat moderately.[174] And at least a couple of children found Hoover's name so ubiquitous that they asked if Hoover was God.[175]

Administration staff, prodded by Hoover himself, discouraged the personal association of Hoover with the Food Administration, and memos went out reminding staff to try to "eliminate such terms as 'Hoover's pledge', 'Hoover's Day', 'Hoover's rules', etc."[176] Staff members avoided such terms themselves, and they occasionally corrected people who invoked Hoover's name inappropriately, but there was little concerted effort at disillusionment. One widely circulated interoffice memo encouraged clerks to preserve the beliefs of those people "who in simple, almost childlike faith, 'write a letter to Hoover,'" because preserving the notion that there was "a kindly personality" running the administration would convert anyone "simple" enough to believe such a myth into a fervent conservationist.[177]

Hoover pooh-poohed odes to his personal power, and he very publicly declined to use the full powers granted his administration. Furthermore, he would later build his political career on his supposed opposition to big government. And yet for all that, his views on federal authority during the war were anything but simple. In a *Saturday Evening Post* interview he gave shortly before accepting the job of Food Administrator in the spring of 1917, he said revealingly that to "carry on war successfully requires a dictatorship of some kind or another."[178] In another interview a few months later, Hoover reiterated, "War is an executive business. It cannot be carried out by committees." Americans had a genius for personal responsibility, Hoover said, but personal responsibility did not primarily mean individualism but rather that "we can lead *and* we can follow." A mass of individuals following no one but themselves meant anarchy, inefficient in peace and suicidal in war. Real personal responsibility meant knowing when to submit to the superior knowledge and organizational capacity of strong, centralized government.[179]

In 1917, the word "dictator" did not carry the same ugliness for most Americans that it would acquire in the following decades, but it was still not a word people used particularly lightly. Instead, it was with genuine gusto, or genuine scorn, that many people continued throughout the war to write letters to Hoover addressing him as Food Dictator. Laudatory articles appeared about Hoover with titles like "In Favor of Autocratic Food Control," "The Autocrat of the Dinner Table," and "Supreme Food Dictator."[180] As individual Americans cultivated their own willpower and exercised control over their appetites and desires, one journalist said their collective contributions would show the immense power of "National Will Power."[181] When it came to willpower, in fact, nations were *like* individuals.[182] Before any nation could conquer another "it must be able to conquer itself."[183] With the will of the nation behind it, some argued, American democracy was strong enough to contain autocratic elements.[184]

In this charged wartime context, the concept of self-control worked as a kind of bridge between desires for free, democratic cooperation and desires for the perceived power and efficiency of autocracy.[185] A nation able to conserve food voluntarily was a nation composed of disciplined individuals willingly following a centrally organized plan, people who did not need external control because they were in control of themselves. Or as President Wilson said in an address to the American Federation of Labor in November 1917, democracy meant "that we can govern ourselves." Although he was calling for union members to work without disruption for the duration of the war, editors immediately connected the tenor of Wilson's words to food control.[186] "If men have not self-control," one quoted him from that same speech in an article on food conservation, "they are not capable of that great thing we call democracy."[187] To merit full political citizenship, adults had to demonstrate self-control, and in wartime that meant submitting to food conservation rules, unhindered by personal preferences or habits.[188] According to this reasoning, if Americans *chose* to submit to federal guidelines, then democracy was still functioning perfectly.

During the public debates over whether or not to impose rations during World War I, food administrators were well aware that to equate voluntarism with democracy was facile, at best. Even while Hoover rallied Americans to the banner of food conservation with his praise of democratic voluntarism, he did so while believing—and saying—that the inefficiency and disorganization of America's "loose democracy" threatened its very survival.[189] Hoover and other food administrators remained willing to use rations to compel Americans to act with the required "self-effacement," if necessary.[190] To resolve the contradictions inherent in this logic, food administrators extolled self-control as a uniquely democratic virtue in itself.

AFTER MONTHS OF URGING MODERATE CONSERVATION, food administrators published a pamphlet in the spring of 1918 encouraging truly patriotic Americans to eliminate all wheat from their diets until the next harvest, six months away. Yes, the pamphlet's author acknowledged, wheatless days were already hard, and giving up wheat flour altogether would be onerous, but that was largely the point. "Now is the hour of our testing. Let us make it the hour of our victory," the author urged—victory not just over the enemy, but also, crucially, "victory over ourselves."[191]

The food conservation campaign of World War I contributed to new and complex beliefs about American food, especially the increasingly central idea that "the secret in eating is to become master of yourself."[192]

Wartime exhortations to change public eating habits came at a time when Americans were already changing the ways they produced, ate, and thought about food. The Food Administration did not introduce radically new ideas about food or consumption, in other words, but its dietary injunctions—loaded with a moral clout of which food advertisers could only dream—gave form and coherence to diverse ideas about food already in circulation in the early twentieth century. At this transformative juncture, a remarkable number of Americans articulated the belief that self-discipline at the table was necessary to temper the country's natural abundance and to control individuals' untrustworthy desires. Those who successfully governed themselves demonstrated their capacity for self-government, the cornerstone of political citizenship in an emerging vision of American democracy whose participants did not need dictatorial control from the outside because they were already dictators of themselves.

2

EATING CATS AND DOGS
TO FEED THE WORLD

The Progressive Quest for Rational Food

To be a good animal is the first duty of the citizen.
—Harvey Wiley, 1915

Herbert Popenoe had to go to police court after neighbors complained to the city of Washington, D.C., that he was killing and eating all the stray cats he could get his hands on. The judge dropped the charges, however, when he was unable to find any law against cat-eating. During the winter of 1918, Popenoe not only ate any number of cats himself—ranging from alley cats to a purebred Angora—but he served them to unsuspecting friends at a series of five dinner parties he gave that winter. At these "cat feasts," as Popenoe called them, he would bring out steaming plates of meat that he had cooked himself, telling his guests it was rabbit or beaver. "Most of them seemed to enjoy it," Popenoe told a reporter, "and after we had pushed back our chairs and lighted our after-dinner cigars, I told them. Some of them said it was as good as rabbit, while others began to get sick."[1] The revulsion of Popenoe's friends did not deter him. Neither did his day in court or a subsequent attempt by the same neighbors to commit him to a mental institution. Popenoe simply dismissed detractors as "less intelligent" and "unscientific," and he said he hoped to continue his experiments on dogs, horses, mules, canaries, and buzzards.[2]

Although he might sound like a crotchety local eccentric, Herbert Popenoe was in fact something of a wunderkind. He was a bright and well-educated eighteen-year-old who was then working as the acting editor of the *Journal of Heredity*, the country's leading publication on eugenics and plant and animal breeding.[3] But if Popenoe was not an elderly eccentric, neither was he a teenage prankster. In fact, Popenoe styled his cat feasts as a vital contribution to winning the Great War, and that is how the national media interpreted them, too. Moreover, Popenoe was joined in his efforts to expand Americans' culinary imaginations by the most eminent food safety authority in the country, Dr. Harvey Wiley. Wiley had spearheaded the fight for pure-food legislation earlier in the century, resulting in the passage of the Pure Food and Drug Act in 1906, and in the late 1910s he was still a household name whose writings on food and health appeared regularly in national newspapers and magazines.[4] When young Herbert Popenoe said Americans should try eating cats, his advice was provocative but dismissible. When Dr. Harvey Wiley said in his wartime speeches, "Cat and dog meat is good eating. Eat up your surplus stock of cats and dogs," he said it as national celebrity and a distinguished expert on nutrition and food safety.[5]

In a nation filled with abundant food resources and populated with pet-lovers, how can we explain this flicker of interest in dog- and cat-eating? Suggestions that Americans should eat cats, dogs, and a range of other seemingly bizarre foods were part of wide-ranging efforts in the first two decades of the twentieth century to establish rational justifications for the foods Americans ate, whether in the interest of health, economy, or patriotism, or—more nebulously but no less powerfully—in the interest of self-control as a moral virtue in its own right. Arguments for rational eating had circulated for decades, ranging from nineteenth-century health crazes to turn-of-the-century fad diets to long-standing attempts to get poor people to spend their food budgets more wisely to efforts to apply science to both agricultural production and industrial food processing.

But the Progressive quest for rational food went further still. The early-twentieth-century revolution in nutrition science gave unprecedented strength to arguments for rational eating, and by the late 1910s, the war's urgency helped to crystallize such feelings and give them broad popular appeal. By 1918, when Popenoe lashed out at critics of his cat-eating by calling them "less intelligent" and "unscientific," he was invoking what had become a Progressive truism: that science, not pleasure, was the best arbiter of wise food choices. In a time of international war, with beef and pork needed for export to Europe, he saw his own willingness to eat cat meat as a mark of his detachment from the childish demands of pleasure and culinary habit. Herbert Popenoe's cat-eating was not only part of a larger argument that truly modern people should not let factors as illogical as pleasure and tradition guide their dietary choices. It was a culmination of that argument.[6]

Besides spreading the gospel of rational eating, the war also helped popularize nutrition science itself. During the war, it would have been difficult to open an American newspaper that did not include some article about trying unfamiliar recipes or ingredients in the name of food conservation. Wartime posters, lectures, cookbooks, leaflets, classes, and news articles instructed Americans how to cook and eat substitute foods like cornmeal and fish and molasses rather than the wheat or beef or sugar needed for export. In this sense, the government campaign served as a significant form of national nutrition education as administrators reassured Americans that what mattered was not that they got beef and bread, but that they got adequate "protein" and "carbohydrates," consumed enough "calories," and ate foods that contained "vitamins." In fact, all of those terms—"strange to the lips of all but scientists" before the war, according to Herbert Hoover—would become commonplace by the end of the war.[7] Although extreme examples of the Progressive quest for rational food, suggestions to eat cats and dogs were an extension of what was becoming a mainstream plea for dietary substitution, bolstered by nutrition science.

RATIONAL DIETARIES AND POVERTY LUNCHEONS

Herbert Popenoe's recommendation of roast cat was not the first time Americans had heard advice to eat seemingly bizarre foods. Attempts to rationalize food had been simmering since at least the nineteenth century, long before young Popenoe was even born. By far the strongest antecedents of wartime pet-eating were the food fads of the late nineteenth and early twentieth centuries—the burst of interest in an array of strange diets with supposedly transformative physical and mental effects, including intensive chewing diets, one-food diets, low-protein diets, all-meat diets, raw food diets, yeast-free diets, forced feeding, fasting, and others. At first glance, food fads look like goofy, irrational approaches to food, precisely the sorts of things that would have impeded the ascent of serious nutrition science.[8] Certainly, much of the eating advice of the era looks absurd in hindsight, and sometimes the proponents of individual dietary regimes were charlatans hoping to cash in on others' gullibility. Taken as a whole, however, food fads of the period were neither irrational nor necessarily exploitative.

Indeed, despite the flawed claims of individual food fads, as a whole they constituted a collective experiment in rational food. Before an elementary consensus on nutrition had solidified, it could be very hard to tell the difference between food science and food fads. Sometimes there hardly was any difference. Guesses were a big part of early nutrition science, and in some cases, one person's guess about how metabolism or digestion worked just happened to be right. For example, one prominent fad of the era was vegetarianism, something most Americans in the early twentieth century considered a bizarre and obviously unhealthful practice. "Vegetarians tell the people to cut out meat," one *New York Times* journalist wrote scathingly in 1910, "and the people tell the vegetarians to go to blazes."[9] Only after nutrition scientists later revealed that moderation in meat eating could actually be healthful did vegetarianism gain some respectability, but its early proponents had no firmer claim to a "Rational Dietary" than those of other fads that scientists later debunked.[10] People may have shown misjudgment when they cottoned on to a fad that seems silly or nutritionally inadequate today. But if people felt better following a certain regime, who can blame them for placing some faith in its particularities, especially when other long-held beliefs about food were crumbling?

Far from two separate developments, in fact, advances in nutrition science actually spurred food fads on, while food fads' popularity in turn contributed to the growing sense that nutrition was both important and accessible to ordinary people. As basic nutrition knowledge reached a wider audience in the early twentieth century, a broad new range of people felt qualified to assert nutrition "facts" based on their own observations.[11] For example, some claimed that meat from young animals was less nutritious than meat from older animals.[12] Some swore that corn was harder to digest than wheat and that white people could not survive without wheat bread.[13] Still others said that invalids and growing children required a steady supply of sugar for good health, or that chocolate was an essential intestinal lubricant, or that deep frying was the most healthful cooking method, or that oatmeal was a wonderfully wholesome food—if and only if it was cooked at least four hours.[14] Such stabs at nutrition science were usually incomplete and often completely wrong. But at a time when formal nutrition science was just emerging, individuals' theories could borrow from its authority.

One of the most famous food fads of the era was Fletcherism, articulated in the late nineteenth century by a man named Horace Fletcher on his fervent belief that *chewing* food, and not swallowing it, should be the focus of dining. Others had sworn by mastication's importance before Fletcher, including the mid-nineteenth-century dietary and moral reformer Sylvester Graham. But Fletcher's energetic showmanship, along with his friendship with dietary entrepreneurs like John Harvey Kellogg, pushed the idea into the mainstream. According to Fletcher, everyone should chew each mouthful of food until it was a tasteless mush, only ingesting those liquids that trickled down the throat involuntarily. When there was no taste left, people were supposed to extract the "fibrous residue" left in their mouths and discretely discard it.[15] By spending so much time with food in their mouths, Fletcher claimed, eaters got complete sensory satisfaction from food without actually eating much at all, and his emphasis on the pleasure of eating inspired some of the most sensual food writing of the era, with his followers claiming that exhaustive chewing offered "a gustatory pleasure almost beyond belief."[16] And since Fletcherizing supposedly provided more satisfaction with less food, people could buy less of it and thus save money. Even while Fletcher's celebrity faded with time, his central point survived well into the twentieth century in lingering popular beliefs that lengthy, thorough chewing was healthful.

Other fad diets relied on the popular conviction that "mixed" foods like soups and pasta dishes were harder to digest than "simple" foods, meaning individual ingredients eaten one at a time.[17] The idea was that human stomachs—or at least white, American stomachs—found commingled ingredients confusing and hard to break down. The Salisbury Diet, for example, which was recommended for victims of gout, arthritis, and chronic flatulence, consisted of nothing but meat and hot water. Because the Salisbury Diet was so simple, its supporters claimed, only a very "small amount of energy was necessary for the digestion."[18] Along the same lines, Ralstonism was a school of thought dictating that people eat only one kind of food per meal, such as a lunch consisting of nothing but potatoes, then a dinner of nothing but cheese.[19] In a similar vein, other people sang the praises of fasting, claiming it gave digestive organs a needed break, freeing up the energy normally spent on digestion for other purposes.[20] By contrast, enthusiasts of "forced feeding," which meant purposefully overeating, claimed that the occasional binge supplied them with a wonderful "abundance of energy."[21]

Interest in most food fads had receded by the mid-1910s, in large part because of the emerging scientific consensus on nutrition.[22] But the retreat of food fads in the face of nutrition's academic enthronement does not mean they had been hollow or irrelevant. Indeed, the eager interest that food fads stoked in a responsive public suggests that the impulses that sustained them in the decades around the turn of the century were far from irrational. Food fads may have been amateur, but in their own way they were hyper-rational attempts to discover the rules underlying how human bodies used food.

Besides food fads, another pillar of early attempts to rationalize food was economic nutrition. By the turn of the century, it had become clear that nutrition science could save money as well as health, and spiking food prices intersected with emerging nutrition science to prompt interest in what contemporaries called the "Pecuniary Economy of Food," as people ranked foods by calories, nutrients, and price to calculate how to get the most nourishment for the least money.[23] Calories were often a central part of such thinking: according to most calculations, the more calories per pound, the higher the food's "fuel value."[24] Calories are not the only factor in nutrition, however, and some reformers worried that economic nutrition oversimplified their message. Thinking only about calories per dollar, for instance, chocolate came out superior to meat, milk, and fruits and vegetables—the cost of which looked exorbitant by this measure.[25] Meanwhile, grains were one of the cheapest forms of energy, and some feared that poor mothers might try to feed their families a nutritionally impoverished diet of bread alone.

Yet the very simplicity of such calculations appealed. Advertisements eagerly played up their products' nutritive bang for the buck, claiming that potatoes were "the cheapest highly nutritious food" or that cornmeal was the most economical grain.[26] Meanwhile, as nutrition scientists increasingly demonstrated that humans could get protein from other sources besides meat, home economists promoted protein-rich vegetarian dishes as economical alternatives.[27] For instance, a meatless cookbook from 1910 was one of several sources that highlighted the "Economic Advantages of Non-Flesh Diet," while newspapers published columns like "Foods Which Will Provide the Most Protein at Smallest Cost."[28] By the time of the war, food administrators would send out a monthly press release tabulating the number of calories available in various foods based on fluctuating food prices.[29] Administrators also promoted peanut butter as an ideal food for the poor, just as peanuts were, conveniently, becoming an increasingly significant crop in the South and as industrially produced peanut butter was becoming widely available for the first time under commercial brand names like Beech-Nut.[30]

Of course, economic nutrition suggested new ways to pacify the poor as well as to feed them, allowing employers to sidestep the question of rising food prices to some extent.[31] If workers could get the same nutrients for less money, and especially if nutrition science proved people did

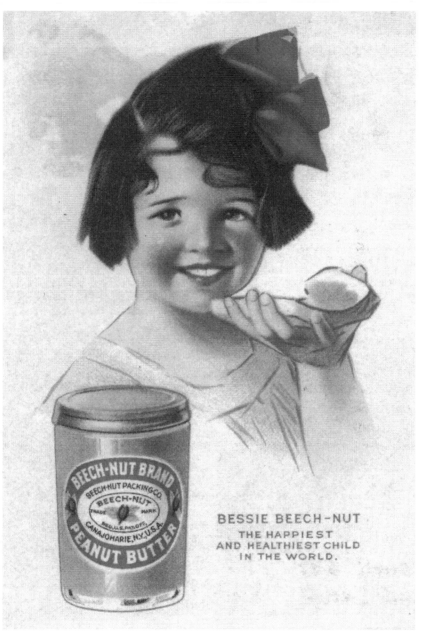

BESSIE BEECH-NUT
THE HAPPIEST
AND HEALTHIEST CHILD
IN THE WORLD.

*"Bessie Beech-Nut," pictured on company letterhead eating
Beech-Nut Brand Peanut Butter, 1917. Peanut butter became increasingly popular
starting in the late 1910s, especially as marketed as a snack and sandwich food
associated with children. Folder "48 Beech-Nut Packing Company," box 299,
Home Conservation Division, General Office, General Correspondence,
1917, RG 4, NARA, Kansas City, Mo.*

not *need* meat to survive, then it followed their wages did not need to be raised. Indeed, some argued they could be lowered.[32] With wages in mind, both nutritionists and industrialists asked: what was the minimum amount of money a person could spend on food each day?[33] Estimates ranged from $.40, less than $5.00 in today's money, to $.10, about $1.20 today.[34] If such economy was possible, according to this reasoning, then poor people who refused to live within such a budget were wasteful, gluttonous, or lazy.[35] So popular was the notion of economical eating that "Poverty Luncheons" became a popular theme party in the early twentieth century, with middle-class women taking turns competing to see who could provide the "the most elaborate meal" on a small budget.[36]

Beyond fad diets and economic nutrition, of course, perhaps the most powerful and far-reaching rationalizing influence on American eating was the industrialization of U.S. agriculture and food processing, which was taking place with dizzying speed in the decades around the turn of the century.[37] Industrial food meant more than Crisco or Cracker Jacks or Corn Flakes, though these products would all be available by the 1910s. Indeed, Americans had eaten some kinds of processed food for centuries, including what now seem lightly processed items like milled flour and refined sugar. But the food industry truly exploded in the last forty years of the nineteenth century, rapidly outpacing even the era's impressive gains in general manufacturing. By the turn of the twentieth century, the food industry was producing a fifth of all manufactured goods in the United States, thanks particularly to expansion of the canning, meat processing, and milling sectors.[38] By the late 1910s, industrially processed foods were twice as valuable a part of the U.S. economy than nonprocessed foods.[39] Many of the products shipped to Europe as food aid during the war would be industrially produced, from canned beans to condensed milk to pasteurized processed cheese, which an American company soon to be called Kraft had just started producing in the mid-1910s.[40] Indeed, as the same basic industrially processed foodstuffs were increasingly available on grocery shelves around the country, the efficiency, standardization, and economies of scale that industrial production enabled would be celebrated both as resounding successes in the quest to rationalize food and as virtues specifically linked to wartime food conservation.[41]

POPULAR SCIENCE

In the nineteenth century, hardly anyone had thought about food in terms of chemical composition. Medical schools had rarely offered information on diet, and the few nutrition texts that existed were dry and erudite.[42] All this started to change, and to change quickly, starting in the 1890s, when the U.S. government started investing in nutrition research through the Department of Agriculture's first formal experiments on animal feed.[43] The popularity of nutrition texts exploded in the next twenty years, and many of those that appeared were filled with illustrations and simple recipes and clearly aimed at nonspecialists. At the same time, cookbooks themselves increasingly included nutrition information as a matter of course, while articles drawing upon nutrition science became common fare in newspapers and women's magazines. In the 1920s and beyond, nutrition would not only be widely considered an important component of good health and preventive medicine, but it would be taught in public schools throughout the country, usually under the aegis of home economics classes.[44] It was during the first two decades of the twentieth century that nutrition metamorphosed from an esoteric subdiscipline into a respected and popular science, one that seemed both uniquely accessible to ordinary people and uniquely applicable to daily life.

By modern standards, of course, the science itself was elementary, and nutrition scientists were often wrong. In this era, for instance, nutritionists argued that stale bread was more healthful than fresh, and that saucy, mixed foods were less wholesome than plain, dry food, or that "brain-workers," farmers, and factory workers all needed totally different kinds of food from one other.[45] Nutritionists' entire obsession with digestibility would come to look misguided to future generations. Meanwhile, they had relatively few tools by which to evaluate the nutrition of specific foods beyond proteins, carbohydrates, fat, calories, and vitamins, the last of which were only very crudely understood at all. Yet even these limited tools offered new and powerful ways to describe food's nutritive content, especially the popularization of calories at the turn of the century, which made food energy readily quantifiable for the first time, and the discovery of vitamins around 1910, which shored up the idea that people had to carefully consider precisely what kinds of food they ate.

Even more radically, those basic tools of proteins, carbohydrates, fats, calories, and vitamins helped nutritionists and other reformers argue that when food was thought of in terms of its component nutrients, educated people could maximize their intake of desired components by substituting one part, or one food, for another. It was an unprecedented way to approach eating, with all sorts of implications. Immigrant fare like pasta with tomato sauce and cheese could *equal* pork chops and potatoes?[46] Lentil curry with rice could equal a steak sandwich?[47] Milk could "take the place of meat," and different fruits, vegetables, and grains could all be rough equivalents of each other, too?[48] By arguing that foods that seemed superficially very different could be vehicles for the same needed nutrients, nutritionists transformed food into a variable in a kind of cultural algebra.

Together, calories and vitamins were crucial in propelling nutrition into national consciousness. The calorie provided an unprecedented way to measure exactly how much fuel people put into their bodies. Invented in the 1820s, the calorie was an arbitrary unit of measure to calculate the energy needed to raise the temperature of one gram of water by one degree Celsius. Scientists only began to apply calories to the measurement of food energy starting in 1896, the year that the nutrition researcher Wilbur Atwater performed his first calorie experiments at Wesleyan University. In these experiments, volunteers entered a sealed chamber called a "calorimeter" from which Atwater could measure the amount of thermal energy expended versus the kinds of foods consumed. After Atwater's experiments, as the historian Nick Cullather has argued, western governments seized on calories as a way to "render food, and the eating habits of populations, politically legible."[49] On a daily level, ordinary people seized on calories, too. The first general cookbook to include the calorie content of its recipes appeared in 1916, and cookbooks increasingly included such calculations.[50] The largest national restaurant chain at the time, Child's, printed new menus in the 1910s giving the calorie content of each dish.[51] "If you want to be fashionable, really and truly fashionable," one columnist advised in the mid-1910s, "you must say, when you go into a restaurant, 'Bring me 200 calories of beef-steak, 100 calories of potatoes, 100 calories of bread,' and so on."[52] By the 1920s, references to calories would become absolutely ordinary in printed discussions of food, especially as they increasingly applied to weight reduction through calorie limitation.

In large part, calories helped redefine Americans' thinking on food because they cemented the notion that food was *fuel*, the actual source of human energy. Although this notion would also become a fundamental and seemingly intuitive way to approach food in the decades that followed, the notion that food was fuel had by no means been universally accepted before the popularization of calories. People had always known, of course, that if you did not eat you got weak and died. But even in the recent past, as the nutritionists Edwin and Lillian Brewster wrote in 1908, "[g]eneral opinion had it that the work of the body is not done on its food. A mysterious 'vital force' was supposed to animate the body and move the muscles.

Heaven supplied us at birth with enough to last us throughout our days, and every stroke of work during the longest life was done on this original supply."[53] The appeal of such vitalist theories, and the popular disconnect between food and energy, makes more sense when considering how complicated calculating food energy really is: it is not intrinsically obvious why a slice of apple should provide less energy than a slice of cheese.[54] Complicating matters further, the calorie amounts in specific foods can range all over the map, depending not only on the size of a portion but on, say, the fattiness of a particular cow. Moreover, the number of calories required for daily consumption by different individuals varies wildly according to an individual's age, size, sex, and activity level.[55] A sedentary person might eat very little and grow plump, while a lumberjack could eat like one and stay lean.

For all of these reasons, the popularization of calories was by no means an obvious or inevitable feat. It was hard to remember what exactly a calorie measured, and seemingly irrelevant even if one could. People joked about applying such a scientific term to daily eating, saying that "Calorie" sounded like a breakfast cereal brand or "a new type of explosive discovered by the War Department."[56] Yet such jokes were jokes, and by the late 1910s a lot of people got them. Reformers worked hard to make calories easier to remember, sometimes showcasing food divided into 100-calorie portions, for instance.[57] By the late 1910s, vitalist theories of human energy had become peripheral, while it had become completely ordinary to think of food as "fuel for the bodily engine" and of bodies as "human motor-cars" that ran on "bread and butter instead of gasoline."[58]

Like calories, the discovery of vitamins revolutionized popular understandings of food and nutrition. They also complicated the idea that calories-per-dollar was the most important food budgeting concern by sharpening the previously hazy notion that it was crucial to control what *kinds* of food people ate. Most crucially, they elevated the importance of fruits and vegetables, which scientists had until very recently decreed to be nutritionally worthless.[59] Westerners had long understood that eating citrus fruits could prevent or cure scurvy, but no one had been sure exactly why that was. Eminent doctors throughout the nineteenth century had denounced the idea that any food contained mysterious minerals or invisible trace elements essential to health.[60] Indeed, as time went on, evidence only seemed to confirm the nutritional insignificance of fruits and vegetables, since nineteenth-century laboratory analyses showed that they contained little besides water and carbohydrates. In 1896, for instance, one doctor and nutrition expert publicly boasted that he had taught his children that fruit had no nutritional value whatsoever and that his sons could walk by fruit stalls without feeling a twinge of temptation.[61] As late as 1911, the U.S. government nutritionist Charles Langworthy argued that fruits and vegetables were nutritionally void, and any faith in their health value was superstition.[62] Of course, Langworthy's line of reasoning indicates that some people did place faith in their health value, in spite of expert pronouncements to the contrary. But to scientists, vitamins seemed improbable. They seemed folklorish.

In the ten years that followed Langworthy's pronouncement, however, those confident dismissals of fruits and vegetables as empty frivolities virtually disappeared. Years earlier, starting in the 1880s, a few scientists had noted that some animals in laboratory settings failed to thrive when given food that was abundant in quantity but limited in type.[63] Almost no one took such data seriously, however, because it did not make sense according to prevailing models of nutritional understanding. In 1905 a scientist in Holland had published an article hypothesizing the existence of some sort of crucial trace element in milk, but his work had little effect in the greater scientific community because he published only in Dutch.[64] Only when a variety of scientists in Europe and the United States started publishing similar findings in the next few years did the idea gain widespread support. One of those scientists was an American named Elmer McCollum, who called the first widely known trace element "fat-soluble factor A" and the second "water-soluble factor B," a lettering system that would eventually be applied to all vitamins.[65] The word "vitamin" itself came from the Polish-born chemist Casimir Funk, who coined it in 1912 as a contraction of "vital amine." Amines, or amino acids, are the building blocks of protein, and Funk's own research centered on protein-deficiency diseases like beriberi, caused by a shortage of what would later be called the Vitamin B complex. The term "vitamin" stuck, even after the final "e" disappeared.[66] Scientific understanding of vitamins remained foggy throughout the 1910s, and popular explanations of them were vague, like one typical explanation in a home economics textbook that vitamins were "substances of great importance" that "scientists do not yet fully understand."[67] But lack of scientific detail did not mar vitamins' mass appeal.

Even as calories and vitamins rocketed into popular understanding in the 1910s, there was real pushback against the incursion of science and metrics into daily meals and daily life. Journalists regularly mocked nutrition science and its devotees, like the newspaper writer in Maine who sarcastically advised Americans to eat with a scale, stethoscope, and calorie table at hand, or the Philadelphia journalist who scathingly observed that humankind had managed to exist "lo, these many generations without any distinct knowledge of the fact that it lived merely because it consumed and absorbed a certain amount of alkali albuminate, aldehyde or ketone alcohols."[68] Bessie Dixon, an African American woman in Norfolk, Virginia, blasted home economists for offering advice on "carbon, oxygen, proportion, etc.," when all real people needed was food at prices they could afford.[69] At the same time, as reformers increasingly depicted educated women as the professional administrators of their families' diets, some women clearly considered new expectations about nutrition mastery a burden.[70] Only a few years before, a woman who could produce appetizing food within the family budget was considered a great success as a cook, but increasingly women who were already stretched thin also felt pressured to calculate things like protein, fiber, calories, and vitamins.[71] As a woman named Mary Gallery pleaded to Hoover from Chicago, "Do call off the scientific crowd—getting awful sick of caloric and percentage of protein at every meal!"[72]

The popularization of nutrition science was remarkably broad during the Progressive Era, but information did not reach everyone and it certainly did not reach everyone at the same rate. Nutrition education generally remained the province of middle-class Americans, and it tended to focus on middle-class concerns.[73] A woman who understood nutrition was supposedly one who could "make a dollar feed the most mouths, who can make a tempting meal out of the left-overs she finds in her refrigerator, and who can see a relishable possibility in a few scraps of meat."[74] By these lights, a cook who scrimped was a better cook than one who did not, although this was scrimping done by someone who could afford a modern refrigerator and who had meat left from one meal to the next in the first place. The poorest Americans often remained ignorant of basic nutrition precepts, and even when they did hear that they should buy milk and fresh produce, they often could not afford to. On the other economic extreme, the very wealthiest Americans were sometimes ignorant of nutrition precepts, too, precisely because they paid other people to buy, cook, and even think about their food for them.[75] For nutrition's middle-class followers, indeed, part of its appeal was the sense that nutrition knowledge was *not* universal. Middle-class writers laughed at people who were not sure whether calories "should be eaten with a knife or with a spoon" and at the dull-wittedness of rural housewives who, according to one joke, threw away their old cookbooks because they did not mention calories: "Twenty years I've been cooking and baking and feeding William and the children on food without any calories . . . and it's a wonder we're any of us alive."[76] In 1922, the creators of a Cream of Wheat advertisement relied on—and sought to heighten—white, middle-class feelings of superiority when they depicted a fictional African American chef holding up a sign that broadcast his ignorance of nutrition science: "Maybe Cream of Wheat aint got no vitamines. I dont know what them things is. If they's bugs they aint none in Cream of Wheat."[77] In contrast to such ignorance, educated white Americans could feel that they were in the know, and that possessing nutrition information itself was an elite form of scientific modernity.

FOOD IN THE COLD LIGHT OF SCIENTIFIC TRUTH

Food reformers in the first two decades of the twentieth century were in deadly earnest about the importance of their task. As they saw it, nutrition was essential to both health and economy, and to both individual and national vigor. Good nutrition habits required continual attention to food choices, and reformers hoped the daily changes they made in people's lives would inculcate broad new habits of thrift and efficiency. Sometimes they even argued that nutrition education would bolster supposedly related virtues of hygiene and temperance.[78] Meanwhile, failure to learn about nutrition spelled decline for individuals and perhaps even for the nation at large. Harvey Wiley, for instance, claimed that childhood malnutrition caused racial degeneration, and he was sure that Americans as a whole were getting smaller and weaker over time.[79] As a remedy, he suggested quite seriously that the federal government should make access to a marriage license contingent upon a nutrition exam to determine if applicants were "competent to feed [their] offspring in a proper way."[80] The argument that poor nutrition threatened national security and national vigor intensified when half a million American men recruited for the Great War were rejected for physical insufficiency.[81]

Indeed, the war magnified nutrition's patriotic implications and amplified those voices arguing that Americans should approach food rationally. Nutrition science made it seem newly important, and newly *possible*, to consider food "in the cold light of scientific truth," to choose foods because they contained the correct quantities of needed nutrients or calories, or because they were cheap, and not simply because they *tasted* good.[82] Eating rationally meant different things to different people, but the common presumption underlying such arguments was that pleasure was a dangerous guide when it came to eating. Highlighting the novelty of this premise, the historian Harvey Levenstein calls the movement that advocated choosing food for its chemical composition rather than for its taste the "New Nutrition."[83]

During the war, reformers met the question of taste head-on. Wartime cookbook authors deemed it the housewife's duty to "purchase for nutriment rather than to please her own or the family palate," and home economists informed adults that eating what they were told to eat, whether they liked it or not, was a moral practice for grown people just as much as for fussy children.[84] Herbert Hoover pointed Americans to their new duty to strip away cultural beliefs about food and "reduce food to its physiologic value."[85] With so much riding on Americans' food choices in the context of wartime food aid, it seemed immoral to prioritize pleasure, and maybe even worse, it seemed base; one Arizona journalist chastised Americans for having too often "followed the lead of a pleasant flavor, much as the lower order of animals do."[86] Only by suppressing animal appetites and eating intellectually could Americans make dietary choices to the maximum benefit of their bodies and their country.[87] To some, really enjoying food at all came to look suspect.

Deterring Americans from eating the calorie-dense staples needed for export to Europe was no easy sell. Today, the dietary changes that wartime food administrations sought to inculcate sound a lot like a health food diet: less beef and pork, butter and sugar, and white flour and more fish and poultry, unrefined sweeteners, whole grains, and produce. The point of the program was not to make Americans healthier, however, and the great majority of Americans did not perceive wartime diet changes as necessarily positive ones.[88] Getting Americans to eat less of the commodities slated for Europe meant convincing them that they could get the same nutrients as usual while eating different and sometimes wholly unfamiliar foods. To do so, wartime food propaganda leant heavily on the doctrine of substitution, the notion that different foods could equal each other in a nutritional sense, and that it was the nutritional sense that mattered.[89] As a result of the wartime emphasis on nutrition substitution, a parade of novel foods enjoyed a temporary place on American tables during the war, from peanut-mushroom loaf to oatmeal jelly to potato cookies to green pea gumdrops.[90] Of course, this supposedly culture-blind nutritional equivalency was only possible by deemphasizing tradition, habit, and, often, the pleasure of eating itself.[91] And it is revealing that many of the recipes inspired by the war—dour dishes like Emergency Biscuits, Economy Pudding, or Battle Pudding, a steamed batter of chopped meat, potatoes, flour, and milk—would vanish from cookbooks as soon as the war ended, a good sign that those who had cooked and eaten them had indeed been inspired more by patriotism than by taste.[92]

Meanwhile, wartime calls to waste nothing, not "one particle," inspired challenges to mainstream definitions of what kinds of food were acceptable for consumption.[93] For instance, one small-town Pennsylvania editor urged local housewives to soak their dirty dishes and then strain out any food particles from the dishwater to use in later meals.[94] Similarly, a Philadelphia man suggested that cafeteria managers should permit diners to return any uneaten food on a special "Conservation Tray," to be resold, though his suggestion fell flat due to new knowledge about the spread of germs.[95] Harvey Wiley insisted that U.S. farmers could support twice as many people if Americans would eat *all* available food—the skins of apples, the peels of potatoes—while failure to do so was "criminal waste."[96] Not everyone approved of such zeal, of course: in December 1917, Wiley received an anonymous package crammed with old potato peelings, with a curt note attached: "This is for your Christmas dinner."[97]

When Progressives talked about alternative meats, that food category most riddled with taboos and prohibitions, an especially keen sense of use-value and efficiency shot through their suggestions. The drive to send meat to Europe, high domestic food prices, and widely shared anxieties about the possibility of future meat shortages all fueled lively experimentation with alternatives to standard cuts of beef and pork.[98] The U.S. Food Administration joined meatpacking companies in encouraging women to cook more often with hearts, lungs, heads, feet, tripe, spleen, and other offal, a revival of cooking practices that had been common in the nineteenth century and before but that had fallen out of favor.[99] Administrators also encouraged the consumption of wild game: venison and rabbit were obvious choices, but they also suggested squirrels, songbirds, muskrat, and, for those in the Alaska territory, reindeer.[100] In newspapers across the country, shark, porpoise, and whale all received glowing publicity, and after about a hundred women approvingly tasted whale steaks at a demonstration cottage set up on Boston Common, some large eastern fish companies ordered carloads of whale meat from the Pacific coast.[101] Various reptiles, frogs, and snails also received attention as possible sources of meat.[102]

Horsemeat was the product that reformers most commonly suggested as an alternative to beef, although it offended American sensibilities almost as much as the thought of eating dogs and cats. A Chicago butcher, for instance, inspired headlines and disgust when he began to sell horseflesh, though some people certainly bought it.[103] One African American man in Chicago brought home horse steaks to his unwitting wife, who happily cooked and ate them but was later furious when she found out what she had consumed.[104] American newspapers reported that horse consumption was on the rise in war-torn France, and while this may have struck American readers as an emblem of hardship, it probably seemed less unpleasant in France itself, where horsemeat had been successfully promoted as an economical and nutritious food since the 1860s.[105] Meanwhile, so many Britons started eating horse during the war that the British Food Controller issued special licenses for butchers and retailers of horseflesh.[106]

EAT UP YOUR SURPLUS STOCK OF CATS AND DOGS

While the thought of eating frog or whale or horse was off-putting, eating dogs and cats felt profoundly, repulsively *wrong* to most Americans in the 1910s. The anthropologist Claude Lévi-Strauss famously wrote that a food must be "good to think" before it can be "good to eat."[107] Cat and dog meat never became good to think for the vast majority of Americans, but for a short time during World War I they became *possible* to think. One reason was the support of scientists, especially of Harvey Wiley himself. In the first two decades of the twentieth century, Wiley was perhaps the best known of all American food experts. For decades, he had served as the chief chemist at the Department of Agriculture, and he had been integral in shaping the pure food legislation passed in the first decade of the century. In the years that followed, moreover, he had continued to publish prolifically on food and nutrition in both academic and popular venues. As one contemporary editorial described his renown, "When Dr. Wiley made suggestions about food they were accepted as the last word in authority."[108] By the late 1910s, Wiley was the author of more than fifty books and the director of Food Sanitation and Health at the Good Housekeeping Institute.

Famous food expert though he was, however, Wiley was conspicuously absent from the ranks of the Food Administration. In truth, Wiley was in an ongoing war with Hoover over the question of whole wheat. Hoover was an engineer and not a nutritionist, but he was convinced that whole wheat caused dysentery, an extension of widely held beliefs at the time that white flour was the purest and most nutritious kind of flour.[109] A prime example of the resiliency of cultural beliefs about food in the face of scientific evidence to the contrary, it was for this reason that the United States shipped mainly white flour to Europe and that food administrators usually did not encourage Americans to eat whole wheat, even as they encouraged them to supplement their white flour consumption with corn, barley, and oat flour. Wiley was passionately angry about the omission of whole wheat from government recommendations, since it meant the U.S. government was diverting a third of the wheat supply away from human consumption. To Wiley, it was an astounding waste in a time of real need. In the spring of 1917, Wiley and Hoover argued heatedly on the point, after which time Wiley was no longer welcome to have anything to do with the Food Administration. Instead, Wiley gave a series of lectures the next winter denouncing Hoover's position on whole wheat. And it was in these lectures that he first proposed pet-eating, something he might well have hesitated to do had he been an official food administrator.

Although younger and far from a celebrity, Herbert Popenoe also had scientific authority on his side. He knew his position as the acting editor of the *Journal of Heredity* gave his actions added clout. His cat feasts attracted national news coverage, and almost all articles mentioned his work at the journal immediately, some referring to him as a "scientist" in their headlines.[110] Popenoe's work at the leading journal of eugenics also gave him access to a network of potentially influential contacts, and he purposefully included government scientists among his cat feast guests.[111] Still, Wiley's backing was invaluable. There is no evidence that Harvey Wiley and Herbert Popenoe ever communicated about cat-eating or anything else, but Wiley's enthusiastic support of the same idea gave Popenoe's cause visibility and lent it a cultural authority it would not have had otherwise.

In staging his cat feasts, Popenoe demonstrated that at least two American culinary taboos were logically groundless: one, that people should not eat carnivores, and two, that people should not eat pets. Although cat and dog flesh was widely assumed to have a gamy taste because the animals were themselves carnivores, taste seemed like a pathetic excuse when talk of self-sacrifice and duty was at a zenith.[112] And refusal to eat something because of emotion or squeamishness was particularly susceptible at this time to charges of sentimentality. Pet-eating seemed to solve several problems at once. To consume otherwise unproductive pets meant utilizing a free, abundant meat source that was easy to catch and that otherwise would itself only require *more* meat from elsewhere.

Indeed, another reason that pet-eating became conceivable was that pet-keeping itself was under siege. It had become prohibitively expensive to feed a pet for many because of soaring food prices, and it had become morally questionable for everyone in light of the campaign to send all surplus food to hungry Europeans. This sense of food waste was compounded by the fact that pets in this era usually ate recognizably human foods like bread, milk, and meat because commercial dog food was still a rarity.[113] Wartime propaganda encouraged Americans to think that feeding meat or bread to a dog meant that there was an *actual* human somewhere—possibly a child—who was not getting that very food.[114] Dogs came under specific attack because they were large animals that ate meat and also because country dogs sometimes killed sheep, threatening wool and mutton supplies. Some state legislatures imposed a tax on dogs, and a bill was introduced in Congress that would have placed a federal tax on all dogs in the country.[115]

For many, the solution to the dilemma of pet-keeping was simply to exterminate their pets, even if they did not eat them. Harvey Wiley forcefully promoted this view himself. "Kill all your pet dogs and cats, but save their hides," Wiley would say in his speeches, and he described an old woman he knew who kept "a mangy, short-winded pup with a bad disposition that eats enough to keep three healthy babies."[116] Newspapers during the war were filled with accounts of people who killed their pets, either because they could no longer afford to feed them, or because they felt it was the ethical thing to do. One California man wrote a letter to the editor explaining that his family had kept six cats, but the week before "we sent three of them to cat heaven, wherever that is, by the shotgun route, and one of the office cats is under sentence." The man calculated that his family had been spending $100 a year on meat, bread, and milk for the cats, the equivalent of more than $1,000 today, and "we might better be giving that amount . . . to help feed hungry people."[117] One letter to the editor in a Fresno paper complained that there had been a "wholesale slaughter" of the city's pets after the paper published an article criticizing pet-keeping in wartime.[118] A poem in the *Los Angeles Times* concluded:

> The bone I gave Ponto bore too much of meat;
> And now we are learning to save.
> So a pup that is gnawing what I ought to eat
> Is better off in the grave.

The editorial that followed praised dogs' devotion and affection, but the writer accepted the logic that *all* food was needed for humans.[119]

Furthermore, while few people relished the thought of killing a companion animal, neither was the prospect morally explosive. Americans' relationships with their pets at this time were quite different from what they would be by the mid-twentieth century. For one thing, small-animal veterinarians were rare and most pets were not spayed or neutered. As a result, many people were thoroughly accustomed to controlling animal populations by killing their pets' unwanted progeny, usually by drowning them.[120] At the same time, Americans were used to living intimately with animals that they later killed and ate. Horses were not the only large animals urban Americans encountered on a regular basis. Well into the 1920s, it was common to keep chickens, pigs, and even cows in American towns, cities, and suburbs.[121] Hoover actually relied upon this practice when he started his "Keep-a-Hog Movement," encouraging suburbanites to replace their pet dogs with pet hogs that they could feed on kitchen scraps and later slaughter and eat.[122]

A final reason that cat- and dog-eating entered the borderlands of Americans' culinary imaginations was that some Europeans were eating them, if only under conditions of extreme scarcity. American journalists pointed out that Parisians had been glad to eat dogs and cats, as well as all the animals in the zoo, during the Siege of Paris in 1870 and 1871.[123] In the current war, Belgians sometimes ate cats and dog meat was a relatively common item in Belgian butcher shops, where it sold at high prices.[124] By the final two years of the war, Germans and Austrians were sometimes eating dogs, too, and it was only when dog meat itself became scarce in the winter of 1918 that American journalists interpreted it as a harbinger of imminent capitulation.[125] The fact that western Europeans were resorting to dog and cat meat spurred Americans to conserve food more strenuously, but it also served as a reminder that such a thing was possible.

WHEN THINKING ABOUT EATING, a favorite metaphor of Progressives was the human engine, a model of rationalization, efficiency, and perfectibility. Harvey Wiley's favorite metaphor, however, was the human animal. To deny humans' animalistic nature was naive, even delusional, he believed. Humans were gloriously omnivorous animals, and whatever preferences they might cling to, they could potentially eat any type of food.[126] This made their food habits infinitely malleable, and in the twentieth century that meant subject to the needs of the state. "'To be a good animal is the first duty of the citizen,'" Wiley wrote, paraphrasing the Victorian writer John Ruskin.[127] His own young sons, he said proudly, were "good animals of the first degree."[128] To Wiley, the needs of an animal were no less regular— or regulatable—than those of a machine. The crucial difference between humans and machines was that humans could *reason*. They could prioritize nutriment, fitness, and the needs of their country. If they were self-disciplined enough, they could slough off habits or personal preferences at will in the name of a greater good.

Herbert Popenoe and Harvey Wiley stepped forward with their modest proposal to eat cat and dog meat at a time when Americans in large numbers were deemphasizing the pleasure of eating, and as a consensus was emerging that even radical culinary experimentation could be at once humanitarian, scientific, and patriotic. Yet despite Wiley's credentials and name-recognition, hardly anyone actually ate their pets, even when they had already killed them in the name of food conservation. For a short time, the food conservation campaign of World War I and the moral zeal it inspired radically expanded American beliefs about the kinds of animals that had flesh acceptable for consumption. However, even as they exemplified rational approaches to food, suggestions to eat pets also exposed some of the limits of Progressive logic. For most alternative foods, in fact, inclusion in daily fare was a temporary expediency, a sacrifice that people happily abandoned when the war ended.

Yet in other ways the Progressive quest for rational nutrition was a great and lasting success. Although it is hard to imagine a century later, many of the foods that got a boost in the war effort and *did* become part of mainstream American diets struck many Americans at the time as objectively nauseating—foods like the sticky, gritty mass produced by grinding a southern legume that American schoolchildren were just starting to clamor for as "peanut butter," or the glutinous pastes that when rolled out and dried became "pasta," or the white, slimy, loose clumps home economists promoted as "cottage cheese." And perhaps most lasting and most successful of all, the industrial food system that emerged in the United States starting in the late nineteenth century was one founded upon the same idealization of efficiency, metrics, and science that underlay Progressive thinking about food during the era of the Great War.

3

FOOD WILL WIN THE WORLD

Food Aid and American Power

It looks, does it not, as if the crowns of Europe were toppling
from the heads of kings. Perhaps you are going to wear them as a halo.
—Ray Wilbur, in a speech to American women, 1917

"Gentlemen, Europe has begun to take stock of us," Herbert Hoover announced in a fund-raising speech in New York in February 1917. Since the
start of the war in Europe, Hoover had led food relief efforts as head of the
Commission for Relief in Belgium. In the months before the United States
entered the Great War as a belligerent, Hoover made a brief trip to the
United States to drum up enthusiasm—and money—for the cause of feeding hungry Belgian and French civilians in occupied areas. He stressed
over and over again in his speeches that America's global position was
changing. In their unprecedented efforts to feed hungry Belgians, he said,
Americans had "laid claim to idealism, a devotion to humanity, and to
great benevolence," but he warned that if they did not increase their support of food relief efforts, their newly minted international reputation for
benevolence would fade.[1] Hoover based his appeals on the idea that Europeans were reassessing Americans: "Europe is *looking* at us; our measure
is being taken."[2] And this was a powerful argument precisely because it
was a moment when Americans were taking stock of themselves anew.

Once the United States entered the war in 1917 and Woodrow Wilson
created the United States Food Administration, Hoover no longer had
to bother with piecemeal fund-raising. Congress allocated $150 million
for the Food Administration, and in the next year and a half it exported

enough food to feed tens of millions of Allied civilians and soldiers.[3] The international food relief project of World War I was America's first formal foreign aid program, and it was unprecedented in its scope.[4] Both the novelty and the ambition of the program buoyed up the claim that in the midst of destruction and death the United States was the one nation whose citizens were devoted to saving lives. Yet although the food aid program was styled as altruism, "aid" in this context is a very complicated term. The U.S. Food Administration was never simply philanthropic. Most obviously, of course, food aid was strategic, and as food shortages worsened on both sides of the conflict, Americans openly considered food shipments a kind of military supply along with guns or gas masks. At the same time, the project was animated by the widely shared hope that food aid would boost the country's international standing in the future, permanently elevating Americans in the eyes of thankful Europeans.

The strategic goals of provisioning America's allies and securing their lasting gratitude were both important factors. They set a precedent for what would become a long-standing U.S. policy of strategically offering—and withholding—food aid, and they also complicated contemporary claims to pure benevolence.[5] But in this case the idea of "aid" is more complicated still. The Allies paid for the enormous flow of American foodstuffs with loans from the United States itself, and those loans helped secure the United States' role as a powerful creditor to Europe after the war. Furthermore, Hoover was proud to run the administration on a business model, and he ran it for profit. After the war, Hoover not only returned the $150 million that Congress had allocated, but he also turned over more than $50 million in profits to the U.S. Treasury.[6] As Hoover put it, "the Administration cost the government over $50,000,000 less than nothing."[7] Feeding hungry Europeans and U.S. soldiers was always Hoover's central goal, in the name of humanitarianism as well as in the name of victory. For example, when it became clear that by bidding against each other for limited food shipments Allied governments were driving up food prices, Hoover urged them to create an inter-Allied food board to dampen competition in the international food market.[8] But that $50 million in profits makes it clear that food administrators could have lowered their prices much further still.[9] Moreover, while administrators stressed to Americans that diets with less meat could be both healthful and economical, it is noteworthy that they continued to prioritize costly meat for their European markets.

Hoover trumpeted the Food Administration's corporate model, in part to defuse accusations that food aid was socialistic, and the U.S. media generally celebrated his entrepreneurial instincts.[10] But in spite of the overtly strategic goals of the program and the fact that it ultimately cost the United States "less than nothing," individual Americans still overwhelmingly described food aid as a great and unambiguously moral accomplishment. After all, there *was* a cost to the millions of Americans who voluntarily ate less, ate differently, and gave up favorite foods in the name of feeding foreigners and soldiers. Moral inducements to save food so that unseen others might eat were powerful tools of mass mobilization on the U.S. home front, and they were the basis of food conservation appeals. Although plenty of Americans chose not to conserve food on any terms, it is little wonder that for those who did practice self-denial in the name of helping others, benevolence indeed seemed to undergird the program. "Do something for other people!" the evangelist Billy Sunday said in a sermon on food conservation, and some people willingly did.[11] Popular perceptions of American generosity infused descriptions of the country's changing international role, and when individuals described their country's new power as one that was predicated on goodwill and good works, those descriptions probably reflected their own moral convictions and willingness to sacrifice at least as much as their naïveté.

Despite widespread pride in the food aid program, Americans generally hesitated, at least far more than they would later in the twentieth century, to assert that they were objectively worthy of adoration. But they eagerly pointed to the existence of food aid to Europe as a powerful sign of how much their country's international standing was changing. Americans had of course measured themselves against Europe since the country's earliest days, but the war gave these comparisons a sharply materialist edge they had never had before. The United States' position vis-à-vis France was an especially meaningful barometer of shifting geopolitics. In part, this was because fighting on the western front devastated French agriculture and because France received more aid than any other ally. Perhaps equally importantly, French culture and French food in particular were long-standing symbols of high European culture. By drawing attention to—and sometimes by simply imagining—how French and other European beneficiaries viewed them, Americans during World War I drew attention to real changes in international power relations while also providing an exceptionally clear picture of the way they hoped to be seen.

THEY WILL EAT OUT OF OUR HANDS

A major reason for reassessing American power in this era was that the European food crisis of the 1910s was making it newly clear that agriculture was vital to geopolitics. Viewed in agricultural terms, with newly justified Malthusian fears about demand for food overtaking supply as a backdrop, the immense size and clearly enormous productive capacity of the United States were crucial parts of the calculus of what world power would mean in the future.[12] The United States had almost 300 million acres under cultivation in the 1910s, more than any other country in the world. And large as that number was, it still represented only a small fraction—15 percent— of the country's total area. In contrast, France cultivated sixty million acres and Britain eighteen million, and even those comparatively small amounts already consumed almost half of France's total area and about a quarter of Britain's.[13] By European standards, the United States' potential to produce food and to support a booming population was mammoth. Already in 1915, one article had crowed that after the war the United States "need be afraid of no nation" because exhausted Europe would "'eat out of our hands.'"[14]

By many lights, in fact, it was already doing so. By the middle of the war, the French had become heavily dependent on American food, and they ultimately received more aid than any ally.[15] The British were not far behind, and by 1918 they depended on U.S. and Canadian imports for almost two-thirds of their total food.[16] British dependence on imported food was not new, and even before the war imports had accounted for more than half of their food supply.[17] But the situation was quite different in France, which had been almost self-sufficient in the years before the war broke out, with French farmers producing upwards of 90 percent of the food eaten within their borders.[18] French agricultural production declined precipitously during the war, due both to fighting on French soil and to the fact that millions of French farmers and workers had been sent to the trenches. Importing and doling out adequate food quickly became a priority of the French government.[19] Plummeting French wheat production was an especially keen source of worry because French people in this era relied inordinately on bread, with contemporaries estimating that bread made up a staggering 70 percent of average French diets.[20] The government subsidized bread heavily during the war and set a price above which the cost of bread could not legally rise, because officials believed that a sharp rise in the price of the national staple would corrode morale and physically weaken those least able to afford it.[21] Yet there were problems with this strategy, and some argued that the low price ceiling for farmers' grain discouraged production.[22] Because of a combination of factors, by 1917 French farmers were producing less than half of the wheat demanded by French consumers.[23]

To induce French people to eat less white flour, in early 1917 the French government outlawed the fresh baguette. Government officials accomplished this by declaring that bakers could only sell stale bread that was at least twelve hours old, and by mandating the partial use of nonwhite flour. If bread was coarse and dry, thinking went, French people might eat less of it. And the strategy seemed to work, with French bread consumption dropping almost 10 percent after the passage of these laws.[24] Practical results, however, did not prevent French people from lamenting the end of "the little golden breads, the crusty flutes."[25] In fact, it was precisely this sort of loving, sensual appreciation of food that the laws aimed to frustrate. And banning the fresh baguette was only the most culturally offensive measure in a suite of prohibitions aimed at limiting consumer demand. The French state also limited how much bread bakers could produce, it ordered pastry shops to close two days a week, and starting with the 1917 harvest it requisitioned all French wheat.[26] In Paris, the Ministry of War took over flour mills and assigned each baker a limited amount of flour.[27] The French minister of ravitaillement, or provisioning, also established a long list of controls aimed at other commodities, including butter, milk, and meat.[28]

There were some food riots in France during the war, though people were spurred to protest more by inferior quality of food shipments rather than by absolute lack of provisions.[29] The agricultural resources devoted to wine emphasize that France was far from a state of famine: wine production in France more than doubled during the war, largely because the crop was recovering from the devastating phylloxera blight of previous decades but also because the French considered wine a war need along with bread and meat.[30] However, what on paper is exactly enough food to feed a population is rarely actually enough, since hoarding, speculation, spoilage, and lags in distribution can all trigger isolated food shortages. For instance, some mountainous regions in France went through stretches of up to two and a half weeks without bread, while German-occupied areas in northern France sometimes went months at a time without certain products, like bacon and salt.[31] Yet despite persistent food shortages, quality of life did not markedly decline for the civilian populations of the major Allies, thanks in large part to infusions of American food. When asked if the Allies were actually dying from hunger, Hoover would answer that it was his job to make sure they did not.[32] In Britain, the overall food supply diminished but quality of life remained relatively stable, and in other democracies, the material comfort of the general population actually improved; precisely because of rationing and state food distribution, the very poorest people often received more food than they had before.[33]

Many Europeans were legitimately and publicly thankful for U.S. aid. During the war, King Albert of Belgium thanked Hoover effusively for the aid he had orchestrated, crediting him with saving Belgium from starvation, and Belgian women, famed for their needlework, embroidered empty U.S. flour sacks with elaborate messages of thanks.[34] Likewise, Belgian ministers said in speeches that only "American efficiency, American sympathy and American devotion" were preventing famine.[35] Of course, a central purpose of such expressions of gratitude was to inspire more help, but not all praise of U.S. aid was intended for public consumption. After Wilson created the U.S. Food Administration, for example, the leader of French food control, Maurice Violette, wrote to the French president, Raymond Poincaré, to inform him that in what he called a "grand gesture" the United States had "just voluntarily imposed veritable privations on itself" in order to furnish its allies with needed commodities.[36] French books written on U.S. food aid in the immediate postwar period described U.S. aid as "a grand and successful food aid experiment," and called Hoover "the great organizer of the economic victory of the Allies throughout the world."[37] An American living in England during the war reported to the Food Administration that "'one hears on the lips of all classes expressions of gratitude to America.'"[38]

According to most American accounts, French civilians, soldiers, and leaders alike openly admired the United States and were painfully grateful for its support. American newspapers brimmed with reports about how much Europeans revered Herbert Hoover, the face of American benevolence abroad. A typical comment came from an editor at the *San Francisco Examiner* who claimed that every Belgian and French child in the war zone "lisps the name of this big-hearted American, morning and night, in prayer."[39] Food aid recipients were supposedly coming to respect and admire all Americans. When the food administrator and physiologist Alonzo Taylor visited the battlefield of Verdun in early 1918, he was shocked to see battle-hardened French soldiers saluting him—an ordinary, middle-aged civilian—until he surmised that they could tell by his clothes that he was American.[40] Likewise, in an article titled "Love for America Growing in France," the *Boston Herald* quoted an American businessman living in Paris who said French people now thought Americans were "the 'nicest fellows' on earth."[41]

In fact, so many Americans living and working in France reported that grateful French people plied them with enormous quantities of food that the Food Administration considered it a public relations problem, since such reports undermined their depictions of savage French food shortages.[42] For instance, when the American nutritionist Graham Lusk received what he considered a disgracefully lavish meal at the Paris Ritz Hotel in early 1918, he complained to U.S. food administrators. One wrote back to assure him that the sense of opulence most likely resulted from a combination of French culinary skill and the gratitude of French waiters who ensured that an American "has all the bread he wants and more," despite national bread regulations.[43] Yet reports like Lusk's were legion, and over the course of the war, the Food Administration released multiple press releases attributing rumors of abundant French food supplies to French pride and hospitality alone, assuring readers that French people preferred their own families to go hungry rather than for Americans to think them ungenerous.[44] Editorials in newspapers across the country scolded American visitors to France for assuming abundance was general simply because they themselves received plenty of pastries. In their modesty and innocence, one North Dakota article deduced, Americans did not realize that the French were emptying their larders in order to express their appreciation for American generosity.[45]

Opinions in Spain, an enemy of the United States in the recent past, also changed because of U.S. wartime activities. As neutrals, the Spanish and Dutch governments interacted regularly with the Commission for Relief in Belgium and the U.S. aid project because they maintained agents in occupied areas to ensure that German forces did not requisition food aid intended for civilian populations.[46] One Spanish writer acknowledged the justified anger over U.S. actions in 1898, but he said Spain now had to concede that U.S. benevolence in the Great War "must be for us as the Jordan in which they wash away their guilt."[47] Likewise, another Spanish author argued that instead of harping on Cuba and the Philippines, Spain should look to the future, which to his mind the United States had come to represent. Until the war, he wrote, "Old Europe was cocky about its tradition and its culture and its ancient scrolls," but it was increasingly clear that the United States was more than just "trusts and financial empires, kings of coal, steel, and railroads, cowboys and boxers; detectives and the robbers from the movies." Its aid work made the United States a country not just of material progress but also one whose citizens were contributing to "the universal work of civilization."[48]

LEAN EUROPE AND FAT AMERICA

Of course, ordinary Americans themselves were not always so enthusiastic about giving up favorite foods like steak and white bread and butter for foreign people they had never laid eyes on, and a major function of government propaganda was to remind Americans to live up to their newly minted reputation as selfless philanthropists. For example, one Food Administration cartoon captioned "The Allied Restaurant" showed a dinner table with a French, English, Italian, Belgian, and American man, labeled by nationality, seated around it. The Europeans all play out their national stereotypes on cue: the Italian is gesturing broadly, the French man is eating, the Englishman is portly and stooped, and the Belgian is small, with downcast eyes. Only the American, sitting at the head of the table, is young, good-looking, and richly dressed, and in the cartoon he leans back lazily to ask the waitress, "What can I have that's *special?*" While the other Allies look on worriedly, the waitress—Liberty herself, as it turns out— takes control of the situation. Hugely muscled, Liberty stands at the head of the table polishing a platter emblazoned with the Food Administration seal, and she answers the American curtly, "Just the same as all the rest, it is table d'hote from now on."[49] Readers at the time would have understood Liberty's reprimand perfectly: table d'hote meant that all guests would be sitting at a common table and sharing from common dishes, and no one would be getting any special treatment.

Even as the lion's share of World War I food aid went very specifically to white, western Europeans, Americans described food relief as a shining example of *global* food management, and the theme of the world sitting to eat at a common table appeared again and again in food conservation literature.[50] As the author of a typical food administration leaflet wrote, "Today Americans have reached a stage of development where they can look upon themselves as citizens of the world—a hungry world—when deciding what shall go on their tables. At the common table a man must stop to ask, 'How much of this should I have?'"[51] And since aid supposedly both preserved advanced civilization and was itself an expression of that civilization, the "stage of development" referred both to the technological and to the moral progress underlying humanitarian food aid. Contemporaries talked explicitly about the world food supply as a single unit, referring to the "world's food reserve," the "world need of bread," or "the world's larder."[52] This new consciousness of a world food supply was one factor helping to develop a larger consciousness of global interconnectedness.[53] The war "contracted our little world," wrote the author of one 1918 press release, creating "a mutual interdependence such as was not dreamed of before."[54]

That sense of global interconnectedness gave meaning and urgency to food conservation, especially the idea that Americans' daily decisions affected people in other countries. Americans heard repeatedly that waste in their own kitchen would lead directly to "starvation in some other kitchen across the sea."[55] But Americans could also do immediate *good* by thinking of others, even when they made seemingly small personal decisions about food. One typical image of American sacrifice on behalf of Europeans came from a Michigan high school student who painted a picture of two American girls talking. When the first suggests they go get some candy, the second replies, "Oh, no when the French babies have'nt enough to eat."[56] And food administrators claimed that whenever a woman bought less cake, or used cornmeal instead of wheat flour, or worked in her garden, *"she is helping to save life in Europe."*[57]

Maintaining that sense of urgency—and of drama—was important because on a daily level food conservation could be awfully boring. Successful food conservation did not depend on heroic feats but rather on an unflagging commitment to very minor sacrifices that no one much noticed except the person making them. Administrators had to battle continually against the mundaneness of saving food, especially since the savings themselves could so easily seem trivial. What difference could half a cup of milk or an extra slice of bread make to anyone? But if those small quantities were meaningless by themselves, wartime articles and exhibitions stressed, it was the collective effort that counted. For instance, one Pennsylvania exhibit demonstrated that if each state resident wasted just half a cup of milk, it would equal a year's output from 500 cows.[58] Another exhibit piled up ninety-one loaves of bread to show how much bread a family of four would free for export to Europe in a year if they each had just one slice less a day.[59] Again and again wartime literature encouraged individuals to imagine their own small contributions magnified many times, and as Hoover said, it "is this multiplication of minute quantities— teaspoonfuls—slices, scraps—by 100,000,000 and 360 days that will save the world."[60] The population of the United States had in fact just recently reached 100 million, and the number gave new heft to Americans' potential effectiveness when they worked in concert.[61]

The collective reckoning common during the war also made the point that many of the ordinary domestic decisions women made were not ordinary after all, because American housewives were now a pivotal part of the world food system.[62] American food systems had always extended beyond their own borders, and as some Americans' culinary repertoires had expanded in the nineteenth century, they had eagerly described themselves as the privileged recipients of the best of the world's food.[63] But the food aid project was different in kind, with Americans, and especially American women, figuring not primarily as beneficiaries but as benefactors, providing sustenance to a world newly dependent on them. For instance, one conservation poster illustrated the long chain of people required to grow, harvest, process, distribute, and cook food in order to "Feed the World," with a housewife pictured as the final, crucial step, spooning food into world's gaping mouth.[64] Journalists gushed about the "infinitely, tenderly, graciously beautiful" contributions of "the woman in her home succoring by her housewifely wisdom those, who far away and unknown, bear the fury of the world's storm."[65]

The fact that this global succoring took place in the domestic sphere was essential. Even as administrators exalted the international dimension of housewives' contributions, the food conservation campaign made crystal clear that American women could really only function internationally by staying home. Similarly, even though young American men made up its volunteer base, the Commission for Relief in Belgium emphatically did not welcome American women as volunteers. Lou Henry Hoover, Herbert's wife—herself frequently described as an exemplary "housewife"—reported firmly that while the commission welcomed the skills of American men, they did not want any women since they already had plenty of "sympathetic, efficient Belgian women to do everything that any woman could do." As far as commissioners were concerned, an American woman in Europe simply meant another mouth to feed.[66] U.S. propaganda continually stressed that women's contributions were no less important or morally profound for taking place in a realm seemingly far removed from conventional statecraft. As the food administrator Ray Wilbur said in a speech aimed at American women, "It looks, does it not, as if the crowns of Europe were toppling from the heads of kings. Perhaps *you* are going to wear them as a halo."[67]

One important way that Americans reconceptualized their standing vis-à-vis Europeans was by contrasting their national cuisines and the women who supposedly oversaw them. Observers called U.S. eating habits the "most extravagant" on earth and drew stark distinctions between weary Europeans, winnowed down to slimness by scarcity and want, and the sleek and easygoing Americans who supposedly had not known real hardship in generations.[68] Americans had always compared themselves to Europeans, but by World War I such comparisons were not simply between Old Europe and Young America, but increasingly between "Lean Europe and Fat America."[69] And precisely because of the elevated place of French cuisine in American culture, these descriptions of European leanness were particularly widespread, and particularly meaningful, when it came to France.

French recipes had been common fare in U.S. print media for generations, even in modest cookbooks and small-town newspapers, but they had never before appeared exclusively as frugal alternatives to rich American foods.[70] Indeed, in the forty years preceding the war, Belle Époque banquets with multiple courses, resolutely untranslated menus, laborious recipes, and baroque presentations had shaped a notion of Frenchness intimately tied to notions of "haute cuisine" and "haute culture," terms whose very meaning derived in part from the fact of their being French. By the 1910s, however, wartime scarcity was helping to drive haute cuisine out of style, at least temporarily, and a recategorization of French food as thrifty peasant fare was taking its place.[71] Reformers urged American women to stretch meat with French casseroles and stews, to cook snails and stringy roosters, and to forego meat altogether in favor of French recipes for potatoes and sauce.[72] "French bread," according to one cookbook, meant wheat-saving potato bread.[73] It is telling that by 1918 an author could blithely say that French recipes did not need to be modified to become conservation dishes because "French cookery is thrifty even in times of peace."[74] As a blanket statement about French cuisine, the notion would have seemed jarringly inaccurate even a decade earlier, and it speaks volumes about Americans' changing perceptions.

In American imaginations, rural French housewives were the custodians of this cheap country cuisine, and throughout the war, images of French women on the American home front appeared almost uniformly as peasants, as in the 1918 propaganda painting asking, "Will you help the women of France?" featuring three rural women in scarves and clogs taking the place of draft animals to lug a cultivating machine through a field.[75] As one magazine writer said bluntly, "Americans are not accustomed to economize with the thrift of the French housewife."[76] Other journalists agreed, praising the French housewife's "native talent for economy" while lambasting American women's supposedly "worldwide reputation for extravagance."[77] A California woman who had lived for two years in cheap European hotels suggested that the government should hire French and Belgian women to "come over here and teach our cooks how to make much out of little."[78] Similarly, Pennsylvania housewives read that they should "[l]earn of the humble everyday French woman to tempt the taste with what costs little."[79] By recasting French cooking as economical rather than extravagant, and French women as necessarily thrifty compared to their lucky American counterparts, writers explicitly contrasted sinking French fortunes with U.S. abundance.[80] The comparison also implicitly encouraged pride that Americans, far from living in a culinary backwater, were on the whole eating more and better than the people of any other nation on earth.[81]

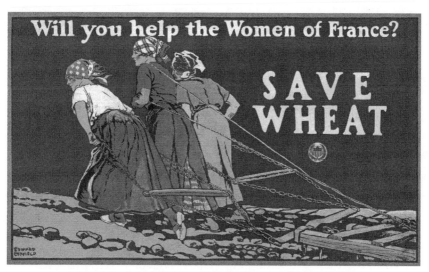

Edward Penfield, "Will You Help the Women of France?," 1918.
The Food Administration's 1918 wheat-saving poster depicted the "Women
of France" not just as peasants but as actual beasts of burden, valiantly working
to scratch out a living from the land in the absence of men and draft animals.
Prints and Photographs Division, Library of Congress, Washington, D.C.

In reality, Americans almost certainly were eating more than people in other countries. According to a range of calorie-based studies performed at the time, average U.S. calorie consumption easily outpaced that of other nations. From 1909 to 1913, the daily calorie consumption of Americans averaged about 3,500 per person, compared with about 3,000 in Great Britain, France, and Germany, and about 2,500 in Italy.[82] These calorie counts seem high—today, the Food and Drug Administration recommends 2,000 calories as the average daily intake for adults—and it is possible that Progressive Era statisticians exaggerated national consumption figures to enhance quality-of-life estimates. But it is also quite possible that these high calorie figures quite accurately reflected the large percentage of physical laborers in the populations who would have needed substantial amounts of food to fuel their daily exertions; today, a manual laborer working a ten-hour day is estimated to need about 4,000 calories.[83] In either case, Americans were increasingly aware that they lived in a singularly abundant country.

Another crucial way that observers highlighted America's changing relationship with Europe was by depicting the recipients of U.S. aid as European children, figures intended to inspire special pity among humane,

Progressive Americans. In an article in the *Atlantic*, for instance, the food administrator Vernon Kellogg assured readers that beneath Hoover's businesslike exterior was a sentimental family man who got misty eyed at the thought of hungry Belgian children.[84] Propagandists' general inclinations to draw attention to the sufferings of European children were intensified by widely shared presumptions that women, the target of U.S. food conservation appeals, were especially motivated by sympathy for children. Administrators and journalists continually made the point that the very survival of foreign children depended upon women's daily decisions.[85] In one publicity bulletin, for instance, food administrators advised women to conjure an image of a European baby stretching out its arms to them as they cooked.[86] And the author of an article in a small-town Minnesota paper went so far as to claim that every time someone refused to join the Food Administration, a European baby, at that very moment, died.[87] Outside of state projects, various private efforts coalesced in the United States to bring aid directly to European children, including a campaign by the Woman's Christian Temperance Union to get its members to "adopt" French war orphans by donating enough money to supply their food for a year.[88]

Of course, another important reason for the focus on children both in U.S. propaganda and on the ground in Europe was the hope that Europe's future citizens would grow up thinking fondly of America. For instance, at the beginning of the war in 1914, Americans had sent a ship filled with Christmas presents to poor French and Belgian children, along with instructions to make sure that both the children and their guardians knew that the gifts came from Americans.[89] One late 1918 story created by George Creel's Committee for Public Information told of Jules and Marie, two fictional French orphans returning to their ruined village at the end of the war. Although they find their house leveled by bombing, a group of cheerful American soldiers builds them a shelter and brings them hot food. The story concludes with Marie declaring that she loves her "friends" the soldiers, and with Jules deciding, "When I am big I will fight for America."[90] Although this story was propaganda aimed at U.S. schoolchildren, hopes of winning the hearts of European children informed more official efforts. After the war, the Children's Relief Fund, an arm of the American Relief Administration founded just after the Versailles conference and run—largely for publicity reasons—as a charity, was motivated by the hope that the children it fed and clothed would grow up supporting the United States.[91]

Appeals about European children were especially poignant because in many cases they were literally orphans, or at least fatherless, as a result of war. They were the children of the lost generation, and Hoover stressed

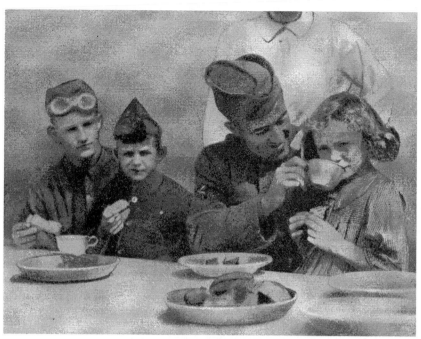

"American Soldiers Sharing with French Children."
American soldiers were photographed literally feeding the children of
France from their own plates. It is possible that the supervisory female figure in
the background was drawn in after the fact to defuse worries about the little girl's
place on the soldier's lap. Photograph reprinted in Marion Lansing and
Luther Gulick, Food and Life *(Boston: Ginn, 1920), 158.*

that the young European fathers who died had sacrificed themselves to protect civilized values Americans shared. Through their international aid program, Americans became foster parents to the European children left behind.[92] Moreover, the overwhelming tendency in U.S. propaganda to depict the recipients of U.S. aid as European children meant that in an important sense they also served as depictions of Europeans *as* children, contributing to conceptions of Europeans at war as disorganized and vulnerable, in need of the aid, efficiency, and guidance of mature Americans.

HUNGER AS A WEAPON

While Americans celebrated their food shipments to their allies, the simultaneous and even central use of hunger as a weapon against their enemies further complicated claims to international moral righteousness. Just as German U-Boats preyed on Allied food shipments, the Allies quite

unequivocally meant for their naval blockade of Germany to make its soldiers and civilians so desperate for food that the country would be forced
to surrender. Although Hoover said he disliked targeting women and
children, he and other U.S. administrators also believed that victory was
"largely a problem of who can organize *this weapon*—food."[93] News articles
appeared in U.S. newspapers approvingly calling hunger "The American
Weapon" or declaring "Starvation Is Weapon to Win War."[94]

While the war lasted, Americans routinely received news that near-
famished Germans teetered on the brink of surrender. Articles described
an emaciated country that could not possibly hold out much longer, and
reports—some of them quite true—circulated of German rations stretched
with ash, starch, kerosene, chalk, and rat meat.[95] While Germans were
not starving, German food shortages were more acute than those in Allied countries, especially starting in 1916. That year, even German soldiers
began to experience shortages, sometimes going for weeks at a time without articles like fat and potatoes.[96] But German civilians generally fared
worse, especially those who could not afford to supplement their diets
with black market purchases.[97] Germans ate animal feed, and livestock
that had not already been slaughtered wasted and died.[98] Meat, dairy, and
fat supplies dwindled, and even when the absolute number of calories
was usually passable, the absence of these culturally important foodstuffs
intensified feelings of deprivation.[99] The U.S. government had of course
launched an educational campaign to convince its citizens that they could
reduce meat and dairy consumption with no physical ill effects by eating nutritionally equivalent foods. But the German government made no
move to inform its citizens that meat and dairy were not biologically necessary, and many Germans believed their wartime diets were harmfully
deficient.[100] Sometimes deficiency was not simply a question of perception; while monthly averages show that the calories available in Germany
were usually roughly adequate for the population, food supply spiked and
fell, with civilians sometimes going days with little or nothing to eat.[101]
Visibly, Germans lost weight.[102]

For Americans, it was a moral tightrope act to justify civilian suffering
in the midst of a campaign that mustered support by spotlighting civilians
as victims. Yet many gamely attempted such ethical acrobatics.[103] For one
thing, they downplayed the pain and hunger the blockade was causing
civilians in the first place by claiming that hunger was actually doing the
Germans good. As one writer for the *New York Tribune* wrote laughingly,
the "War diet in Germany has accomplished a greater reduction of the
corpulency of the average German than all the Marienbad cures, Russian

baths, and drastic courses of exercise" combined.[104] Some also argued that Germans simply deserved what they were getting. One Iowa article, for instance, insisted that Germans who attacked women and children in the areas they occupied were far more barbarous than Americans could ever be.[105] Most often, to reconcile the United States' discordant positions as both munificent food provider and, along with its Allies, calculating food withholder, U.S. propaganda and media expressed the idea that the only thing keeping Germany from immediate surrender was the diabolical discipline of German soldiers themselves.[106] For example, one war correspondent wrote that the Russian front collapsed because Russian men were worried about their hungry families, while German men relentlessly continued fighting even as they knew their families were slowly starving at home.[107]

By the spring of 1918, the German army was so short of supplies that it requisitioned food from civilian farms, and American journalists enthusiastically described German soldiers plucking food from the hands of hungry German children.[108] Commentators also argued that civilization—or lack thereof—affected the body and its needs, and overall eugenic fitness did *not* necessarily make for physical toughness, especially for women and children. A common argument was that Belgians and other allies especially needed certain kinds of food *because* they were a delicate, civilized people who could not withstand much physical hardship.[109] Extending this sinister logic, the fact that Germans had managed to resist the blockade for so long contributed to portrayals of them as uncivilized automatons, heedless of their own hunger and indifferent to the hunger of others, whose very ability to withstand the blockade justified its continuation.

The use of hunger as a weapon only sharpened after the war. When the combatants finally signed the Armistice in November 1918, Hoover did not pause for breath. Instead of talking about "victory," he referred to the "change in the foreign situation," estimating that more than 200 million Europeans still needed American aid.[110] Food administrators kept up the drumbeat of conservation, urging Americans that they would need to continue conserving food for months, and maybe longer.[111] But predictions that Americans would keep cheerfully Hooverizing indefinitely soon proved too optimistic.[112] War sacrifices had been acceptable when there was a war, but they seemed much less so in peacetime. "America no doubt likes Mr. Hoover for what he has done," one journalist smirked just days after the Armistice, "but most Americans are willing to struggle along in the confidence that he has already done enough."[113] Flagging domestic food conservation turned out not to be Hoover's biggest problem, however.

With the signing of the Armistice months earlier than Americans had anticipated, the Allies suddenly had access to cheaper markets for foodstuffs in South America, Australia, and Asia, and they no longer wanted to buy relatively expensive U.S. commodities. This unexpected rejection of U.S. goods left Hoover responsible for a surplus of U.S. food three times greater than normal. Furious and bitterly disappointed, he later described the cool willingness of the Allies to see U.S. financial markets collapse as a betrayal of the meanest kind.[114]

U.S. financial markets did not collapse, however. Even after the Armistice, ninety million "enemy peoples" still did not have enough to eat because the Allies refused to lift their blockade of the Central Powers.[115] England and France intended to continue the blockade until the peace treaty had been signed, and they meant for the blockade to compel terms very favorable to themselves. Hoover, who of course considered the vanquished enemy a prospective market, was at the forefront of those arguing that food relief would be a practical as much as a humanitarian good.[116] All winter, Hoover lobbied vehemently for permission to liquidate his surpluses—especially a huge supply of high-priced pork—in Germany. As the months went by, the prolonged blockade inspired increasingly loud objections on moral grounds, and the Allies finally granted Hoover permission in March 1919 to sell the U.S. surpluses to their former enemies. The Food Administration delivered almost $300 million worth of food to Germany, all they could afford, though considerably less food than German officials estimated they needed. Administrators also delivered $200 million worth of food to Poland, $145 million to Austria, and $115 million to Czechoslovakia.[117]

The decision to provision former enemies before the formal signing of the peace was obviously pragmatic, but it was also conveniently consistent with the supposed U.S. ideal that no one should starve for political reasons when the food existed to feed them. It was also pragmatic in another crucial way: as anti-Bolshevism and pro-democratic capitalism. Hoover was adamant that as pitiful as the millions of skinny and stunted European children were, they also represented a future "menace to their nations," and unless they received aid, and quickly, "their distorted minds were a menace to all mankind."[118] Hoover was fond of repeating that "famine breeds anarchy" and that anarchy was infectious.[119] Still, government food aid did not survive long into the postwar period. Hoover had always wanted the Food Administration to be only a temporary agency, but he was angered by its dismantling in 1919: too soon, in his opinion, to deal adequately with postwar food relief in Europe, even with the creation that year of the American Relief Administration, a private, surrogate relief organization.[120]

For Germans, conditions in the winter of 1918–19 were bad, though not much different from the previous two years, which is to say that food supplies were meager and shoddy but usually calorically adequate, especially when supplemented with purchases from the black market. Much worse for German morale was the fact that after the Armistice such misery seemed pointless.[121] Even with American food shipments starting early in the spring, it was a hunger winter, one that seemed all the crueler to Germans because it happened after they had already asked for peace. Those months of hunger were crucial in compelling Germany to sign the war guilt clause and to agree to crippling reparations at the Treaty of Versailles, and the Allies' use of hunger as a weapon in those circumstances bought capitulation at the price of deep and lasting resentment.[122]

ONE OF THE FOOD ADMINISTRATION'S GREATEST TRIUMPHS was making Americans care about food aid, at least for the duration of the war. About 70 percent of U.S. families actively participated in food conservation, and a major reason that they did so was that food administrators convincingly linked Americans' daily habits to the fates of other people and to their own country's changing place in the world.[123] Obviously, U.S. interests lay in having its allies fed, but for some Americans aid revealed a national greatness of character that transcended such strategic concerns. As one journalist wrote in a Kansas newspaper, "Possibly no other nation in all the world would do what America proposes to do—refrain from using the food that is so plentiful for all our needs, in order that people we have never seen may have some of our stores."[124] Americans romanticized their food program, preferring to think of it as humanitarian aid rather than as a function of geopolitics; even as the Allies went into deep debt to buy U.S. food, few contemporaries lingered on the contradictions of an "aid" program run for profit.

Postwar realities dampened Americans' exuberance about the United States as a beloved and benevolent world power, but they did not change the growing belief that the United States had a leading role to play in the young century. Wartime food aid was one of the country's first forays into Europe as a modern bureaucracy, and the United States became a rising world power during the war and because of it. To a great extent, ordinary Americans experienced America's rise to power both imaginatively and in their everyday lives through international food aid.[125] Indeed, by the end of the war, the Food Administration had retracted its motto, "Food

Will Win the War," and had suggested instead a drastically more ambitious slogan, "Food Will Win the World." The United States' new brand of power was both economic and moral, resting not just on the country's vast resources but also on its supposedly benevolent intentions. In many ways, this rehearsed the grand theme of subsequent American incursions into the world in the twentieth century: the desire and consent of those who accepted American goods and values into their markets and their lives.[126]

World War I food aid inspired the utopian vision that modern technology and advances in civilization itself made it possible, as one Philadelphia journalist put it, "to move the world's supply of foodstuffs wherever it may be needed."[127] Even as the European food crisis underscored the vulnerability of large food systems, some Americans were only increasingly confident that they were developing the very technologies needed to produce, transport, calculate, and organize food on a global scale. Indeed, the fact that Americans launched an international program on the scale of World War I food aid bespeaks their confidence in a whole range of technologies on which it depended, from communication and transportation systems, to food production, preservation, and distribution technologies, to statistical information gathering, to nutrition science. With careful planning and proper funding, some optimistically suggested, they might actually be able to feed the world.

But it was clear well before the war ended that truly feeding the world required more than surplus crops and global transportation networks. People were also suffering from hunger during the war years in the Ottoman Empire, the Middle East, India, and elsewhere, and those people rarely received attention in the U.S. press or aid from the U.S. government.[128] From 1917 to 1919, for instance, there was a catastrophic famine in what is now northern Iran, but the Persian government got no U.S. aid even after direct appeals.[129] Many eagerly adopted new language about "world food" during the world war, but feeding the world was always too tall an order when the time frame for such sacrifice was indefinite, and when the potential recipients included every person on the entire, insatiable globe. The experience set a powerful precedent for what would become a routine practice of the U.S. government during the twentieth century: the strategic—and highly selective—use of food aid as an arm of foreign policy.[130]

4

A SCHOOL FOR WIVES

Home Economics and the Modern Housewife

Cooking is an art, and should be a labor of love.
—Mrs. Ada Buxton, 1917

On Valentine's Day in 1912, a West Virginia farmer sat down and wrote a letter to the president of Cornell University. "My Dear Professor, I have red of your women students," he wrote. "I would like to correspond with One . . . For the purpose of Matermonial." The farmer provided his economic prospects as well as a physical inventory: "I am 44 years old weig 210 pounds, high 5 ft. 10 in. Never was sick, nor never was married. Please give this your student."[1] There is no record that Cornell staff replied. Six years later, in 1918, a surgeon in New York wrote to the Cornell home economics department to inquire about hiring a graduate as a cook. "I am establishing a 'Rest Cure' for patients," he wrote, "and wish to obtain a good reliable woman who has taken a course in domestic science to do the cooking and take charge of the kitchen end of the house."[2] This time a member of the Cornell staff did reply, but she wrote a discouraging response. The founder and co-chair of Cornell University's home economics department, Martha Van Renssalaer, reminded the doctor that *her* students were college women, and the "position as *cook* as it is generally understood does not seem to satisfy them after they have spent so much time and money on a professional course."[3]

Both the West Virginia farmer and the New York surgeon misunderstood what exactly a woman studying home economics might hope to do with her life. But of the two, it was the farmer who was closest to the mark. For these college-educated women, servant work was unthink-able. But marriage and housework, precisely because of the preprofes-sional study they had undertaken, were the very futures many of them sought.

It had not always been the case that highly educated, relatively privi-leged women were eager to take on full-time housework. Nor had such women always conceived of such work as a profession. On the contrary, it is hard to grasp now just how closely middle-class Americans at the turn of the twentieth century associated housework with servitude. When most people today think about American families in the past, they tend to assume that from this country's earliest days up through the 1950s, virtu-ally all women were housewives, performing the bulk of their families' housework by themselves and not working for pay outside the home. But the "housewife" has never been as homogenous or as unchanging a role as popular culture suggests. American women in significant numbers have always worked outside the home, and in the first two decades of the twen-tieth century, about a quarter of American women had paying jobs.[4] Fur-thermore, even those women who did not work for wages did not neces-sarily spend their days cooking and scrubbing; domestic servants allowed a significant minority of American women freedom from the physical de-mands of housework.

Through the late nineteenth century, indeed, domestic servitude had been the practical basis upon which elite U.S. womanhood was defined. There had been efforts throughout the nineteenth century to ennoble housekeeping and to call attention to its social value, especially in popu-lar books like Lydia Maria Child's 1829 *The American Frugal Housewife* or Catharine Beecher's 1841 *Treatise on Domestic Economy.*[5] Yet even as some nineteenth-century Americans had exalted women's moral and managerial oversight of the domestic sphere, they generally deempha-sized the physical work that went into housekeeping. If the wife was to make the home a haven, the husband should not observe her toiling, if possible. The labor that went into producing middle-class homes was supposed to be done with discretion, ideally by servants or slaves. The middle-class devaluation of housework was linked to general Victorian devaluations of physical labor, and new definitions of the middle-class family came to be based in part upon the idea—and it always was more an idea than a fact—that middle-class women and children did not work. On a practical level, servitude's centrality to middle-class culture was made possible by a steady supply of people, many of them recent immi-grants, willing to do other people's housework for money. By the 1880s, almost a quarter of the families in American cities employed at least one servant.[6]

Yet just a few decades later, by the 1910s, a majority of the white, middle-class women whose families had paid servants to cook and to perform heavy housework began to perform that work themselves. This required a significant cultural shift. For women in the 1900s and 1910s, housework had very recently connoted not just servitude but also slavery, and to some degree middle-class women who did housework risked muddying their own social standings, even their class and racial identities, with those of servants and slaves.[7] It was in dispelling these fears that the home economics movement succeeded most brilliantly, as practitioners worked tirelessly to bring prestige to work that had been "a symbol of bondage," as one home economist put it.[8] Throughout the first two decades of the twentieth century home economists confidently asserted that the modern housewife's combination of native intelligence, genuine familial love, and professional education made it impossible to compare her to a servant.

The motor driving this reinvention of housework was the novel idea that far from drudgery best performed by a paid underclass, housewifery was a vital public service, crucial to the health of American citizens and the American nation, and an intellectually challenging profession. This new view of housework was part of an ethos of professionalization that was sweeping a variety of middle-class fields in the early twentieth century. Like their counterparts in increasingly feminized occupations like secretarial work and nursing, home economists stressed the importance of pre-professional training, schedules, and standardization. But when it came to housework, reformers were not genuinely professionalizing it at all. Because housewives remained unpaid, rhetoric about professionalization remained just that. In fact, the glaring irony at the heart of the movement is that it was precisely by raising housework's prestige with a vocabulary of professionalization that reformers truly and effectively *deprofessionalized* it, by finally making it widely accepted as work that was best performed by unpaid female family members rather than by paid servants.

In the midst of growing feelings that it was possible that housewives could be modern, educated, and even fashionable women, the food conservation campaign of World War I accelerated changes in ideas about housework even further by turning housework unequivocally into patriotic service. Together, the discourse of intelligence and expertise emerging out of the home economics movement and the elevation of housewives in the wartime food conservation campaign helped make middle-class housewifery seem like an important and intellectually rigorous profession, one that had only seemed like servility because Americans had not known enough about it.

SERVANT PROBLEMS

Keeping servants had been central to middle-class culture in the nineteenth century, but the institution of domestic servitude was withering by the twentieth. Middle-class Americans were increasingly vocal about what they called "the servant problem," as fewer and fewer women and men proved willing to accept positions as servants, with the unexceptional pay, long hours, relative dependence, and low status they entailed.[9] One writer in the 1910s claimed to have heard the despairing wail of "My cook is gone!" thousands of times, and joked, "Perhaps there is a sort of Pied Piper who walks the city streets, invisible to mortal eye, and calls enticingly to the cooks to follow."[10] Of course, privileged people despairing when servants quit and panicking about having to do their own housework sounds alarmist, even ridiculous. Most U.S. families had never had servants, and there had always been more men and women working as servants than men and women employing them. Moreover, the "servant problem" was anything but a problem for individuals who had previously been servants and managed to get better jobs.

Yet although the so-called servant problem was more ideological than demographic, alarm about retaining servants was more than whining. Those American women who employed servants in this era often genuinely depended on the work their servants did to make possible their own middle-class status and even their own physical freedom and mobility outside the home.[11] Servitude had been a robust American institution from the country's earliest days, and its decline sent tremors through other areas of American life, affecting family structures, the kind of work that women did inside and outside the home, and views of women themselves. In practice, when middle-class women lost servants and were unable to hire new ones, they usually began to do their families' domestic work themselves. Taking up the demanding, physical tasks that had recently been the paid work of servants meant directly confronting the nineteenth-century stigmatization of women's bodily labor. Even more to the point, some women were genuinely incompetent when it came to housework. In most cases this was not pretended feminine helplessness but a reflection of the fact that women who had spent their lives in households with servants often possessed few or none of the wide array of skills required to make an early-twentieth-century household and kitchen run.[12] Like Francis Griffin, a wealthy New York woman who lost her two cooks on the same day in 1917, women whose servants left were sometimes forced to cook a meal for the first time in their lives.[13]

In many ways the entire discipline of home economics was a response to the servant problem.[14] In the late nineteenth century, home economists had pushed women to make the home more businesslike, in large part because they believed that a modern, standardized environment would help attract and retain servants.[15] But by the 1900s and 1910s, as people in large numbers continued to leave domestic service for better jobs, home economists more often argued that the answer to the servant problem was simply not to have servants at all. Instead, they made the case for women to take on housework themselves as a full-time job.[16] On a practical level, they said, middle-class women *could* take over the work that servants had previously performed because a home economics education would equip any woman with the skills to do it. And on a cultural level, women *should* take it over because it was nationally important and intellectually challenging work that middle-class women were uniquely suited to do well.

Resignation to the decline of servitude was aided by the fact that servants had simply become less essential to the functioning of U.S. households by the 1900s and 1910s than they had been in previous decades. For one thing, some of the work that servants had performed within the home in the nineteenth century took place outside its walls in the twentieth. Americans increasingly bought ready-made food like bakery bread and commercially canned food, which had been invented a century earlier and was finally consistently reliable by the 1910s. Meanwhile, the practice of keeping boarders and lodgers to supplement family incomes began to disappear around the turn of the century.[17] Another important factor was that many household chores were less onerous than they had been, thanks to technological improvements like modern plumbing. Iceboxes had been improved, and early electric refrigerators were manufactured for domestic use starting in the early 1910s, a development spurred by the rapid electrification of American homes beginning that decade.[18] Methods of food preparation also underwent vast improvements, and by the late 1910s gas stoves were becoming common even in rural areas, replacing more laborious coal stoves. According to Progressive logic, labor-saving devices were not luxuries for the lazy, but rather achievements in efficiency that modern women should demand.[19] For example, an advertisement for Hoover vacuums featured a woman who told her husband that she "needed and deserved mechanical aids for just the same reasons he used them."[20]

Incidentally, Hoover vacuums, a company founded in the first decade of the twentieth century, had nothing to do with Herbert Hoover, although some people assumed that the food administrator had allowed his name to be used by the company in order to promote efficient housekeeping.[21]

Labor-saving technology eased discomfort with the notion of middle-class women performing household chores, but new appliances and other innovations only partially explain housework's recategorization as a form of loving familial nurture in this era. Housework was still laborious, and in some cases technological shortcuts could actually lead to more work as they heightened standards of cleanliness. Some of the Victorian stigma attached to physical work had faded with early-twentieth-century exultation of masculine vigor and the "strenuous life."[22] Praise of athleticism and physical prowess still extended only tepidly to women in this era, but it was becoming increasingly unpatriotic to cling to any old-fashioned notion that ladies needed servants because they themselves should not perform any kind of physical labor, even inside their own homes. If anything, the growing acceptance of women's physical activity only set the stage for a host of other factors that would justify this sea change in the organization of women's labor.

Most strikingly, home economists and other reformers argued that educated middle-class women were not just adequate replacements for servants but actually made vastly superior housekeepers. As one food administrator claimed, homes run entirely by "the *intelligent* women of America" would be healthier and more efficient than homes run by hired help.[23] Indeed, intelligence was coming to be seen as the touchstone of successful housekeeping, and the term was rampant in discussions about housewives. At this time "intelligence" meant two different but related things. First, intelligence signaled the *innate intellectual capacity*— or "real, honest-to-god brains"—that middle-class white women could supposedly bring to bear on questions of housework.[24] This special intellectual aptitude contrasted implicitly, and sometimes explicitly, with what some presumed to be the limited intellectual capacities of those people who had previously performed housework as servants, especially working-class women, recent immigrants, and African Americans. As one leading home economist said baldly in 1907, servants were "apt to be of limited mental resources."[25] But intelligence also had another common meaning at this time, and that was to be *informed*, in the same way it was later used in the "Central Intelligence Agency." For housewives, information meant education, specifically an education in home economics. This two-pronged notion of intelligence, meaning both white, middle-class women's supposedly natural intellectual capacity and their preprofessional education in home economics, helped reinvent the modern housewife.

Home economics had emerged in land-grant institutions in the 1870s upon the growing belief that domestic work was vitally important and that it could be studied scientifically. Starting in the 1880s, home economics movements also took off in western European countries including France, England, Germany, and Sweden.[26] By 1908, when the American Home Economics Association formed, practitioners confidently described their field as a middle road between women's reform work and the otherwise male-dominated social sciences.[27] By the 1910s home economics was expanding rapidly, helped by strong support from federal legislation. In 1914 the Smith-Lever Act created the Cooperative Extension Service, based on the idea that farmers and farmers' wives needed scientific training. Extension programs, overseen by land-grant institutions, sent men and women trained in agriculture and home economics to rural areas, where they visited small communities and often people's homes to teach new farming techniques or to provide information about health, hygiene, and scientific food preparation. In 1917, the Smith-Hughes Act provided more federal funds to land-grant colleges to train teachers in vocational fields, including home economics.[28] Partly spurred by the surge in trained home economics teachers, domestic science classes expanded in public and private institutions and at all educational levels, in universities, in high schools, and even in elementary schools.[29]

Until recently, historians paid little attention to home economics, perhaps because many of them grew up fighting against "Home Ec" as a bastion of rigid gender roles.[30] But ironically, the very denigration of home economics in the late twentieth century resulted in part from the resounding success of its early mission. Home economics and popular nutrition were triumphant Progressive reforms, and their health and hygiene doctrines became so completely accepted throughout the twentieth century that they started to sound obvious instead of innovative. But far from conservative, antifeminist homebodies, the women who had run domestic science programs in the early twentieth century were business-minded, iconoclastic professionals who demonstrated home economics' bearing on social and political questions. Of all things, they were not traditionalists; one of their central points was that young women should ignore older women's domestic advice. As one touring exhibit pointedly explained, home economics stood for "ideal home life for to-day unhampered by the traditions of the past."[31]

Home economists also worked to demonstrate that their discipline was a scientific one. Even the names that now seem commonplace—domestic *science*, home *economics*—were chosen because the terms implied that the subjects they encompassed were serious ones.[32] Martha Van Rensselaer co-chaired Cornell's department with Flora Rose, and the two women, who were also lifelong domestic partners, shared a conviction that hard sciences gave their discipline "a scientific foundation which placed it on a basis of equality with other college departments."[33] Home economists embraced hard science in part because it gave them academic credibility, yet even as the discipline gained respectability and prestige, there remained strong currents of mistrust, dislike, and mockery of the discipline and its practitioners.[34] The tone of domestic science advice could be moralizing, classist, xenophobic, and self-righteous. The advice could also sound controlling, sometimes to a seemingly irrational extent, like commands that food should *never* be highly seasoned, or that children should be taught *never* to comment on food, or that bowel movements should take place *only* before or after breakfast.[35] A writer in the *Bellman* magazine in 1918 dismissed home economists as "well-meaning old maids who never kept house" and whose unsolicited advice was often impractical or absurd. Their own cooking experience, he sneered, "consists in having fed themselves out of a paper bag and their visitors with homemade fudge and marshmallows toasted over a candle-end in a two-room flat." At base, this may have been an antifeminist and an antilesbian argument, but the author's emotional reaction illustrates a common discomfort with the all-knowing tone and physically intimate nature of home economists' directions.[36]

Yet resistance to home economics advice was wearing down, in large part because so many of its suggestions were not impractical or absurd at all. Science was not just window dressing for home economists, and advances in hygiene and food safety meant they had hard answers to real problems. Home economists offered immediately useful, and in some cases life-saving, information about hygiene and nutrition. In earlier generations, women who had worked in their own homes without the aid of servants had toiled for long hours, frequently in filthy conditions. High child mortality rates through the end of the nineteenth century resulted not only from malnutrition and lack of vaccines, but also because of ignorance about the spread of germs and basic food safety principles.[37] Home economists provided novel information about washing hands, preventing food spoilage, and obtaining pure food. Academically demanding university home economics departments required students to take a variety of science classes because it was thought that to truly understand cooking and hygiene students had to understand the chemical, biological, and bacterial processes underlying them.[38] Popular culture picked up on the scientific threads running through new descriptions of housework, like the 1911 *Good Housekeeping* story that called the kitchen the "laboratory which supplies our table," or the 1917 cartoon that pictured a housewife combining a "chicken wing," "last night's peas," and "prunes" next to a male scientist surrounded by beakers, with a caption pointing out that they were both producing "war inventions."[39]

Meanwhile, home economists also popularized dramatic recent advances in nutrition science. In some parts of the country protein and niacin deficiencies made pellagra and its attendant dementia and mucous-caked skin lesions commonplace, while widespread vitamin D deficiencies softened and bowed the bones of rickets victims. Home economists provided information about basic nutrition science and preached the message that fruits and vegetables were not luxuries for the rich but rather important components of healthy diets that all families should try to prioritize in their grocery budgets. At the same time, they also saved people money by assuring them they could buy less meat and still get the same nutrition from foods like milk, peanuts, and beans.[40] All in all, a home economics education included a suite of domestic reforms with the power to tangibly improve the health and the quality of life of the people they reached.

PROFESSIONALIZING HOUSEWORK

In this context, *not* training for homemaking seemed increasingly old-fashioned, even perverse. A fundamental principle of the home economics movement was that housekeeping was a profession, just like medicine and the law, and it likewise required formal preprofessional training.[41] Housewives in the 1900s and 1910s described home economics in explicitly preprofessional terms, and many of them eagerly acquired the trappings of professionalism, including schedules, unions, and even uniforms. Women formed professional organizations for housewives, including the National Housewives' League, which became a powerful consumer organization.[42] While housekeeping advice had been a standard part of nineteenth-century cookbooks, a new professional style of housekeeping manual appeared by the dozen in the first two decades of the twentieth century, with titles like *Practical Homemaking: A Textbook for Young Housekeepers* or *Wanted, a Young Woman to Do Housework: Business Principles Applied to Housework*.[43] In a typical manual from 1917, the author argued that the housewife's job was in need of the same standardization as that of any modern worker, and she advised readers to frame a daily schedule of chores listed in half-hour increments from six in the morning until the last dinner dish was put away at night.[44] Other authors advised women to think of their homes as businesses, using accounting ledgers and reducing waste as carefully "as the man in the big business stops small leakages."[45] Home economists also enthusiastically applied motion studies to housework to find the most efficient methods of accomplishing domestic tasks.[46]

The Progressive Era was the heyday of professionalization, and the professionalization of housewifery fell in line with the era's general emphasis on distinguishing between experts and nonexperts.[47] In this sense, the new conviction that being a housewife required formal training was not particularly unique; the number of women undertaking professional training in fields like education, nursing, social work, and stenography also rose exponentially in this era.[48] But some felt that homemaking was simply *different*, and they disapproved of its professionalization. In a letter to the editor of *Good Housekeeping* magazine, one woman wrote, "Whenever I hear an appeal to apply system and business organization to home making I shake my head. Must we always live on a schedule and keep our belongings in pigeonholes? In the new dignity with which education has taught us to regard our housekeeping, I sometimes fear that the pendulum will swing too far and that we shall lose sight of the home comfort in our effort to organize the home."[49] Others criticized efforts to get housewives to wear uniforms, especially after U.S. food administrators created what they called the "housewives' uniform," a tent of a dress with big pockets to hold housekeeping supplies, topped off with a white cap.[50] Some notable Washington ladies had formal portraits taken wearing the uniform, with captions clarifying that they wore it "as a reminder that [they] signed the food pledge" rather than in preparation for actual physical labor.[51] Women who actually did housework day in and day out were less than enthusiastic, and some of them thought the uniform ridiculous. In a Georgia editorial, one woman called housewife uniforms "childish foolishness" and said people should be able to do their chores without "play-acting."[52]

As middle-class Americans rethought what housework was and who should do it throughout this era, there was tension between the home economics principle that housework required preprofessional training and the popular idea that housework was women's natural work, something they were innately skilled at and instinctively drawn to. The idea that housework might be "fun" dodged this apparent contradiction, and popular descriptions of modern housework in this era said its fun derived from

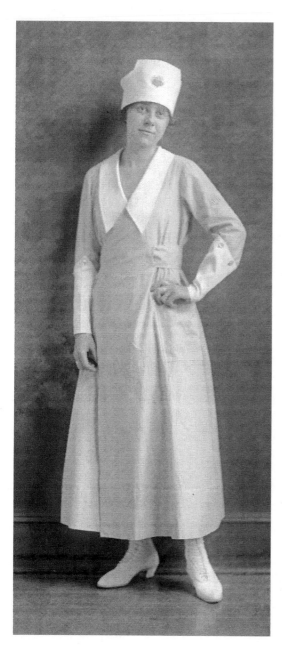

A woman wearing the Food Administration "housewives' uniform." Food administrators encouraged women to make the uniform and to wear it at home while doing housework, and the sewing pattern for the uniform was available to anyone for ten cents. Building upon home economists' argument that housewifery was a profession, administrators also hoped the uniform might instill a sense of group identity among conservationists. "Very Important Historic Material," folder "Pictures," box "H6–37, 21," American Association of Family and Consumer Sciences Records, Division of Rare and Manuscript Collections, Cornell University, Ithaca, N.Y.

the fact that it required such sharp intelligence; housekeeping problems became puzzles that supposedly appealed to women's natural feminine curiosity.[53] During the war, articles like "Fun in the Kitchen" and "Cooking for the Fun of It" argued that precisely because wartime food conservation was so difficult, it made cooking "more fun than fashion shows or solitaire."[54] Cooking took brains, reformers stressed, a fact that heightened both its prestige and its potential pleasures.

Still, the eagerness to apply a rubric of professionalization to domestic work hints at the stakes involved. Homemaking *was* different from other professions because its practitioners were not paid, and most home economists actively affirmed housework as unpaid labor outside the market.[55] Its professionalization, in this sense, was purely imaginative. Of course, home economics training did lead to paying jobs for a small percentage of women who went on to teach it and an even smaller percentage who got related jobs in industry. But even as home economics served as a back door into college for thousands of women who otherwise would not have been accepted as regular undergraduates, many college women found that their home economics training led back home after all.[56] Reformers were only able to professionalize housework on an imaginative level because they so convincingly decoupled it from servants' work—which had truly been professional housekeeping. In reality, reformers did not professionalize housework, but deprofessionalized it.

It was not inevitable that the modern housewife evolve in this way. Individual women doing the bulk of their families' domestic work by themselves and without wages was neither a natural nor a particularly efficient system. Instead, it was a tragically wasteful one, according to the writer and feminist Charlotte Perkins Gilman, who had become the leading spokesman for a radically different model of housekeeping by the 1910s.[57] Gilman detested the fact that millions of individual women spent long hours every day planning, preparing, and cleaning up after individual meals, which tethered women to the home and turned them, she believed, into "over-worked, ignorant, unpaid mother-servant[s]." If anything, a housewife's lot was worse than a servant's, Gilman pointed out, because a servant could at least leave if she did not like the people who employed her. Housewives were simply trapped. Instead of settling for empty exaltation, Gilman said, women should *truly* professionalize housework, starting by transferring cooking outside the home to community kitchens, where women or men could go at the end of the day to pick up reasonably priced hot meals.[58] Unlike individual home kitchens, community kitchens could take advantage of economies of scale, saving a little money for everyone and enormous amounts of time for women who would otherwise focus their waking hours on cooking food.

Although Charlotte Perkins Gilman became the most vocal proponent of community kitchens, she was hardly their first or only supporter. Women's magazines had discussed the merits of cooperative housekeeping since at least the 1860s, and one way that home economists in the late nineteenth century had responded to the servant problem was by suggesting that cooking could take place in community kitchens.[59] In the same era, Edward Bellamy's famous 1888 novel, *Looking Backward*, had imagined a future socialist utopia in which domestic labor was outsourced to places like public kitchens and public laundries.[60] Throughout the late nineteenth and early twentieth centuries, socialists and other reformers argued that food should be produced outside the home both as a way to save women from needless domestic labor and to ensure that the poor received adequate nutrition.[61] Some of them did more than argue, too. In 1890, reformers in Boston started the New England Kitchen, which charged minimal prices for hot meals designed to be picked up by the urban poor and eaten at home. Although neither the Boston New England Kitchen nor its New York successor lasted more than a few years, workers at settlement houses like Chicago's Hull House looked to it as a model.[62] Even seemingly mundane reforms of the era, like widespread calls for women to buy bread from bakeries instead of baking it at home, were related to ideas about the social virtues of bulk food production.[63] Of course, consumers did not have politics in mind every time they bought bread or anything else; among other factors, it was starting to become cheaper in some cases to buy industrially produced foods than to pay for the ingredients and fuel needed to make them at home.

Public interest in community kitchens reignited during the Great War, with the heightened emphasis on efficiency, reduced waste, and economies of scale. In Britain, hundreds of "national food kitchens" operated during the war, and government administrators there credited them with contributing substantially toward feeding the population.[64] American government officials discussed ways of replicating the British model in America, and food administrators commissioned a formal study of community kitchens.[65] The authors of the resulting report observed that Americans seemed to be keenly interested in community kitchens, which they believed were "a logical outgrowth of war emergency conditions."[66] Indeed, they noted that wartime community canning kitchens staffed by volunteers had already sprung up around the country in order to help people preserve the surplus bounty from war gardens.[67] While government-funded community kitchens never became a significant part of Americans' eating habits, restaurants and food-delivery services did. Food delivery would become very ordinary over the course of the twentieth century, but in the late 1910s the concept of hot meals delivered to individual homes seemed vividly connected to politically charged questions about the servant problem, women's roles, and food conservation. For example, when the for-profit American Cooked Food Service Company debuted a popular food-delivery system in New York City in 1918, observers celebrated it as a community-minded system combining "English, Socialistic and American ideals."[68]

In contrast to community housekeeping schemes, home economists by the 1910s were arguing quite uniformly that what was needed was not *shared* housekeeping or even *less* housekeeping, but rather "better housekeeping," performed according to their methods. And they criticized feminists' suggestions that women would want to give up housework in order to "slav[e] for money in a factory or office."[69] Women working for wages outside the home: *that* was slaving. Unpaid housekeeping, in contrast, was nothing like servitude or slavery precisely because it was a labor of love. This argument made sense to many women, especially given their employment options at the time. Of the almost 25 percent of American women who were gainfully employed in the 1910s, few had white-collar jobs, and even those who did generally faced long hours, low-status positions, and little chance for advancement. In 1915, for example, one former stenographer published an autobiographical sketch called "Housewifery vs. Stenography," describing how her paid job, tyrannical boss, and jealous coworkers had made her miserable. After a few years of glum employment, however, she got married and became a housewife, and as a result, she wrote, "I'm, O, so happy! I'm healthier, too, because of the exercise my housework gives me. It's a positive joy for me to cook and see John's cheeks stick out with good living. I'm proud that my little boy has never had a sick day and that it's my efficiency that keeps him well." She employed a maid for a short time, she said, but she soon chose to do without the intrusions of a servant and to simply do all the housework herself.[70]

Although plenty of people casually described housewifery as a profession, those who could afford to think in such terms regularly claimed that being a housewife was better than mere paid employment because a home was not simply a workplace but a place imbued with "affections," "inspirations," and "spiritual values."[71] Another crucial pillar of home economists' case that women could and should do their own housework was that housewives, unlike servants, genuinely loved the people they served, an argument that built upon and transformed older associations between housework, servitude, and familial affection. During the nineteenth century, Americans who had employed servants or owned slaves had only increasingly used a vocabulary of familial duty, paternalist concern, and even love to describe and justify relationships between slaves or servants and their masters or employers, an argument slave owners in particular intensified in the face of the expanding abolitionist movement.[72] By the early twentieth century, however, the notion of loving servitude was fading, and home economists advised women to treat mistress-servant relationships as purely economic ones.[73] Instead, they insisted with growing boldness that the people best equipped to serve families' needs were those with authentic family love. As one woman in Washington, D.C., put it, American women needed to realize "that cooking is an art, and should be a labor of love, and be proud to be their own cook."[74] The same familial and paternalist discourses used to justify slavery and servitude in the nineteenth century also made it possible in the first decades of the twentieth to imagine that a loving, unpaid mother and wife should take over this sort of work. Servants were not family, after all, and housewives were.

GENERAL HOUSEWIFE ON A FOOD CRUSADE

On a cold January night in 1918, Martha Van Renssalaer prepared to give a speech at Cornell University's "Agricultural War Dinner." If the group of women and men gathered for the dinner missed prewar plates filled with steaming roast beef and soft white rolls, they did not say so. Instead, they ate their fill of fruit cocktail, baked kidney beans, stuffed potatoes, and cabbage salad, with squares of barley bread on the side. For dessert, they had a choice of cocoa, vanilla ice cream, or cookies made from rye flour and oatmeal, to conclude a meal scrupulously in line with meatless and wheatless wartime food guidelines. As the diners slowed down, only munching occasionally on the peanuts placed in little bowls on the tables, speakers began their presentations. When Martha Van Rensselaer finally rose to speak, audience members knew that she was about to leave for Washington to become co-chief of the Food Administration's Home Conservation Division, the highest-ranking position of a woman scientist in the U.S. government.[75] Her talk was titled "Women and the War."[76]

Home economics expanded furiously in the 1910s, thanks not only to federal funding but also to America's involvement in the Great War and the wartime food conservation campaign.[77] Once it became clear that food would play a crucial role in the war, home economists rushed to demonstrate the relevance of their discipline to the project, creating new recipes accommodating wartime substitutes, designing conservation courses for universities and high schools, and using their experience with home extension programs to teach housewives and farm women how to apply food conservation techniques in their own kitchens.[78] Even before it became an official agency, the Food Administration formed a Committee on Home Economics, and home economics directors, always women, were appointed in every state.[79] Herbert Hoover wrote a letter to all university home economics departments in the country, predicting that home economics graduates "will find themselves called to places of usefullness far surpassing . . . anything heretofore thought possible."[80]

Besides boosting home economics directly, the war also helped make servitude unfashionable, especially because keeping servants in wartime meant taking laborers away from war-related work on farms or factory floors. Resentment toward people who still kept servants became more open during the war. For instance, one of the paintings the Food Administration circulated at state and county fairs in 1918 pictured a servant in a formal black dress with white apron and cap, bringing a tray of food to an already overburdened table while in the background the shadowy ghost of a trench soldier gnawed on a crust of bread.[81] As a Baltimore journalist implied when chastening anyone "who still holds to the *luxury* of a dark-complexioned menial," employing a servant had become an extravagance no matter how much money you had.[82]

Others feared that servants, besides representing luxury and waste, themselves impeded efficient food conservation. In fact, precisely those privileged people who still employed servants by the late 1910s often argued that while they themselves supported food conservation, their servants did not. For instance, the prominent antisuffragist Alice Chittenden said, "Between many a willing housewife and the accomplishment of her desire is that Chinese wall of indifference—the servant slacker." According to her, the average servant was "a marvel of incompetence, wastefulness, indifference, absolutely unamenable to discipline," and opposed to anything resembling food conservation.[83] Negative pronouncements about servants in this era were regularly imbued with racist and classist assumptions, but stereotypes about the natural ineptitude of servants appeared with particular venom when the servants were African Americans.[84] When white women complained that it was impossible for them to conserve food as long as they had "a negro cook in the kitchen," however, they opened themselves up to an easy retort.[85] As one Alabama editor shot back, "If your cook is extravagant, oust her and do your own cooking! If you cannot cook, begin to learn now!"[86]

Plenty of women resented food conservation's special focus on their food decisions. Some took offense at the implication that all women had wasteful habits to curb when so many women had conserved food all their lives by necessity.[87] Others said they could not eat less than they always had because they did heavy manual labor all day and needed every crumb for sustenance.[88] To others, the focus on women felt unfair when men's appetites seemed like larger obstacles to effective conservation. One El Paso housewife suggested in a handwritten letter that a "word to the men-folks about demanding certain foods, cooked only certain ways will assist the women, Mr. Hoover."[89] Another woman wrote from Wisconsin about the meatless and wheatless days: "I am sorry to say, men seem to respond to it the least."[90] While administrators continued to aim most of their messages at women, a few addressed fears of men's reluctance to sacrifice, like one poster picturing a stout man feasting on an enormous restaurant meal, with the plea spelled out below: "Sir—don't waste while your wife saves."[91]

Yet other women felt empowered by the idea, as one Washington, D.C., woman expressed it approvingly, that the "little hands" of the women of America held the fate of world democracy.[92] Wartime rhetoric described the housewife as a strong, even martial figure who provided nation-building sustenance and international succor.[93] When food administrators proclaimed that food was crucial to winning the war, their next proclamation was usually that the U.S. housewife was on the frontlines, in her own "Amazon Army of Food Conservers."[94] Militarizing women's contributions raised the stakes. To waste any food whatsoever represented a housewife's failure to fulfill her "part in the great world struggle," while successful changes to family eating habits meant the housewife was "doing her bit toward making the world safe for democracy."[95] Posters declared that "Food is ammunition," and images paired domestic objects with weapons, demonstrating that hogs were worth more than shells, or that home canning was a literal weapon against Germany. Gender lay at the heart of appeals to Americans to save food, and it was supposedly the U.S. housewife whose personal food choices and domestic thrift figured as the bulwarks between the Allies and hunger. Images of warriorlike women—"General Housewife" on a "food crusade"—both acknowledged and enlisted women's contributions to the state and the war effort, although this brand of state participation was based upon women's actions in the private sphere.[96]

Because of home economics' successful professionalization of housewifery and its elevation as national service during World War I, the housewife in this era was taking on new, self-consciously modern meanings. *Today's Housewife*, a magazine that started appearing under that name in

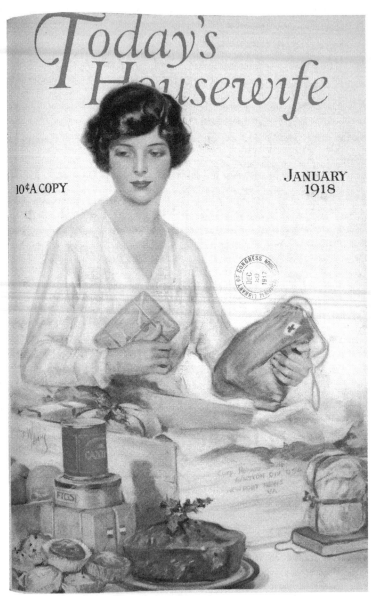

The cover of Today's Housewife, *January 1918. This modern housewife, well-groomed and evidently financially comfortable, packs holiday foods and Red Cross supplies into what is presumably a care package intended for soldiers abroad. Library of Congress, Washington, D.C.*

February 1917, epitomized this sense of the roles' renewal and modernization.[97] Yet while "housewife" remained the most common term to describe a woman who worked in her own home without servants and without wages, it was by no means the only one. Beliefs about this role—the sort of work it entailed and the sort of people who did such work—were shifting, and a battery of terms attempted to respond to these changes. Besides "housewife," other terms in general use during this era included "housekeeper," "homemaker," "home woman" "house-mother," "householder," and, with their air of administrative competence, "home manager" and "house manager."[98]

Those who hoped to elevate the status of professional housework tended to favor terms like "house manager" and "housekeeper" because they used the businesslike "house" instead of the emotionally charged "home" and because they were potentially gender neutral. After all, men sometimes needed food advice, too, like the widower in South Dakota who wrote food administrators to point out that he had been doing all his own cooking since his wife died three years before.[99] Yet too businesslike or too masculine a connotation could also be off-putting, and writers frequently paired terms like "housekeeper" with softening qualifiers to emphasize that the person it referred to was a wife and mother, such as "the American mother and housekeeper" or "Mrs. Housekeeper."[100] However, there was a big problem with the attempt to promote "housekeeper" as the general term to describe women who did their own housework, and that was that "housekeeper" could also refer to a paid servant.[101] In fact, in the U.S. Census for both 1910 and 1920, "housekeeper" was supposed to refer only to servants, and census keepers were dismayed when enumerators also listed women doing housework in their own homes as *housekeepers*," making a mess of their statistics.[102]

Of the possible terms to describe women who did their own housework full time, the ancient, conservative, Old English "housewife" remained the most popular one, with all its implications of marriage fully intact.[103] Top food administrators hated "housewife" because it seemed to apply only to married women whose main occupation was unpaid housework in their own homes, excluding servants, women who employed servants, women who worked in other jobs outside the home, unmarried women, and, of course, all men.[104] When James Montgomery Flagg, the illustrator who created the iconic World War I image of the pointing Uncle Sam, sent in the first draft of a propaganda poster he had created for the Food Administration, administrators angrily sent it back because Flagg had used the word "housewife" in his painting. Of the most "exceedingly great importance," an administrator admonished Flagg, "we want to stop the use of the word Housewives."[105] Yet no one could stop it. While "housewife" had always been popular, it was becoming unrivaled, and its dominance only increased in the decades that followed. And that was largely because of its implications of love, femaleness, and family, and not in spite of them.

In early 1918, an article titled "War Restoring Kitchen to Its Pioneer Place as Center of Home" appeared in newspapers across the country, and in a sense the headline was right.[106] The whole idea of respectable house-wifery signaled a return to some of the domestic ideals of the early republic, when women's domestic work seemed plainly of a piece with societal and national well-being. Furthermore, wartime rhetoric about women as the overseers of national sacrifice was a revival of older beliefs about women's special capacity for abnegation and piety. But in other important ways, the housewife model cast in the 1910s had no real precedent. The image of the housewife as an educated, powerful figure whose informed domestic decisions were a crucial part of international welfare and national victory was conspicuously modern.

SUFFRAGE AND THE ENLARGEMENT OF MUNICIPAL HOUSEKEEPING

The decline of domestic servitude and the professionalization of housewif-ery took place alongside the campaign for woman suffrage, and the movements intertwined in significant ways. Suffragists generally supported home economics, believing that domestic science demonstrated women's intellectual competence and their capacity for higher education. Many also hoped that by modernizing housework and lessening its burdens, home economics could serve as a liberating force for women generally. At the same time, concerns about woman suffrage spurred its supporters to respond definitively to the "servant problem" because they knew their opponents could and did use confusion over housework as evidence against women's problem-solving skills.[107] One antisuffragist, for example, said women could hardly claim the right to help steer government while "in the management of her own household, where her authority is absolute, she had failed to convince the world of her power to govern."[108]

Most meaningfully, the political exigencies of wartime food conservation provided suffragists with dramatic evidence that even traditional women's work was linked to politics. Suffragists rightly feared that the war's glorification of martial manhood threatened their cause.[109] Yet the war also magnified feminine virtues in ways that were potentially useful for the suffrage movement. By the late 1910s, women had been arguing for decades that management of the home was related to politics, describing city sanitation, waste removal, food safety regulation, and a host of other public issues as matters of "municipal housekeeping" that were both integral to the general welfare and natural extensions of women's conventional domestic concerns.[110] By placing food preparation and homemaking in national and international political contexts, the Great War allowed women to push this argument further, and suffragists quickly aligned themselves with the campaign for this reason.

Most directly, supporters of suffrage argued that women could most effectively deal with problems of food now and in the future if they had full political citizenship.[111] As one Wisconsin woman wrote in a letter to the Food Administration, she hoped "that we shall soon be able to vote for men and women who will give us adequate food legislation."[112] Others saw the government's reliance on women to conserve food as a bargaining chip. A Chicago woman, for instance, pledged to cooperate with the Food Administration but asked in the same breath whether Hoover in turn would cooperate with her by working for woman suffrage.[113] Other women simply refused to assist with food conservation at all until women were enfranchised, like the Massachusetts farm woman who would not sign the food pledge because as "a being with no political rights . . . I fail to see why my signature on one of your cards would have the slightest weight."[114] To suffragists and their sympathizers, the food problem made woman suffrage a more pressing issue than ever.

Administrators were apparently eager to enlist influential suffragists in their campaign, and leaders like Harriet Stanton Blatch and Helen Guthrie Miller toured the country giving speeches linking food conservation and the elevation of housekeeping to women's political freedom.[115] Administrators also tried to get Carrie Chapman Catt, president of the National American Woman Suffrage Association (NAWSA) and perhaps the best-known suffragist in the country, and Laura Clay, a leading southern suffragist, to volunteer as regular speakers, but both women declined because of their busy schedules. In fact, had the food conservation campaign started at any time *but* the summer of 1917, the high point of U.S. suffrage demonstrations and activity, suffragists almost certainly would have taken an even greater role.[116] As it was, NAWSA's weekly periodical, the *Woman Citizen*, issued a special edition on food conservation, and NAWSA produced a home economics textbook.[117] Local suffrage associations all over the country held conservation lunches and garden fairs and suffrage markets, where they sold produce at reasonable prices.[118]

Food also came to play a highly symbolic role in the suffrage campaign itself. Led by Alice Paul, the head of the more radical National Women's Party, suffragists started picketing in front of the White House in January 1917. The demonstrations continued unabated after the United States entered the war in April, and by the fall, the protesters' continued presence and their pointed reminders of the emptiness of claims about universal American liberty were becoming an international embarrassment. Finally, in October, police arrested and jailed dozens of women. Thrown into dank and vermin-infested cells and given food that was disgusting and sometimes inedible, the jailed women used their mistreatment by the state as proof they needed political rights.[119] Hunger strikes were by no means unprecedented in the international suffrage movement, but it is still significant that when Alice Paul and other suffragists imprisoned in the fall of 1917 chose a symbolic act that would simultaneously communicate the righteousness of their cause and their capacity for political self-government, they chose to fast.

While some refused food altogether, others publicized the gross inadequacy of the food they did receive. As it happened, Nan Wiley was among the women imprisoned that fall, and suffragists eagerly sent her husband, the famous food expert Dr. Harvey Wiley, meticulous descriptions of the food they received at every meal, noting whenever the items were rancid or contained worms or insects.[120] Wiley used his status as a nutrition expert to publicize the fact that the food fed to jailed suffragists was degrading and even dangerous.[121] Against the backdrop of intensifying federal pleas to American women to help with food conservation, headlines about the suffragists' mistreatment infuriated many Americans who had previously been indifferent to their cause. For instance, even though she was "not a suffraget" herself, one Philadelphia woman refused to sign the food card because of suffragists' mistreatment: "How did you treat the women of Our Country when they came to you for their rights? You all put them in Jail. Do you expect them to help you now"?[122]

Yet other people, including many other women, protested suffragists' public involvement with food conservation and their attempts to turn the new spotlight on food toward their own cause. Antisuffragists said lobbying for suffrage was wasteful, destructive, and unpatriotic at a time when the domestic work of all women was needed for wartime food conservation.[123] For instance, a farmer's wife in Minnesota, her hands "full of blisters yet" from threshing grain, wondered angrily "if those women that are bothering our executive officers at the capital with their banners would not be ashamed and quit" if they knew how urgently real women's work was needed in the nation's fields and homes.[124] Similarly, antisuffragists like Alice Chittenden chastised women for trying to tackle "mannish" political problems under the guise of "public housekeeping," when they should be attending to *actual* housekeeping.[125] To contrast the usefulness of their own nurturing domestic skills with the presumed extradomestic activities of suffragists, antisuffragists in Boston held a "Thanksgiving pie-fest" for servicemen who could not return home for the holiday in 1917.[126]

Others described even women's well-intentioned wartime activities outside the home as dangerously counterproductive to war aims. For example, in a special wartime cartoon from the creators of *The Outbursts of Everett True*, a popular comic strip of the era, a woman approaches the truculent Everett True and tries to sell him war savings stamps. In the next frame, only her skirt is visible as she flees, while he shouts after her, "I will gladly buy, madam, but I now want to give you a lesson in practical patriotism. Go home and stop your children from trailing half-eaten cakes and cookies wherever they go, and you will not be undoing the good work you are accomplishing by selling War Savings Stamps!!"[127] In a similar vein, the author of a Baltimore article made a devastating comparison between two well-intentioned housewives. The first, Martha, was highly organized, efficient, and energetic—and she stayed home all day attending to her home and her family's food needs. The second, Emily, prided herself on her patriotism because she volunteered for hours every day making surgical dressings outside the home, but in reality her hours away from her domestic duties meant she made poor choices and was perennially wasteful. Emily's attempts at patriotism failed because she neglected her home.[128]

Even as suffragists claimed that the international pressures of food conservation showed that educated women could be uniquely capable state actors, antisuffragists used the charged discourse about domesticity as powerful proof that women's place was in the home.[129] Food administrators as a group never officially endorsed woman suffrage, and administration literature generally evaded the question of women's political enfranchisement. While administrators recruited prominent suffragists as lecturers, some prominent antisuffragists also numbered among their speakers, like the muckraking journalist Ida Tarbell.[130] Instead, administrators compromised by describing housewives as strong, capable, and even martial figures whose political citizenship was, for the moment, irrelevant.

"I AM NOT A COOK," a Georgia woman named Seaton Taylor Purdon declared in 1917. "I don't like the word. It sounds greasy and smutty . . . hard and scrubby." Purdon had been married for a decade, and she had never cooked a single meal. Presumably an actual "cook"—a servant—had done that work. By the time the Great War began, however, food preparation was rapidly coming to seem important and even prestigious. New slogans like "Kitchen Conservation" and "Patriotic Housewife" filled the newspapers, and Purdon said those slogans appealed to her because they sounded "clean and intelligent and patriotic." In fact, the new wartime language about housewifery convinced Purdon to start cooking for the first time in her life. Or, as she revealingly put it, it convinced her "to enter my kitchen laboratory and to begin scientific research there to help Hoover."[131]

Questions about who did housework were tense ones in the first two decades of the twentieth century, and the images of bodily hygiene, or lack thereof, that Seaton Purdon invoked when she rejected cooking as greasy, smutty, and scrubby comprised a discourse on class. Home economists met such associations head on by investing housework with middle-class markers of prestige, arguing that doing housework well required high intelligence and a professional education based in science. The home economics movement further reframed women's roles by renewing housework's social value and giving it a sense of urgency that the U.S. experience in World War I compounded.

The vision of the modern housewife that emerged in the era of the Great War celebrated women's competence, yet it offered women an ultimately limited role. The very prestige granted to modern housework effectively silenced more radical alternatives to housekeeping while sidestepping the question of whether competent housewives could also be full political citizens. Even as home economists applied a vocabulary of professionalization to housework, they also clearly affirmed that housework could never be an actual profession because it was an extension of a woman's supposedly natural family role as a caregiver. Home economics made housework a challenging and dignified role requiring intelligence and preprofessional education, and in so doing it made it clear that it could never be a challenging or dignified job. Housework was both prestigious *and* unpaid, on both accounts making it seem reassuringly unlike the labor performed by servants.

5

A CORN-FED NATION

Race, Diet, and the Eugenics of Nutrition

In the interest of the race, of its mental as well as physical development,
there is no subject which should occupy the attention of educators comparable
with that of food. —Ellen Richards and John Norton, 1917

In 1917, the cuisine of the Old South arrived in New England. Southern
food was already there, of course, in the recipes and products and techniques carried north by generations of migrants and travelers. And of
course most "southern" foods themselves had been carried south in the
first place. It was Native Americans and colonial New Englanders who
had first experimented with the cornmeal recipes at the heart of the early-
twentieth-century version of southern cooking.

Yet from 1917 to 1919, in front of packed crowds at dozens of venues
around New England, an African American woman named Portia Smiley
demonstrated how to cook southern foods.[1] A college graduate, a published scholar, and a teacher, Smiley gave these southern food exhibitions
dressed up in the kerchief and full skirt of a mid-nineteenth-century slave
woman. As her audiences saw it, she was instructing them in the cuisine of
the antebellum South, cheerfully showing them how to make foods from
"Befo' the War."[2]

The ostensible purpose of these southern food demonstrations was to
increase the use of cornmeal, which most of Smiley's recipes contained.
During World War I, the U.S. government strenuously promoted corn as
a substitute for wheat, needed for food aid shipments to Europe. For white
audience members, however, it was Smiley's own southern blackness—as

much as the foods she cooked—that was on display. The wartime context of the food demonstrations only lent patriotic prestige to a kind of voluntary minstrelsy. The problem was that the thousands of people for whom Smiley performed did not recognize her clothes as the costume they were. Rather, they saw the "genuine bandanna turban" and the "voluminous white apron" of an authentic "Southern mammy."[3]

In the midst of the Great Migration, as hundreds of thousands of African Americans moved permanently from the South to the North, journalists emphasized Smiley's essential and unwavering southernness. She was "a genuine southern cook," a "typical southern cook," a "paragon of Southern cooks."[4] And lest anyone question what such a confirmed southerner was doing north of the Mason-Dixon line in the first place, they stressed she had come "north *solely and only* to disclose the secrets of just how to turn corn meal into the 'eatins' that have made southern hospitality and the southern table the envy of every cook in the land."[5] Writers described Smiley's southern accent and imitated—or invented—her speech in print: audiences could learn to make "the mos' appetizing things" with corn, "the kind of eats that just naturally slip down and might nigh carry your tongue along with them. Um yum, you all jus' watch Aunt Portia mix these dodgers!"[6] Her white sponsors and the northern journalists who reported on her food demonstrations did not refer to her as "Miss Smiley" or even simply as "Portia Smiley." Rather, they called her "Aunt Portia," using the falsely familial and presumptively familiar title that elite white southerners had favored for older black women.[7]

The fact that white northern food conservationists hired a southern black woman to instruct them in corn cookery was not an accident. Race and regionalism were integral to their understanding of corn, as well as other foods. For many Americans in the Progressive Era, race and food were intimately connected, even mutually constitutive. For decades, various Americans had expressed the idea that people of certain races ate certain foods, while people of other races ate other foods. Yet these assumptions about food and race were starting to come under greater scrutiny in the era of the Great War. Portia Smiley's wartime cornmeal demonstrations took place amid changing ideas both about nutrition science and about diet's implications for racial identity. Progressive zeal for social control assumed its most extreme form through eugenics, whose practitioners attempted to manage the "evolution" of national populations. By the early twentieth century, however, a new science called euthenics was complicating eugenicists' claims that sexual reproduction was the all-powerful instrument of racial change. Even as they maintained the conception of race and the importance of racial fitness, both black and white euthenists argued that environmental factors profoundly influenced physical and intellectual development. Food was one of their supreme tools.

Popular understandings of diet's effect on race were already changing when the United States entered the Great War in the late 1910s. But the war pushed these changes even further. The wartime campaign to forego familiar foods like wheat and beef—regularly described as the "natural diet" of white people—meant favoring other foods, some of which white Americans had previously thought of as fit mainly for people of other races.[8] In other words, in the midst of shifting beliefs about the nature of biological race and the meanings and limits of racial change, transformations in what was patriotic to eat coincided with new scientific advice on what was possible to eat.

THE EUGENICS OF NUTRITION

The notion that people could consciously guide racial development was not new. By the 1910s, eugenicists in Europe and the United States had been enthusiastically discussing racial transformation via sexual reproduction for decades. Eugenics was an ersatz discipline that had emerged in the final decades of the nineteenth century in response both to the popularization of Charles Darwin's theory of evolution by natural selection and to the recent successes of plant and animal breeders.[9] As it became clear that species changed over time, it seemed logical that humans might try to improve their own species. More specifically, it seemed desirable that whites might try to improve their own race, while ensuring its demographic dominance. Where natural selection was messy and slow, "artificial selection" seemed marvelously efficient.[10] Eugenicists openly described human reproduction as *breeding*, as they encouraged supposedly rational decisions about which human traits should be propagated and, ultimately, which people deserved to reproduce.

But how could something like diet affect the supposedly genetic process of racial change? Heredity dominated thinking on race throughout the era, but by the early twentieth century even fervent eugenicists recognized that parentage was not the only factor affecting health, intelligence, and appearance. Clearly, sanitation, exercise, nutrition, air quality, and other factors also profoundly shaped human development. As one race reformer put it, eugenics' narrow focus on heredity could "carry the race toward perfection" only so far; it needed the help of "its sister science, euthenics."[11]

Euthenics was a new discipline that emerged at the turn of the century to address environmental effects on race, and the feminized description of it as a "sister science" was consistent with broader perceptions. Although women were often ardent eugenicists, euthenics seemed to many to be an explicitly feminine field since its focus on hygiene and food overlapped with domestic concerns. Indeed, euthenists were often women active in the home economics movement. Before the term "Home Economics" had gained common currency, early practitioners had even debated adopting the term "Euthenics" for the title of their discipline as a whole.[12] And some urged white women to study home economics precisely because they were "the future mothers of the race."[13]

Of all the environmental factors that seemed to affect race, food was preeminent. If one knew how to read them, food's effects on the body were everywhere: in the larger statures of immigrants' children who received ampler diets than their parents had as children, in the crippling ravages of dietary diseases like rickets and pellagra, in the miraculous physical improvements claimed by adherents of fad diets, even in the physical and temperamental characteristics of different peoples, attributed to their diverse national cuisines.[14] Some people swore that anyone with a little experience could tell what kinds of food people ate by looking at their facial features.[15] Some even suggested that a new, superior race would result from the radical dietary improvements made possible by modern nutrition science and self-control.[16] Whatever the fantasies and misperceptions that led to the revelation, diet's immediate sway on the body made it seem like an especially potent factor in directed racial development.

Like eugenics, euthenics was a confused movement, a pseudo-scientific rubric under which diverse theories competed, the bulk of which served mainly to buoy up the theorists' self-aggrandizing conjectures about their own racial fitness.[17] Instead of a single, unified theory to explain how diet affected race, people instead offered sundry and sometimes contradictory suggestions. At times contemporaries drew stark distinctions between whites' supposedly delicate digestive tracks and the cruder digestive abilities of other peoples, as when a doctor in 1897 had argued that white people would literally die if forced to eat nothing but Chinese food, or when a journalist in 1900 claimed poor African Americans could eat anything "from horse-shoe nails and billy-goat tin cans up to elephant hide."[18] At other times, observers claimed that European and white Americans' penchant for rugged fare like beef made them uniquely strong, martial, and adventurous, in contrast to Asians, whose meek vegetable diets were thought to make them passive and philosophical.[19]

According to current theories, indeed, meat-eating had a profound effect on race.[20] Commentators asserted that it was meat that had nourished white intellectual and linguistic development over the course of evolution and that it was reliance on meat that had given Britons—nicknamed "beefeaters"—Anglo-Saxon racial traits.[21] In contrast, the "lower races" allegedly ate mostly vegetable diets, and some said vegetarianism itself accounted for their humble place in the racial pecking order.[22] According to the rather confused logic surrounding these discussions, meat had made whites the superior race that they were, and in turn, their superior racial identity made meat their natural food: wheat and beef were "the natural diet of the white man in the temperate zone," and white Americans were supposedly "born" with a desire for meat.[23] The association between meat-eating, whiteness, and power helps to explain the wartime vitriol toward vegetarianism. Even as the government urged its citizens to eat less meat, those who exalted the martial virtues went out of their way to link vegetarianism to inefficiency, effeminacy, and cowardice.[24]

Yet for all the attention focused on white meat-eating, plenty of non-whites also ate a lot of meat, and not all those people struck white Americans as particularly advanced. "Most of us believe that the flesh-eating nations are the leaders of civilization," wrote two nutritionists in 1915, but they ticked off an inventory of other peoples—from Turks to Maoris to Koreans—who also ate a lot of meat and yet were "neither civilized nor efficient."[25] At the same time, others pointed out that many of the "hardy peasants" emigrating from Europe to the United States had eaten little meat in their home countries and yet demonstrated remarkable strength and skill.[26] Even more problematic, throughout the era nutrition scientists were suggesting with growing confidence that protein could be obtained from a variety of nonmeat sources and that meat itself was less necessary either to mind or to body than once believed.

Simultaneously, traits that many had taken to be indelible racial characteristics increasingly seemed to result from diet. For instance, a white American man who had lived in Mexico for over a decade claimed that the greasy food there had made him mentally and physically sluggish but that after switching back to an American diet he found himself once again able to do advanced thinking and hard labor.[27] Similarly, a nutritionist suggested that while vegetarianism might account for low intellect among some races, those people became immediately more intelligent whenever they started to eat meat.[28] Instead of debunking the notion of biological race itself, however, many interpreted diet's supposed physical and mental influences to mean that races could simply change more quickly than previously imagined. For example, in 1912 a professor named Edward Steiner spoke from personal experience when he claimed that an immigrant arriving in the United States "becomes a member of a new race in a single generation." He himself had been born a Hungarian Jew "with only Semitic blood in me," but he claimed the new environment and abundant food in the United States had made his once-Semitic blood "pure American."[29] These new ideas about diet's powerful effects on race were one factor helping to revive Lamarckism—the idea that acquired traits could be passed down to children—in this era: if parents ate well and grew tall and strong and smart as a result, it seemed logical to many that their children would be taller and stronger and smarter, too.[30]

Eugenics and euthenics were deeply entwined. For instance, the renowned diet reformer John Harvey Kellogg was also an avid eugenicist, and he argued that a national registry of "human pedigree" should guide Americans' reproductive choices. In his vision, anyone planning to marry could consult the registry in order to investigate the genetic background of his or her potential spouse.[31] The federal government made no move to start such a registry, but in 1916 a group of eugenicists and euthenists did. At Kellogg's urging, his own Battle Creek Sanitarium housed the registry, designed to catalog "human thoroughbreds." The first person to register was Miss Susan Myrick, a physical fitness teacher from Georgia described by journalists, and by herself, as a "perfect woman" who climbed trees and slept outdoors all year long. Writers made clear that Myrick's perfection resulted from her environment as well as her genes; she was a devoted athlete who had "been taught to care for her body since she was a little girl."[32] But eugenics and euthenics were not always harmonious. Environmental effects on race defied the eugenic obsession with sexual reproduction as the cornerstone of race health. And some eugenicists cautioned that euthenics was risky business because by encouraging better food and hygiene, it promised to "conserve the life of even the most wretched human being," thus preventing what some considered the desirable deaths of the unfit.[33] Yet euthenists themselves promised to do more than preserve members of diverse races; many of them aimed explicitly to improve the white race.

Euthenics' intellectual vacuity did not prevent people from believing that diet and other environmental factors had racial results. If individuals ate poorly, they were unable to develop physically and mentally, and if diet affected individual health and disposition, then the food choices of a nation—or a race—could transform it in the future.[34] In an era saturated with racial theories, it came to seem that much more than dinner was at stake in deciding what to eat.

A HIERARCHY OF GRAINS AND RACES

White Americans supposedly had an obligation to their race to think very carefully indeed about diet, and the Great War only deepened this sense of racial obligation.[35] The slaughter of swaths of England's middle and upper classes—with whom some white Americans imagined an Anglo-Saxon kinship—exacerbated fears about racial survival. To make it worse, many assumed that in both Europe and America, those men who had volunteered for the army instead of waiting to be drafted were "the cream of the population."[36] According to this perspective, while the "finest types of physical manhood" went off to face machine guns, the less fit "were left at home, to father their kind."[37] One leading American eugenicist described the war as a "calamity"—not for humankind, but for the white race.[38] To make matters worse, the U.S. Army's rejection of half a million American men because of physical or mental unfitness sparked new worries about racial degeneration and the effects of nutrition on health.[39]

Shifting beliefs about food and race permeated efforts to change American diets during the war. When they sought to reduce wheat consumption, food administrators encountered particularly strong prejudices about the racial nature of food customs. This was a time when bread accounted for almost a third of all the food an average American ate, and when wheat was widely believed to be fundamental to national health.[40] The food expert Harvey Wiley even proposed establishing a federal minimum wage pegged to the price of wheat, so that workers would always be able to afford at least a minimum amount of bread.[41] As they tried to reduce wheat consumption at home, food administrators emphasized that wheat was only one of the many grains that could be used to make bread, along with corn, rice, oats, rye, barley, millet, and other cereals, and they publicized recent nutritional research demonstrating that other grains could offer nutritional advantages over white flour.[42]

Despite expert reassurance, however, many Americans remained adamant that wheat was superior to all other grains and that white flour was the highest, purest form of wheat.[43] According to this thinking, American soldiers *deserved* white bread: "Eat husks, if necessary, but send white flour to the fellows that are facing hell for you and you!"[44] People also routinely described wheat as a food that was both uniquely good and uniquely necessary for white people. In a commonly quoted phrase of the day, wheat was "the most sustaining food grain of the great Caucasian race."[45] Eating other grains flew in the face of popular, racialized hierarchies that placed wheat incontestably *above* all other cereals, followed by corn, oats, and finally rice.[46] Why did so many Americans consider wheat to be exceptional? Some argued, speciously, that it required more delicate cultivation than other grains and thus highly cultivated peoples were naturally the ones who ate it.[47] But for the most part, faith in wheat's superiority was simply descriptive. Because white Americans and western Europeans already relied more heavily on wheat than on other grains, and because so many of them considered themselves to be superior people, it made sense to them that their own staple grain was the best one.

Yet changing food habits complicated the racialized hierarchy of grains. Americans were eating more nonwheat cereals like corn and rice on a regular basis in the 1910s, and as they did so their racial associations with these grains shifted, if they did not altogether disappear. Rice cultivation had been widespread in colonial America, and it was common knowledge in the early twentieth century that white and black southerners had eaten rice for generations.[48] Americans outside of the South also ate rice occasionally, with Americans on average annually eating somewhere between eight and seventeen pounds per person.[49] U.S. rice production was rising steadily in this era, with the domestic acreage devoted to rice tripling in the first twenty years of the century.[50] Yet despite rice's centuries-long history in America and its contemporary visibility, its most vivid identity in the early twentieth century was as a foreign food.[51] Popular depictions of rice concentrated on its centrality to "the oriental races"; Asians were estimated to consume three-quarters of a pound daily per person.[52] Recipes containing rice often nodded to the East, like Oriental Stuffing, Calcutta Rice, and Japanese Eggs, and at least one recipe author gave rice-cooking instructions in the imagined voice of a Chinese cook: "Boil quarter of an hour or little more . . . keep him covered near the fire, then rice all ready. Eat him up!"[53]

Rice's eastern associations were strengthened by popular depictions of rice as an Asian supergrain, capable of fueling the prodigious labor of Chinese, Indian, and Japanese people.[54] White Americans who had grown up on the truism that meat was essential to health and strength marveled that anyone could toil for hours on nothing but rice and vegetable foods.[55] For instance, the author of an editorial in one small-town

Ohio paper was amazed that the Japanese had "fought and financed a great war"—the Russo-Japanese war of 1906, which the Japanese won—and were growing into "a great industrial nation, on a diet mostly of rice, root crops, barley, vegetables and fish."[56] But even if rice were a sort of miracle food, some believed its powers were accessible only to Asians. And those powers could be turned against whites. Around the turn of the century, Yellow Peril rhetoric had suggested that white men who supposedly required meat could not compete against Asian workers who could live cheaply on rice.[57] In 1906, the American Federation of Labor had gone so far as to frame labor problems in terms of dietary racism, publishing a booklet called *Meat vs. Rice: American Manhood and Chinese Coolieism.*[58]

By the 1910s, however, nutrition science was demonstrating that rice could be a healthful food for people of all races. After all, some white Americans, especially southerners, did eat rice, and they seemed to do just fine. One joke of the era laughed about this unlikely concurrence: South Carolinians were like the Chinese because they both "'eat rice and worship their ancestors.'"[59] One food administrator reported that at a Filipino boarding school for sons of U.S. army officers, each white American boy energetically performed his schoolwork and played baseball on a diet of curry and rice, "never realizing that he has had not only no bread but also no potatoes."[60] If anything, emerging evidence suggested that Asian diets might actually be *more* healthful than standard American ones. By the late 1910s, in the midst of rapidly rising U.S. rates of heart disease and other chronic diseases linked to diet, one journalist expressed the increasingly widespread concept that "rice-eating Orientals who rarely have steak or roast" out-lived Americans who lived on meat and bread and pie.[61]

Meanwhile, corn's even more prominent role in wartime food conservation was helping it to shed strong associations with poverty and provincialism.[62] Like rice, corn had been a staple of American diets in the colonial era. Unlike rice, corn had been absolutely ubiquitous in nineteenth-century cookbooks, too, starring in recipes like Cornmeal Gems, Indian Fritters, and Johnny Cakes. But by the late nineteenth and early twentieth centuries, middle-class Americans were eating less of it, favoring the industrially milled white flour that was increasingly available in towns and cities. Although American farmers in the 1910s produced a large corn crop, the bulk of it went to domestic livestock feed, and on average Americans ate less than one bushel of corn per person annually, with most of that consumption concentrated in the South.[63] Some southerners proudly discussed corn's staple role in their diets, like the Tennessee woman who described how for supper her family always ate "corn-bread and either sweet or sour milk and the children and Hubby and I sit round the fire and eat our milk and bread (the bread is baked in an old time oven) and enjoy our selves. The children sleep better on it than anything we can give them and the corn is nurishing and healthy."[64]

But by the 1910s many southerners were neither so open nor so enthusiastic about corn. Indeed, embarrassment about corn was most acute just where corn consumption was most prevalent.[65] Southerners knew "all about cornbread," as one journalist in an Alabama paper put it, but "some may timidly deny their knowledge and understanding of it, having become biscuit-proud."[66] Some white, middle-class southerners candidly discussed their wheat flour pride. For instance, a Missouri man admitted that he was raised on corn bread but "escap[ed] from it to Wheat bread at the first chance," just as a North Carolina woman explained that she and her family did not like corn bread because people "of the old South" preferred white flour biscuits.[67] Never mind that in the antebellum South itself, cornmeal had been vastly more prevalent than wheat flour. Southerners generally had the most to gain by distancing themselves from corn, but Americans around the country rejected corn as the food of "red necks and poor people," fit for those "whose tastes are common and whose associations must be low."[68]

Regional and racial prejudices had strengthened negative associations with corn inside and outside the South, but such associations were not purely imaginary. Until the mid-1910s, nutritionists had forcefully condemned southern diets, and Americans had real reasons to fear that there was actually something wrong with corn, and perhaps something physically inferior about corn-eaters. Pellagra—a potentially fatal disease whose victims' skin erupted in painful, weeping lesions—had been prevalent for decades throughout the South, just where corn was most commonly consumed. This coincidence fueled suspicions that corn itself caused pellagra. In truth, pellagra was related to diet, but it was the *absence* of protein and niacin that caused it, not the presence of corn or anything else. Only in 1914 did the epidemiologist Dr. Joseph Goldberger decisively challenge long-standing theories that corn-based diets triggered pellagra by running a controlled study of the diets of Mississippi prisoners who suffered from it. Those prisoners who received plenty of meat and milk got better, while prisoners who remained on a low-protein diet continued to suffer. When the newly healthy prisoners returned to their former low-protein diets, their pellagra also returned.[69] It was only after these medical studies in the mid-1910s that doctors were finally able to assert definitively that corn had nothing to do with pellagra or any other known disease, and that it was in fact a healthful grain.

While fears about corn's unhealthfulness faded, its regional associations held on. Just as the presence of rice inspired Asian recipe titles, so too did recipes with corn as their main ingredient often receive southern names like Virginia Spoon Bread, Dixie Gingerbread, or Southern Bisque.[70] Northern food administrators swore that, for southerners, eating a meal without cornbread was "like eating food without salt."[71] And in the name of wartime wheat conservation, writers urged northern women to "take a peep into a Southern woman's cookbook and try her favorite recipe for cornbread."[72] But despite such imaginative descriptions, corn had never been an exclusively southern food. New Englanders pointed out that corn was an old-time favorite of theirs, too, appearing in older dishes like hasty pudding, brown bread, and fried mush.[73] Meanwhile, people sent in cornbread recipes to the Food Administration from places like Iowa, Michigan, Pennsylvania, Baltimore, and New York City.[74]

Beyond corn's broad southern connotations—as well as its associations with southwestern and Mexican cuisines—many connected corn most strongly with southern African Americans.[75] Portia Smiley's "Befo' the War" cornmeal demonstrations were only one example of this connection. Two decades earlier, for example, the African American poet Paul Laurence Dunbar's popular poem "When De Co'n Pone's Hot" had affirmed corn's centrality to southern black diets and culture.[76] And in an era when both southern and nonsouthern whites assumed that African Americans had gained expertise over corn cookery as the longtime cooks of the South, many suggested that African American cooks might teach others how to do it as well as they did.[77] Early in the war a Florida man had anticipated Portia Smiley's work by advising the government to seek out "some black mammy" to teach northerners how to make corn pone, and Herbert Hoover himself had wanted to hire a "negro" cook to teach Washington chefs how to make corn bread.[78] Typically, a New Jersey cornmeal recipe pamphlet promising to teach corn cookery "the Good Old Southern Way" featured a black woman in a kerchief on its cover.[79] When food administrators encouraged Americans to eat corn bread in place of wheat bread, one journalist translated the directive into imagined African American dialect: "Eat 'Cohn Pon.'"[80]

Corn's strong regional and racial associations also inflected decisions about what foods were shipped to Europe. U.S. food administrators focused on grain exports because European diets leaned heavily on bread, but administrators could have chosen to export the relatively abundant U.S. corn crop instead of prioritizing wheat. There were some pragmatic obstacles to shipping large amounts of corn, since corn's natural oils can go rancid in transit and because there were few of the special mills in Europe needed to grind corn. But at least as much as these pragmatic concerns, wheat took priority because of food culture on both sides of the Atlantic. Early in the war, volunteers for the Commission for Relief in Belgium had made sporadic efforts to get Belgians to appreciate corn, and in 1916 one white American volunteer supposedly kidnapped a "regular American darky" he happened to stumble upon in a small Belgian town, driving him back to the commission kitchen and "turn[ing] him loose in the corn" without bothering to ask if he had ever cooked before in his life. According to an article later published in the *Saturday Evening Post*, the man cheerfully rose to the occasion, attracting a crowd of Belgians and winning them over with homemade "corn cakes, corn muffins, and every kind of corn joy that a negro ever loved."[81] Such reports were dubious at best, however, and most efforts to turn Europeans into corn lovers were ineffective. French people, who ultimately received the bulk of American food aid, proved especially resistant. The renowned nineteenth-century French chef Alexandre Dumas had dismissed corn as heavy, hard to work with, and only digestible by people with strong constitutions, and his disdain still typified French attitudes.[82] Virtually no French bread was made with corn in the 1910s, and the little corn grown there went exclusively toward animal feed.[83] Unlike potatoes, tomatoes, and tobacco, corn was one native North American crop that had yet to become a major hit in Europe, except among some polenta-eating Italians. The United States ultimately sent only a negligible amount of corn to Europe during the war.[84]

Instead, administrators focused on converting Americans into corn-eaters themselves, though this was no easy task either. Propaganda focused on the idea that corn was a *uniquely* American food that all Americans should be proud to consume. In one cartoon published in U.S. newspapers, a portly French chef, complete with a pointy moustache and a white toque, faced off against an African American woman in a kerchief and a hoop skirt. Confronted with a few ears of corn, the French chef throws up his arms in bewilderment while the woman cradles an armful of ears, saying, "You all jus' give that co'n to me. Ah knows what's good!"[85] It was wasteful to spend energy proselytizing to Europeans on the virtues of corn, food administrators urged, especially when U.S. recipes used corn to its best advantage. But government efforts to boost corn's status marked an uncomfortable departure for people who had grown up thinking of corn as inherently inferior.[86] In response to optimistic descriptions of corn as the national grain, a Los Angeles preacher spoke for many when he wrote angrily that corn was "the prevailing grain food among the Southerners, and especially among Negroes, but it is not the standard American food and never was."[87] Those Americans who were proud that they had never eaten corn bread often had no intention of starting, whether it helped the Allies or not.[88]

Yet in spite of resistance, more people in this era were coming once again to think of corn simply as an American grain, sometimes even as *the* American grain—one that was, after all, native to the Americas.[89] Indeed, instead of obscuring associations between corn and southern or African American diets, administrators shrewdly turned food prejudices on their head by highlighting those connections as authentic links to the U.S. past. They amplified such associations, in fact, by also emphasizing corn's links to American Indians and the colonial period. Corn was regularly described as the food of the "Indians, hardiest of races," a culinary expression of the widespread romanticization of Native Americans in the early twentieth century.[90] Writers pointed out that "hominy" was an Indian word, and they routinely referred to the grain as "Indian Corn," maintaining a designation that had been common in earlier centuries.[91] Wartime literature played on this association, like one corn-boosting poster that pictured an impassive Indian chief holding a fistful of corn.[92] At the same time, corn also connoted early white pioneers, who had "adopted the diet and conquered a continent."[93] Corn *had* been paramount to colonial American diets, forming the major exception to colonists' efforts to eat like the English, and some claimed that it was precisely because of corn that "our pioneer forebears thrived and grew greatly in body, and purpose and brain."[94]

Cornmeal products might seem old fashioned—like something "our grandmothers used to bake"—but that was not necessarily a bad thing.[95] As some twentieth-century Americans turned nostalgically to what they saw as a simpler past, magazines and newspapers printed colonial recipes that made use of corn, while recipes like "Old-Time Corn Bread" emphasized corn's age and authenticity.[96] Others called corn "American in every grain," "America's Own Food," a "distinctly American" food, a "REAL AMERICAN FOOD," the "Food for Americans," the "Nation's Mainstay," and the "true American food."[97] In fact, it was just at this time that the term "corn-fed" was coming to mean quintessentially all-American, with a midwestern—not a southern—slant.[98] By the mid-1920s, a popular song called "She's a Cornfed Indiana Girl" would pay tribute to the wholesome charms of an all-American country girl from the heartland.[99]

Corn and rice were only two of several grains that got a boost in the war era from federal attempts to convince Americans to eat less wheat, efforts that had to confront popular racialized hierarchies of the day that had placed wheat and wheat-eaters above other grains and the people who relied on them. Yet whereas rice and corn had once primarily suggested the exotic East or the backward U.S. South, the wartime food conservation campaign and the emerging nutrition science it relied upon offered powerful arguments that consumption of these grains posed no threat to anyone's racial identities and that, if anything, they might be a boon to health. As Americans all over the country began to eat more rice and corn, they started talking about these grains, and sometimes about themselves, in new ways.

AFRICAN AMERICANS, FOOD, AND A
NEW KIND OF UPLIFT

During the Great War, African Americans generally embraced food conservation as an opportunity to prove their patriotism and to dispel racial prejudice, operating on the optimistic theory that when "men fight together and work together and save together, this foolishness of race prejudice will disappear."[100] Off the battlefield, food administrators promised that black men and women who conserved food would bring "glory" to "the race."[101] For the most part, African Americans responded by taking up food conservation with gusto. In southern states, prominent black men, often the presidents of African American colleges, led local food conservation efforts.[102] African Americans held a 5,000-person food conservation convention in Atlanta and smaller meetings throughout the South, pledging money to support Belgian babies and growing and canning thousands of pounds of food at black orphanages, secondary schools, and colleges.[103] The Food Administration's bureaucracy included a "Negro Press Section," led by a black man named A. U. Craig and staffed entirely by African Americans, which printed special bulletins aimed at blacks. Section workers received so many requests for their pamphlet "How the Negro Can Help Make Food Win the War" that they had to order extra print runs.[104]

Unsurprisingly, racism and condescension permeated attempts to direct African American food conservation. White women regularly took it upon themselves to hold educational food conservation meetings for black women, sometimes purposefully including music to draw them in as they apparently assumed both that music would be uniquely appealing to black women and that conservation information would not be draw enough on its own.[105] One black woman in Washington, D.C., was outraged after attending a food conservation meeting for "colored women" run by white people, after one speaker imitated her "'old black mammy'" and another speaker told a joke about an "old darkey down South."[106] Food-saving literature aimed at African Americans was often intentionally simplistic in tone. For example, the middle-class African Americans working in the Negro Press Section clearly suspected the details of food conservation might confuse uneducated readers: "If there is anything in reference to the saving of food that is not clear to you," they wrote in one bulletin, "call upon your county director, and he will cheerfully help you."[107]

Meanwhile, African Americans were increasingly working as extension agents in the South.[108] This was less because of expanding job opportunities and more because whites believed African Americans needed more uplift than anybody but hardening segregation prohibited white extension workers from entering their homes.[109] By the summer of 1918, the Department of Agriculture had trained more than 200 African American home demonstration agents, while southern states appointed dozens of additional African American agents to visit local homes and farms.[110] The leading black intellectual W. E. B. Du Bois noted irately that the government was "spending more money today in helping Negroes learn how to can vegetables than in helping them to go through college."[111]

In spite of African Americans' individual and collective contributions to food conservation, many whites persisted in the racist fancy that African Americans were incorrigibly wasteful and greedy when it came to food. One white Virginia man harped on the wastefulness of black chefs, while a North Carolina man blamed any waste in southern kitchens on "carelessness and lack of training of the Colored cooks."[112] This was at a time, of course, when middle-class southern whites did not do much cooking themselves. Other whites claimed that African Americans were relentlessly pleasure-seeking and thus powerless to resist the lure of their favorite foods. Patriotic food conservation appeals would be futile, they were sure. One magazine writer suggested that the only way to ensure black southerners' loyalty in wartime was to bribe them with "a string of catfish and a wagonload of watermelons."[113] And while *they* had enough self-discipline to conserve food voluntarily, many whites swore African Americans would "never enlist for voluntary efforts of food saving."[114] Typically, in an article printed in Arizona, a journalist joked that if food administrators could "get a culled pusson to look at three fat po'k chop and decide to eat but one because of the necessity for war economy we shall admit that the age of miracles began with Hoover."[115] Of course, these racist assumptions served the double purpose of throwing into relief whites' supposed mastery over their own appetites.

In white imaginations, African Americans *cared* more about food than whites did, and black cooks were more concerned with the social status that "proper" food conferred on the people who ate it than their white employers were. Thus, wrote one Baltimore journalist, wartime conservation would mean big changes to black cooks' "lavish ideas as to the proper preparation of a Maryland dinner."[116] Likewise, the Hoovers' African American cook supposedly had "very definite ideas" about "what 'quality folks' ought to have on their tables," and Mrs. Hoover supposedly had trouble convincing her "that meatless meals and hoecake" were "quite the thing for Mrs. Hoover to offer to her guests."[117] It is significant in this narrative that it is the African American servant herself who seeks to protect her white employers from the effects of a culinary transgression; meatless meals and hoecake were poor southern—possibly black—foods. And yet at the same time, the very fact that it was a black servant erecting these cultural borders emphasized for white audiences how childishly folklorish such borders really were. The idea that African American servants were more sensitive to their employers' social standing than they were themselves was a reiteration of an old theme, beloved by elites, that it was in fact the socially disadvantaged who cherished class differences. In this case, whites imagined that food conservation would confuse and disturb black cooks who "didactically held to cherished ante-bellum recipes," slyly implying that it was African Americans themselves who clung to antebellum ways, which included most distinctly, of course, slavery itself.[118]

Throughout the Progressive Era, educated, middle-class women were more and more relying on printed cooking instructions in cookbooks and magazines and on formal training from home economics courses. And in this context it is all the more telling that whites clung more fiercely than ever to the racist trope that African Americans cooked by instinct. In 1903, for instance, one former slave owner wrote that the source of slave cooks' good cooking had not been knowledge or experience but rather black magic and "kindly incantations."[119] Likewise, the staff of a girls' school during the war said they would love to supply the government with the recipe for the wheatless war bread made by the school's

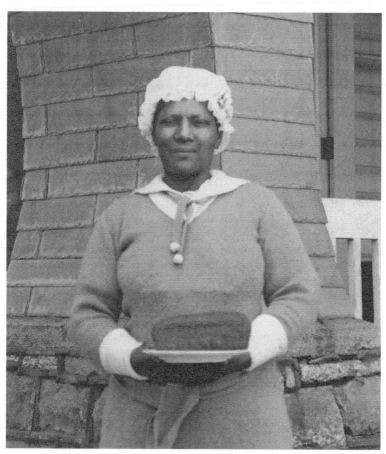

This woman was identified only as "Mammy" by administrators of the
Bremestead School in Lake George, New York, where she worked as the head cook.
School administrators reported that "Mammy's" war bread was exceptionally good
but her recipe was unavailable because, they said, she cooked only by "instinct."
Folder "58 Bremestead School," box 300, Home Conservation Division,
General Correspondence, RG 4, NARA, Kansas City, Mo.

cook, whom they called "Mammy," but they could not because she cooked only "by instinct."[120] In the same way, after a foreign guest staying with the Hoovers asked for their cook's corn bread recipe, the cook supposedly had to cook the corn bread all over again "to find out just how 'twas I did make it," consciously measuring for the first and only time to discover what quantities she had used.[121] At a time when many African Americans knew how to cook out of necessity and when many middle-class and upper-class whites did not know how to cook at all, whites translated

African Americans' authority over food into evidence of their lack of authority over other areas of life. If African Americans were good at cooking, they reasoned, then it was because they were instinctively drawn to food preparation instead of to more intellectual work. In turn, this supposedly inborn attraction to food made African Americans uniquely fitted to *be* cooks.[122]

If some believed African Americans were instinctively skilled at cooking food, they also thought they were naturally good at farming it, and many whites assumed that the biggest contribution African Americans could possibly make to the war effort was in a field.[123] Instead of working in "Northern 'war' plants," a *Washington Post* writer quipped, African Americans "would better be cultivating Southern food plants."[124] As critics saw it, of course, the problem was that more and more African Americans were heading toward those very factories in the North. During the 1910s African Americans were leaving the South in staggering numbers to take better-paying northern jobs.[125] Between 1916 and 1918 alone, half a million black southerners moved northward, many of them eager to secure industrial war jobs, and all of them anxious to flee the segregation and violence of Jim Crow.[126] The northern migration panicked white southerners who saw a plentiful and dirt-cheap labor force streaming away, and they did what they could to discourage mass departure, painting the migration as a fool's errand and the North as a fool's paradise.[127] Despite such self-serving pessimism, and despite sometimes violent efforts to force African Americans to stay, however, migrants continued to pour into and remain in the North.[128]

As destructive and baseless as the racist evolutionary theories rampant in the early twentieth century were, they influenced blacks as well as whites.[129] Even the *Crisis: A Record of the Darker Races*, the preeminent African American newspaper founded by W. E. B. Du Bois, contained stock racist gags in this era, including images of stereotyped mammies, dialogue of poor blacks written out phonetically for comic effect, and references to African Americans' supposedly natural sense of music and rhythm. Even when rebutting scientific racism, African Americans regularly used a vocabulary of race difference and race development, sometimes by turning vituperative reprimands against poor and uneducated African Americans. At this time, black infant mortality rates were significantly higher than those among other groups, while life expectancy was significantly lower.[130] Bolstered with such data, some whites claimed that African Americans were actually degenerating as a race—a devolution that some said would lead to their eventual extinction. While African Americans scorned such genocidal suggestions, they sometimes met the underlying racism half-way, agreeing that their race had far to go but arguing that it was making great strides instead of going backward. For example, some black writers conceded that African Americans fell short of "the full modern standard," but they claimed that African Americans were undergoing a "rapid evo-lution."[131] And even if blacks were somehow "behind" as a race, some in-terpreted this positively to mean it was a "young race, developing into its prime."[132]

Guiding that development was crucial, and socially ambitious African Americans in the early twentieth century talked openly about sexual re-production as a way to advance the race.[133] But increasingly, influenced by the euthenics movement, some also began to talk about directing racial development by improving environmental factors.[134] If black health and fitness were currently less than ideal, one journalist argued, that was the result of bad food and unwholesome surroundings, *not* "inescapable he-reditary ills."[135] To improve themselves physically, another journalist ad-vised, individuals should eat "strengthening food, sleep with the windows open, and get out of the alleys and swamps."[136] Black writers sometimes chastised others for their food habits. For a long time, ran an editorial in the *Crisis*, "it has been known that we as a race eat too much meat, espe-cially pork, and are ruining our digestions with hot bread made daily."[137] Mothers read in the *Chicago Defender* that the food they fed their children influenced the structure of their faces: if a child's chin looked too big, then parents should give the child less starch, and if parents considered a child's lips too full, they should provide less sugar.[138] "Food—reasonable food" was what African Americans needed to "win health and efficiency," not eugenic breeding.[139]

To refute charges that they were degenerating racially, some African Americans also energetically provided evidence of their physical health. Observers claimed that race health manifested in black men and wom-en's "remarkably beautiful figures, strong, well-developed, beautifully molded."[140] As they saw it, physical vigor was a tangible sign of racial vi-tality, proof that black racial degeneration was a fiction. From a racial perspective, physical health and beauty were particularly important in children, the flag-bearers of racial change, and "Better Baby" contests flourished during the 1910s and 1920s as both whites and blacks enthu-siastically evaluated children with external measures of physical vitality. The contests extolled children's looks as the ultimate indicators of indi-vidual and racial fitness, and it is notable that they thrived even as medi-cal science increasingly demonstrated that appearance was not a reliable measure of health.[141] Similarly, starting in the early 1910s, the *Crisis* published a yearly children's issue, by far its most popular of the year.[142] The special issue included dozens of photographs of sturdy black children, some of whom—"Perfect Children"—had won prizes in Better Baby contests.[143] *Crisis* editors were confident that even a cursory examination of the photographs of the "well-nourished, healthy, beautiful children" would dissolve the charge that African Americans were incapable of advancing physically.[144] Although editors acknowledged that the children pictured came mainly from financially comfortable families and that plenty of poor children were less robust, they still insisted that the number of healthy black children was growing, not shrinking.[145]

IN THE PROGRESSIVE ERA, it seemed clear to a remarkable number of people, both black and white, that the best way to produce a "better race" tomorrow was to produce "stronger individuals today."[146] Good nutrition, sound hygiene, and other environmental factors clearly seemed to affect racial fitness as well as individual well-being; more and more, the two kinds of health looked inseparable.[147] Newly bolstered by such euthenic claims, many rejoiced that nutrition science had handed them a powerful tool to direct racial progress, and by the time the United States entered the Great War, some proposed that the austerity demanded by food conservation itself could improve racial stock: "We eat less, fewer and simpler now. We'll be a stronger race as a result."[148] The euthenics movement capitalized on emerging nutrition science to promote a new kind of racial uplift.

Euthenics and eugenics were interwoven, and euthenic assessments of diet and race fed upon the same self-glorification that fueled the eugenics movement. The intersection of racial theories and nutrition science deeply affected the wartime food conservation campaign, particularly efforts to get Americans to eat less wheat and more rice and corn. The Progressive Era was the high point of euthenics, and in the decades that followed, Americans decreasingly thought about food as a category that fell along strict racial lines or of racial traits, as such, as being determined to any great degree by diet. Still, euthenic ideals survived in surprising ways. In the late twentieth and early twenty-first centuries, Americans in large numbers continued to attribute some parts of intelligence, stature, physical health, and personality to genes, but they generally saw genetics on an individual or familial scale, rather than on a racial one. Meanwhile, a century after the height of the euthenics movement, Americans' fascination with the ways environmental and cultural factors like diet, exercise, sanitation, and education shape intelligence and health shows no sign of diminishing.

It was at euthenics' peak, just as common understandings of both nutrition science and the so-called racial sciences were shifting, that Portia Smiley toured New England teaching white northerners to cook with corn. Smiley's success as a culinary authority, gained while she was dressed as a slave, points to the perversions at the heart of the era's dietary racism: her ability to present herself as an expert on corn depended precisely on racial prejudices that her knowledge and expertise themselves challenged. Yet however incoherent such prejudices may have been, Smiley still lived in a world that they shaped. She had apparently been born in South Carolina in the late 1850s, presumably as a slave. By the time she was in her early twenties, she was working as a servant in Georgia, living in the home of her white employers, an illiterate housewife and an auctioneer.[149] Then, somehow, she was able to leave servitude behind and move to Virginia, where she attended the Hampton Institute. For thirty years afterward, she was a popular teacher at a variety of black secondary schools around the South, and it was during these decades that she started to publish scholarship, writing and contributing to several journal articles about African American folklore.[150] Then came the Great War and her celebrity as a cornmeal demonstrator. In 1919, she authored an entire edition of the *Journal of American Folklore*, and by 1920 she was living in Boston, where she worked as a cooking instructor and lived as a lodger in a boardinghouse, the only African American in a house filled with white people.[151]

But Smiley's relative prosperity did not last. By 1930, she was no longer working as a cooking instructor and no longer able to afford a room in a boardinghouse. Instead, she was once again a servant, living in the Boston home of the elderly white woman who employed her.[152] Smiley appears in no censuses after that, presumably because she died. After all, she was an older woman herself by 1930—probably in her early seventies. But probability is all historians have in the case of Portia Smiley. Early censuses reported that she was born in 1857, but starting in 1920 Smiley seems to have claimed that she was born twelve years later, in 1869.[153] While nineteenth-century census records frequently contained errors, it seems probable that the birth year given for Smiley when she was a young woman was more accurate than the one she reported in 1920; in other words, it seems unlikely that in 1880, for instance, she could have passed for twenty-three if she were actually eleven, whereas it seems plausible that as a sixty-three-year-old in 1920, she could have passed—and may well have wanted to pass—for someone in her early fifties. Perhaps she shaved a dozen years off her age out of vanity, or out of pragmatism as she sought to renew her career. Or perhaps Portia Smiley simply wanted to play a new role, that of a woman born after the Civil War, a woman who had never been a slave to anyone.

6

AMERICANIZING THE AMERICAN DIET

Immigrant Cuisines and Not-So-Foreign Foods

Not only do we meet strange foods when we travel,
but if we are patriotic, we have them when we stay at home.
—Harvey Wiley, 1918

Around noon one day in the early 1910s, a home economist paid a visit to an immigrant family's small home. She found the family in a stuffy room, eating lunch while a large cat perched on their dirty table, begging for morsels. The cat, the filth, and the airless room were bad enough. But much worse was what the family was eating, and how. Crowded around a single common bowl, the family members squeezed in together in order to scoop stew into their mouths with their bare hands. To the woman reporting on the incident later, it was a revolting sight, one that revealed many of the problems with immigrant eating and, by implication, many of the virtues of the way she and like-minded Americans ate.[1]

Today, the idea of a family shoveling stew into their mouths with their hands seems strange, but it is their bare hands that surprise us, not the fact that they were eating stew in the first place. That immigrants to the United States in the early twentieth century often ate things like stews or other mixed, saucy dishes seems utterly unremarkable. But people remarked on it all the time in the Progressive Era. For years, doctors, home economists, and efficiency experts had warned that to eat gloppy, mixed foods containing many ingredients—a style of cooking some native-born Americans had come to define as inherently foreign—was to imperil digestion and to deviate from white people's so-called natural diet. The conjoined nature of these mixed foods seemed unwholesome and inscrutable, and fears of the unknown combined with fears of dirt, disease, and contagion.

During the era of the Great War, Americanization—the movement to induce foreign-born people and their children to adopt "American" customs and habits—reached the height of its power. By 1910, more than a third of the U.S. population had been born outside American borders, and food had become an important part of Americanization efforts.[2] Reformers worked to convince immigrants to eat the plain meat and starch pairings that they considered the model American meal, and the physical foundation of American efficiency and success. While immigrants were the focus of such efforts, however, it was not just the foreign born who were hearing advice to eat plainer, more insipid meals: reformers were urging everybody to "cultivate a taste for simple foods" in the name of a supposedly authentic American diet.[3]

Yet even as Americanization efforts crested in the late 1910s, the whole concept of Americanization itself was changing. In the context of wartime food conservation and out of a growing realization that many immigrant dishes actually offered nutritional and economic advantages, reformers increasingly sought to modify immigrant diets rather than to revolutionize them. And when made with familiar ingredients and adjusted to become less spicy and less saucy, these "foreign" dishes themselves became more acceptable for consumption by native-born Americans. Meanwhile, more native-born Americans than ever were eagerly seeking out exotic tastes.

Indeed, at the very high point of Americanization efforts, self-evidently foreign foods were appearing more often in ordinary American newspapers, cookbooks, and kitchens. These two processes seem counterintuitive, but they were not actually at odds. Foods like hamburger casserole, chicken noodle soup, and chili struck many in 1910 as obviously foreign foods. Yet only a few decades later they would strike their grandchildren as comfortingly all-American dishes. In a way, both generations were right. The process of making foreign foods widely acceptable meant producing blander versions using ingredients with which native-born Americans were already familiar. In so doing, Americans domesticated the very foods they thought of as the basis of their newfound culinary cosmopolitanism.[4]

It is always impossible to identify precisely why or when something as nebulous as the food preferences of millions of people changed. But during the 1910s, 1920s, and 1930s, large numbers of Americans—particularly middle-class, white Americans—*did* increasingly seek out what they considered obviously foreign dishes like pasta, goulashes, stews, and casseroles. In part, new interest in the pleasures of the exotic and in foreignness itself was a top-down trend, fueled by the reassurances of nutritionists, World War I propaganda, the urgings of recipe authors and magazine editors, and the enticements of corporate marketing. A broad range of Americans had expressed interest in foreign foods and foreign ways of eating for decades, but these foods attained a level of popularity in the 1920s and 1930s that was truly unprecedented. And that popularity resulted from a combination of factors, not all of them suggested by experts or advertisers, ranging from changing beliefs about the relationship between food and race, to anxiety about the homogeneity of an industrializing food supply, to nostalgia for simpler times and peasant fare, broadly construed, to the fact that immigrants themselves seemed less of a threat as immigration rates receded during the 1910s and plummeted after the Immigration Restriction Act of 1924.

Americans became vastly more receptive to so-called foreign foods in the era of the Great War, as they domesticated them by using familiar ingredients and as they recast them as both appealingly exciting and fundamentally unthreatening. In this era, fewer Americans found foreign foods to be inedibly exotic, and more than ever came to find them uniquely modern and uniquely desirable. These changes in Americans' attitudes happened over decades, and they happened unevenly, as individual perspectives changed haltingly over time. But by the 1920s and 1930s, enthusiasm for foreign foods would become mainstream in a way it had never been before, and that enthusiasm would continue to inform definitions of modern American eating for decades.

THE AMERICAN COOK AND PURE FLAVORS

To many in the first two decades of the twentieth century, the United States felt awash in foreign-born people. About thirty million European immigrants had entered the country during the nineteenth century, and the pace of immigration had only accelerated since the turn of the twentieth, as immigrants poured in from southern and eastern Europe.[5] Immigration helped push the U.S. population from 63 million people in 1890 to 100 million by the late 1910s.[6] By the time of the Great War, a third of all Americans primarily spoke a language other than English.[7] Fearing that foreign influences would swamp collective American customs, some Americans—mainly white, native-born people—turned with zeal to the project of Americanization.[8] Proponents of Americanization shared a faith in their own superiority, and they sought to convince immigrants to adopt what they saw as a superior "American culture," which could refer to anything ranging from beliefs about time and money, to ideas about democracy or women's roles, to the adoption of the English language, to health and hygiene practices, to styles of dress and hair.

In fact, the sense of superiority that fortified Americanization efforts was more than cultural. It was racial. Like most Americans in the early twentieth century, Americanization reformers generally believed that immigrants represented *races* that were as distinct from each other as they were from the white Anglo-Saxons who supposedly made up the U.S. majority. When they thought about race—and they thought about it a lot—Americans in the early twentieth century did not just see blacks and whites, Hispanics and Asians. Instead, as the historian Matthew Jacobson has described, they saw a gallery of races: there were Slavs, Hebrews, Irish, Finns, Poles, Italians, Latins, Nordics, Alpines, Teutons, and Anglo-Saxons, among others. And that was just among people of European origin, not including a dizzying array of Mongols, Malays, Negroes, Orientals, and more.[9] At the turn of the twentieth century, race meant much more than color, and beliefs about nationality, religion, and language all inflected American racial taxonomy.[10] As a direct result of racial beliefs, food became a pillar of Americanization efforts.[11] It is not only that racial beliefs informed thinking on food, however: ideas about food also influenced changing ideas about race. Indeed, the intimacy of eating and the materiality of food itself made it a substance that embodied race and difference in a uniquely tangible way. The foreignness of immigrants could seem most acute when Americans thought about the strange—in some cases, the disgusting, almost unimaginable—things they ate.

Yet, in a peculiar counterpoint, many Americans at this time also thought of foreign food as the pretentious diet of the American upper class. Throughout the late nineteenth century, wealthy Americans and their emulators had eagerly replicated European styles of cooking and dining, particularly the rich, sauce-based dishes and elaborate multicourse meals of French haute cuisine.[12] By the 1910s, however, enthrallment with fancy European cooking was fading. Elaborate and unpronounceable French dishes seemed elitist, and middle-class Americans were increasingly vocal about their objections to foreign phrases on American signs and menus.[13] In New York, for example, one pure-food organization launched a national campaign to eliminate French from American bills of fare, including the use of the originally French word *ménu* itself, arguing that "Americans are entitled to the privilege of ordering their dinners in English."[14]

A cartoon that appeared in a trade publication for American bean growers illustrated the supposedly enervating effects of a fancy French

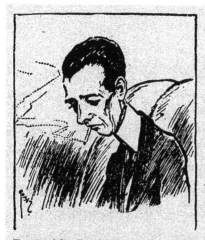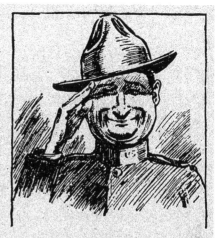

Reginald Looked Like This While His Chef Fed Him Caviar, Filet Mignon, Paté de Fois Gras, etc.

But Now That He Gets Plain Baked Beans and Fresh Air He Looks Like This

—*From Life.*

This cartoon shows the positive transformation wrought in
"Reginald"—and potentially in American manhood as a whole—by the
combination of fresh air and plain American food to be found in army life.
From The Bean-Bag *1, no. 2 (East Lansing, Mich.: Little, 1918), 44.*

diet and the restorative potential of plain, American food. The cartoon's first panel depicts a man called "Reginald" at the time when "His Chef Fed Him Caviar, Filet Mignon, Paté de Fois Gras, etc." On this diet, Reginald is the very picture of an effete neurasthenic. He slumps in an armchair, his neck is bowed and his shoulders stooped. He looks emaciated and spent: his cheeks are sunken, his eyes are downcast, and he barely manages to hold a drooping cigarette between his lips. In the next panel, however, "Plain Baked Beans and Fresh Air" have completely transformed Reginald. Now he stands erect, facing the viewer squarely and smiling while he salutes. Dressed in a U.S. Army uniform, he looks fifty pounds heavier.[15]

Whether referring to the food of impoverished immigrants in U.S. slums or to fancy European haute cuisine, white, native-born reformers generally described foreign food as objectively inferior to their own. But what *was* their own food? For a long time, the United States had not seemed to have a clear national diet, largely because Americans' diets had looked so hopelessly diverse.[16] While the country had relatively distinct regional cuisines, the borders of those cuisines had always been blurry, smeared by nonstop migration among people, food products, and recipes alike. Around the turn of the twentieth century, however, a newly articulate version of American national cuisine began to emerge in direct response to the rising tide of immigrants. In the absence of a clearly unified national diet, reformers around the turn of the century invented one, and they did so by looking very selectively to the past. According to them, a true American diet was a historical amalgam of pioneer simplicity and white New England staples, especially wheat, beef, pork, dairy products, and boiled vegetables.[17] One of the hallmarks of the version of national cuisine that emerged in the first two decades of the twentieth century was the sense that real American food was by nature plainer, simpler, more honest, and less convoluted than food from other countries.

In practice, plain food meant foods with few constituent ingredients and with those ingredients generally visible. With no sauces and few spices, no scraps of this and that, people could see and *know* what they were eating, and their bodies could better absorb what was put into them. By this logic, a beef and vegetable soup was by its very nature less digestible than plain beef with cooked vegetables on the side. This middle-class idealization of plain food contrasted sharply and purposefully with the diets of poor people. Whether they were born in the country or not, poor people tended to mix their foods together as they cooked in order to heighten flavor, stretch costly animal products, and help to use up every crumb. Associations with poverty and poor health helped to tar mixed foods in the minds of food reformers, and that was especially true when those mixed foods came from poor immigrants. As some middle-class, native-born whites saw it, immigrant food *meant* mixed food—"foreign mixtures" like stews, pastas, noodle kugels, stir fries, casseroles, sausages, and sauces.[18] The very mingledness of such foods seemed suspicious. Who knew what such "strange compounds" really contained?[19]

Indeed, while saucy French-inspired dishes differed markedly in spirit from rough immigrant fare, in this respect they did not differ much in fact. As middle-class Americans increasingly rejected French culinary elitism, they put French food in the same category of unwholesome mixed foreign foods, describing French sauces as deceitful concoctions or as "camouflage" deployed to cover up food's natural taste and perhaps to make edible something that otherwise was not.[20] For example, one journalist claimed, incorrectly, that medieval cooks had used spices to cover up the taste of rotted meat and that the "modern complicated cookery" of France evolved out of this deceptive tradition.[21] Of course, food reformers were selective in their description of what mixed foods meant. For instance, while saucy foods were clearly foreign and clearly bad, familiar goods like biscuits or cookies or puddings, which also contained many constituent ingredients that had been mixed together, were almost wholly exempt from the scrutiny brought to bear on other kinds of mixed foods.

In an era saturated with racial theories, it seemed logical that race might influence how the body absorbed food, and many assumed that whole races of people had distinct and predetermined dietary needs. In some cases, reformers argued that eating mixed foods was tantamount to racial transgression. As one doctor wrote in 1914, "[d]ifferent races" needed "different foods differently prepared."[22] Accordingly, reformers sometimes described mixed foods not only as un-American but as un-white, as "nauseous messes which a white man could not eat."[23] They meant that literally, believing that white people's stomachs actually could not digest combinations of mixed foods, while the stomachs of other, less civilized people could.[24] Meanwhile, spicy and highly seasoned food might be harmless enough for those "in the tropics," but they would do positive ill to Americans.[25] In contrast to the mixed and pungent foods that characterized the cuisines of so many other parts of the world, white American cuisine was supposedly plain, pure, and easy to digest.[26]

Digestibility was indeed a driving concern in this era, part of broader preoccupations with the body's economy of energy.[27] Much more so than people today, Americans in the Progressive Era tended to see ingestion and digestion as two distinct processes, stressing that it did not matter if people were swallowing nutritious foods if their digestive tracks were hindered from absorbing what they ate. And all sorts of things could supposedly foul the digestive works. In the name of promoting digestion, people chewed food for minutes at a time and boiled food for hours, and they stayed away from sour foods, spicy foods, heavy foods, and foods that were very hot or very cold. They avoided eating too quickly, eating too much, or eating in a bad mood.[28] Attitude supposedly had such a profound effect on digestion that Harvey Wiley feared that the food forced down the throats of protesting suffragists in the 1910s—ingested with violence, in other words—might actually kill them as it moldered, rank and undigested, in their intestines.[29] Digestion was hard work, food reformers emphasized, and it was important not to tax the system with food that was difficult to incorporate. Moreover, they said that energy that went to digestion did not go other places, like the brain or the muscles: adherents of the fasting fads that swept the United States around the turn of the century had praised fasts as a way to rest the digestive organs and therefore enhance mental and physical vigor.[30]

Preexisting fears about the unwholesomeness and indigestibility of foreign foods also influenced dietary research in the first two decades of the twentieth century. As nutritionists and home economists brought laboratory data to bear on the question of mixed foods, they clearly expected to find evidence that dishes containing many different ingredients that had been combined before being consumed were harder to digest than plainer foods. And when they looked for this evidence, they found it, or at least they thought they did. For example, a group of doctors in 1906 wrote a series of essays arguing that they had witnessed firsthand that meals combining too many ingredients made people unhealthy. One of the doctors assured readers that, horrified as they might be at the thought, he had some patients who ate meals consisting of up to eighteen different ingredients, and he said disgustedly that their stomachs reminded him of a "garbage pail."[31] A study in the early 1910s backed up such claims when it concluded that animals were most vigorous when they were fed a plain and limited diet.[32] As one journalist typically warned readers, eating "all kinds of otherwise proper food in one meal" turned a stomach "into an acid and gas factory."[33]

Likewise, some native-born Americans feared that the strong flavors and spices they associated with immigrant foods also made digestion more difficult, and reformers insisted that food "should *never* be over-seasoned."[34] One home economist, for example, urged cooks to approach herbs and spices with the utmost caution: "not too much, not too many kinds at once, and not applied indiscriminately to foods which need them and foods which do not."[35] A typical recipe for chicken curry from the mid-1910s instructed cooks to season the sauce with either a scant teaspoon of curry powder *or* a little mushroom and celery—but certainly not both.[36] For years, doctors and home economists harnessed nutrition science to support their idealization of plain, supposedly all-American food, insisting that simple, minimally seasoned foods were the most healthful.

Of course, the fact that authorities continued to devote so much energy to telling all Americans—not just immigrants—to eat simple foods indicates that many people were not already doing so. And most people never had. Food reformers who fancied themselves traditionalists were, like all fundamentalists, highly selective in their historical vision. Americans had always eaten foreign foods. Most nineteenth-century U.S. cookbooks alluded to far-flung geographical origins as a matter of course, and it was completely commonplace to find a scattering of self-evidently foreign recipes like Chicken Pillau, Mullagatawnee Soup, and Irish Stew in even the most mundane cookbooks.[37] Meanwhile, many of the nineteenth-century recipes that look blandly all-American at first glance were in fact filled with ingredients that would have been carried across the country or across the ocean, like pepper, sugar, cinnamon, nutmeg, cloves, curries, almonds, figs, oranges, lemons, coconuts, bananas, chocolate, coffee, tea, and tapioca, among many others.

Moreover, the idea that mixed and strongly flavored foods were somehow un-American was a profound departure from historical eating practices.[38] Although Progressive reformers nostalgically held up colonial American cuisine as the apogee of simple, unmixed fare, prerevolutionary Americans had in fact mixed foods all the time for the sake of taste as well as economy—stretching meat, reinventing leftovers, and using up odds and ends in an inexhaustible variety of stews, hashes, mushes, souses, scrapples, meat pies, and puddings. And this very American reliance on mixing foods did not go away. While popular American cookbooks throughout the nineteenth century were dominated by English-style preparations heavy on boiling and baking, they also contained a wealth of mixed foods, including soups, soufflés, timbales, and croquettes, and all manners of food doused in gravies and floury sauces. What was more, it was practically obligatory for American cookbooks throughout the nineteenth century to include long sections on homemade pickles, ketchups, vinegars, sweetmeats, slaws, and other pungent relishes. Yes, Americans had eaten plenty of boiled meats and vegetables in the old days, but they had also eagerly deployed an arsenal of highly seasoned condiments to enliven them at the table.

It was not that food reformers in the early twentieth century had come to find sauces, stews, and highly seasoned foods unappetizing. Most often, in fact, they expressed the belief that such foods were *too* appetizing.[39] Spices aroused the appetite unnaturally, they claimed, inducing people to eat too much or to eat the wrong things.[40] Eating highly seasoned food was another form of gluttony, and spices were a culinary warning sign that the eater was more concerned with flavor and enjoyment than with nutrition.[41] Spices and sauces could also be dangerously addictive. As the cookbook author Mrs. Norton wrote in 1917, spices "pamper perverted appetites," making people dependent on strong flavors in order to eat anything at all.[42] In the same vein, one wartime press release claimed that Filipinos *needed* curries, because nothing else could stimulate their "jaded appetite[s]."[43] The addiction-inducing propensities of flavor supposedly transcended food, in fact. During the high point of the temperance movement in the 1910s, many claimed that excessive spices and sauces led to alcoholism and drug abuse. "Condiments create a desire for narcotics," one doctor typically asserted, explaining that sauces masked the real taste of food, leaving people mentally unsatisfied and thus thirsting for stronger stimulation.[44]

American eating around the turn of the century can look utterly bipolar. On the one hand, there were deep strains of culinary conservatism, both among immigrant groups and among native-born Americans, as a variety of people looked to the past for food they considered comforting, wholesome, and in some cases more authentically American.[45] On the other hand, there was a consistent and growing appetite for culinary novelty and exoticism—an appetite for the idea of foreignness itself.

AMERICANIZING TO WIN THE WAR

The push and pull of the era's different culinary impulses influenced nutrition science and shaped efforts to Americanize immigrants. Armed with a newly coherent vision of their national cuisine as one that was plain, honest, and lightly seasoned, reformers throughout the early twentieth century aggressively sought to Americanize immigrants' diets by convincing them to eat blander, simpler, and less saucy food. Reformers chastised immigrant mothers for letting their children "indulge in the vicious practice of sopping," that is, dipping their bread in liquid before eating it.[46] They railed against the relatively common practice of feeding coffee to children.[47] Others accused immigrants of feeding their babies nothing but spaghetti, or nothing but sausages and beer.[48]

Although the term "Americanization" had been around for decades by the 1910s, its meaning as a proactive project to assimilate immigrants really solidified during the Great War.[49] Americanization activities around food were particularly charged in wartime, in part because Americanization seemed to some to go "hand in hand with food conservation."[50] For instance, members of the National Liberal Immigration League, which advocated Americanization instead of immigration restriction, distributed food conservation pamphlets to immigrants preparing for U.S. citizenship.[51] Food conservation activities also seemed like an ideal way to reach immigrant women. While immigrant men often had frequent contact with native-born Americans and the English language, immigrant women were less likely to work outside the home and less likely to have regular interactions outside their neighborhoods. Food brought Americanization into the usually inaccessible private sphere. The Woman's Defense Committee suggested that each native white woman should "adopt" a foreign woman to Americanize in conjunction with the war effort.[52]

Wartime food conservation materials appeared in dozens of languages, including a special poster that the Food Administration printed in multiple languages aimed at different immigrant groups. The English version of the poster read, "You came here seeking Freedom / You must now help to preserve it." The Food Administration produced bulletins in Yiddish, Russian, Polish, Slovak, Czech, Hungarian, Norwegian, Swedish, Finnish, Portuguese, Spanish, Greek, Italian, French, Japanese, and Chinese.[53] Food administrators in the "Vernacular Press Section" also sent food conservation materials to the editors of foreign language newspapers, asking them to translate and publish the copy. In this way, food conservation information also reached readers of German, Croatian, Lithuanian, Serbian, Romanian, Dutch, Slovenian, and Danish, among other languages.[54] Despite objections from some Americans, especially southerners, to the idea of government food cards printed in foreign languages, multilingual efforts intensified during the war.[55] In food exhibitions—which volunteers, home economists, and other reformers set up throughout the era in a variety of venues as a form of public education on food—demonstrators sometimes enlisted the aid of bilingual volunteers to interpret their speeches.[56] Reformers also sometimes called upon translators when they went out to teach canning and other skills to immigrants in their homes.[57] The Department of Agriculture encouraged American schoolchildren who were learning a foreign language to take part in the Americanization cum food conservation campaign. After receiving training from demonstration agents, children went out in teams of three to immigrant neighborhoods, where they gave demonstrations on how to can or dry foods, first in English, and then, when possible, in the foreign language.[58] Sometimes native-born reformers also learned a little of the language of the immigrant groups they hoped to reach, like the women canvassing for food conservation in Boston who learned a few Italian sentences to help ease open tenement doors.[59]

Immigrants' children were often the ones to translate English-language literature for their parents. In fact, volunteers canvassing for pledges in neighborhoods with a high percentage of immigrants sometimes asked for extra time, because they had to wait for children to return from school so they could translate for the adults.[60] Because so much information aimed at immigrant families had to pass through children, administrators knew their conservation bulletins had to be pithy.[61] One twelve-year-old translated the food card for his mother, then signed his mother's name for her because she could not write. When asked if he fully understood what food conservation meant, the boy said it meant he and his brother should eat

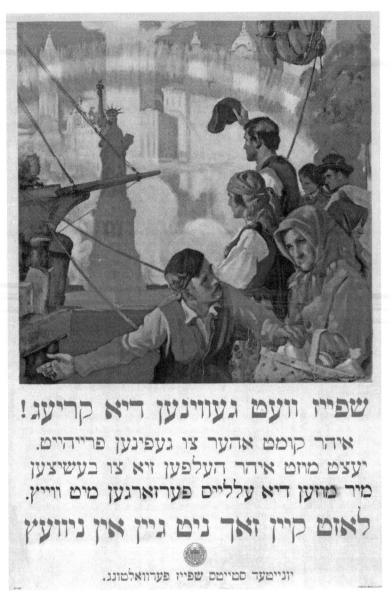

*Charles E. Chambers, "Food Will Win the War—You Came Here
Seeking Freedom, Now You Must Help to Preserve It." This Food Administration
poster argued in multiple languages—Yiddish, in this case—that food conservation
was part of immigrants' obligations as new or prospective American citizens. New
York: Rusling Wood, Litho., 1917. Prints and Photographs Division, Library
of Congress, Washington, D.C.*

less candy, but he added that they could not eat less meat because his family could almost never afford to buy any in the first place.[62]

Some reformers worried not just about immigrants' comprehension of English but also about their intelligence. A fictional Italian American in one Pennsylvania newspaper, inspired by Hoover, whom he calls "Herb da Hoove," decides to conserve meat. But when his wily butcher tries to convince him to buy expensive beef instead of cheaper fish, the gullible immigrant gets confused and gives up on buying meat altogether: "So we have da spaghet for da supper."[63] Similarly, when another fictional immigrant, an Irish woman in a 1917 skit published in the *Chicago Examiner*, hears that the potato peelings she has been throwing away for years contained good nutrients that have gone to waste, she looks around for the policemen she is sure must be coming to arrest her, and she exclaims, "I'll have to be addin' a new sin the next time I go to confession!"[64] Whereas native-born Americans supposedly went about solving problems rationally, immigrants were, by some lights, fatalistic and superstitious. One journalist claimed that if the child of a Greek immigrant refused to eat something, "it is all on the knees of the gods, and the swarthy parent shrugs his shoulders, casts up his dark eyes, and says to the social settlement worker, 'O, you can't do anything with those little ones.'"[65] Because of language barriers and because of racial assumptions about immigrants' intelligence, reformers believed Americanization lessons had to be elementary.

Besides questioning their comprehension and their intelligence, people also questioned immigrants' loyalty to U.S. plans. As one Buffalo, New York, woman declared, "Aliens" were apt to "slide easily away from obligations readily assumed by the *real* American!"[66] Others wrote to the government to report that the foreign-born people they knew were disinterested in food conservation, or openly antagonistic to it.[67] In Los Angeles, one observer reported that foreign restaurant owners "not only made no pretense of observing meatless Tuesday but loaded their bills of fare with meat orders, and profited by the patriotism of the neighboring 'white' cafe keepers."[68] When a Chinese American restaurant owner in Denver asked the state food administrator how new food legislation would affect the food he served, journalists described him as more anxious to avoid punishment than he was to help the nation: "After a severe struggle with nouns and verbs, Quong Wah managed to ask if he would get in jail if he put pork in his chop suey."[69]

A major weakness of Americanization campaigns was that immigrants often had little interest in taking up American ways, and that was especially true when it came to food. First-generation immigrants were often conservative in their dietary choices, and in the strange new places they found themselves they eagerly reproduced familiar and comforting foods they knew from home—or, when they could afford to, richer, meatier versions of those foods.[70] Mary Schapiro, a native-born Jewish woman and a zealous Americanization reformer, criticized the "defects" of Jewish immigrants' diets as she saw them: they were "overrich," "overseasoned," and short on fruit and vegetables. However much their diets needed to be changed, however, Schapiro predicted that an immigrant housewife would "smile at the suggestion that any young American woman can teach *her* how to cook."[71] Schapiro's prediction turned out to be pretty accurate. Few immigrants were eager to give up familiar cooking styles, especially in exchange for the plain, flavorless fare advocated by Americanization reformers. One frustrated reformer, having encountered one too many foreign-born women who was incomprehensibly content to keep cooking "in the same old unwholesome way," compared herself to a skilled doctor whose patient had determined to die anyway.[72] Reformers accused obdurate immigrants of capitulating to their own "racial prejudices," but historians have found that, in reality, many immigrants simply thought their own food was better.[73]

Increasingly, Americanization strategies focused less on the wholesale transformation of immigrant diets and more on modification. In growing numbers, Americanization reformers believed they had to respect and work with immigrants' traditions and, as one home economist wrote, "to take and use the elements offered by the foreigner." For example, even as dieticians working with Italian Americans continued to urge them to drink more milk, they acknowledged that they might as well let alone Italians' fondness for whole wheat bread, olive oil, and greens, since new science showed that such foods were nutritious, even if they still seemed distinctly foreign.[74] During the first three decades of the twentieth century, immigrant communities throughout the United States were also becoming less isolated and less conservative when it came to food. Americanization reformers were quick to attribute any such changes to their own efforts, but in truth the changes were largely a result of diminishing numbers of new immigrants entering the country and the growing availability of mass-produced commercial foods.[75] Department of Agriculture research had long suggested that older immigrants tended to cling to familiar foods while their children were quicker to pick up American food habits.[76] Yet what had once been viewed as favorable steps toward full assimilation seemed less desirable in the context of high food prices and growing popular willingness among a variety of Americans—foreign born and not—to try foreign foods.[77]

Indeed, some reformers even encouraged second-generation immigrants to eat the dishes of their parents' home countries on occasion. For example, when extension workers assembled simple "American dishes" that they wanted foreign-born people to adopt, they also included a handful of dishes from immigrants' countries of origins so that "the young people would learn to appreciate the elders' dishes."[78] Similarly, in 1919, a highly educated Jewish man named Nathan Isaacs, who was a former U.S. Army captain as well as a lawyer and a Ph.D., argued passionately against Americanizing immigrants' diets. Writing in the *Menorah Journal*, an early forum for Jewish intellectuals and a setting for ongoing discussions of assimilation and identity, Isaacs told a story about a U.S. Army camp where men from different immigrant groups had been at each other's throats until the officers finally organized everyone into "foreign-language units," complete with their own cooks. Morale perked up immediately. "If Italians want spaghetti and Hungarians goulash and Jews 'gefillte' fish," Isaacs asked, "why sicken them all with pork and beans? It really does not make better Americans of them." On the contrary, eating familiar foods and surrounded by people who spoke their language, the men became happier and supposedly all started learning English.[79] Encouraged to retain some degree of their ethnic identity, in other words, they became *more* American, not less.

At the same time, others worked with growing enthusiasm to convince *all* Americans to try a limited repertoire of foreign recipes, especially those that stretched meat and wheat. The idea that seemingly different foods could be nutritionally equivalent was a foundational one in nutrition science, and it helped to lessen the stigma of foreign foods. In 1901, the distinguished home economist Ellen Richards had proposed the term "food synonyms" to describe foods whose ingredients and nutritional content were virtually identical from country to country.[80] By 1917, two food reformers created a chart of their own "food synonyms" so that readers could see at a glance that the vegetable soup on the white American table, the minestrone in the Italian home, and the pot of gemüsesuppe on the Jewish woman's stove were really one and the same. The argument that the ingredients of foreign dishes were "practically the same as those that enter into our recipes" was increasingly common and also increasingly accurate, as native-born Americans and immigrants alike relied on ingredients readily available in U.S. grocery stores to cook "foreign" foods.[81]

The comparatively light use of meat and wheat in many foreign recipes also made them more acceptable in the 1910s, both because they tended to be cheaper at a time of high food prices and because they freed up commodities needed for food aid to Europe during the war. "Not only do we meet strange foods when we travel," Harvey Wiley wrote pointedly, "but if we are patriotic, we have them when we stay at home."[82] As a result, wartime food fairs around the country highlighted foreign cookery.[83] At a Cleveland food exhibit, for instance, visitors sampled macaroni and spaghetti and then learned how to cook them.[84] The most popular booth at New York City's Conservation Food Show was the International Demonstration Booth, where a variety of immigrant cooks took turns demonstrating how to make their national dishes.[85] Others published foreign-recipe leaflets in English and other languages, with the idea that the recipes would teach English to immigrants while at the same time broadening the use of conservation-friendly foreign foods among native-born Americans.[86]

In the same vein, the Food Administration sent out a press release at the end of 1917 claiming that to conserve food, it was imperative that Americans become familiar with the cost-saving food of "European peasants."[87] Others said housewives should learn to cook European dishes because U.S. soldiers might well return home having developed a taste for the foods of the countries where they were stationed.[88] Although a popular cookbook called *Allied Cookery* had appeared on both sides of the Atlantic in 1916, Americans did not confine themselves to foods of the Allies, and in some cases they even turned a spotlight on Germanic and central European cooking, with some food conservation fairs teaching women how to make sauerkraut.[89] Feeble attempts to get people to call it "liberty cabbage" flopped, supposedly because sauerkraut was already widely known and widely liked.[90]

Meanwhile, the government actively promoted potatoes as an alternative to wheat. While potatoes were native to the Americas, they had not been particularly prominent in U.S. diets in the nineteenth century, and in the early twentieth many Americans were just as apt to describe them as a hardy pan-European peasant food than as a specialty of their own country.[91] Some highlighted the Irishness of so-called Irish potatoes, while others speculated that potatoes were the secret of German strength and efficiency.[92] Still others described potatoes as a predominately French food, like one American man who recommended that all Americans try a delicious potato dish he had sampled in France, "'Pom de Tare Souffle.'"[93] Yet by the 1910s potatoes were becoming much more of an American mainstay than they had been in the nineteenth century, and they increasingly served as the basis of everyday meat-and-potato meals.

As eaten by immigrants, mixed foods worried Americanization reformers because they seemed cryptic and indigestible. But mixed, self-evidently foreign foods—in the form of casseroles, chilies, stews, and pasta dishes— were coming into fashion with remarkable speed. Americans knew that foods like stews were popular in Europe and among immigrant groups in the United States.[94] But people grudgingly acknowledged that similar dishes were also part of an older American heritage that modern Americans had forgotten or ignored. For example, one article in a small-town Illinois newspaper stressed that people "of all nations have used combinations of foods cooked together in one dish," including people of the United States—possibly even "your grandmother."[95] Some liked to say that the return of mixed foods meant a return to the honest American frugality that had characterized the country's youth.[96]

At the same time, since the turn of the century, middle-class Americans had been giving up on multicourse meals that required the help of servants and long stretches of time to eat, although for the most part they still ate meals consisting of multiple dishes, usually a meaty main course supplemented with grain and vegetable side dishes.[97] Yet given the decline in servants and the emphasis on housewifely efficiency, rising numbers of Progressive women were turning away from separate dishes altogether and toward what they called one-dish meals or, increasingly, casseroles.[98] One-dish meals, hearty mixed dishes that contained most or all of the food a family would eat for a meal, were usually relatively straightforward to prepare, quick to eat, and easy to clean up.[99] Their streamlined simplicity was appealing in Taylorist terms, and as home economists studied housewives' movements in the kitchen, one-dish meals promised, literally, to save steps.[100] Their efficiency was enhanced by the fact that the recipes increasingly called for canned goods, which by the 1910s were finally both reliably safe and widely available. One-dish meals also eliminated nutritional guesswork: a meal consisting of many separate dishes might be well balanced as a whole, but individuals could end up eating too much of one dish and not enough of another.[101] One-dish meals solved this problem, because by serving a hearty bean stew or a hot dish combining meat, grains, vegetables, and cheese, a housewife could satisfy all the nutritive needs of her family in a single stroke.[102] And thus one-dish meals also routed the dangers of excessive "freedom of choice" at the table.[103]

Recipes published in newspapers and magazines in the 1910s demonstrate the widespread interest in foreign cooking among food writers as well as readers. Some one-dish meals were recognizably American, like chowder, hash, scrapple, or the southern Brunswick stew.[104] However, many of the saucy dishes and one-dish recipes American women were encountering by the Great War era were obviously and proudly foreign. There were Italian recipes such as Roman Meat Pudding with Macaroni or numerous recipes for risotto.[105] Economical French recipes printed in newspapers and magazines included Pilau, Salmon Souffle, and Cheese Fondue.[106] There were also more specific nationalist recipes, like Belgian Baked Potatoes, Norwegian Pudding, Russian Stschi, Scotch Broth, Hungarian Goulash, and Hungarian Polenta.[107] And there were recipes for southwestern and Mexican foods like Mexican Corn Pudding, Mexican Stew, Tamale Pie, and Hominy and Red Peppers.[108] Recipes for one-dish meals and soups also appeared advertising a South or East Asian provenance, including Mulligatawny, Indian Dal, Indian Curry, and Mongol Soup.[109] Far from downplaying their foreign ties, the creators of many one-dish recipes by the 1910s chose titles that waved their foreignness like a flag.

SPAGHETTI À L'AMERICAINE

Americans have always been interested in foreign foods to some extent, and that interest had intensified in the final decades of the nineteenth century. But the years between the late 1910s and the mid-1930s saw the blossoming of widespread, self-conscious interest in foreign foods among a wide variety of Americans. Of course, what "foreign food" means depends on who is asking. And it also depends on when. Decisions about which foods get classed as foreign and which do not shift enormously over time, most obviously as different national or ethnic groups come to be considered more or less foreign themselves.[110] For instance, as German Americans became more assimilated in the early twentieth century, so too did previously "German" foods like hamburgers, wieners, and pretzels. But the cultural logic behind popular designations of foreignness is not always obvious. Why had macaroni and cheese thoroughly shed any ethnic associations by the 1930s, when Kraft started marketing its boxed dinners, while spaghetti—canned and mass-produced decades earlier—remained recognizably Italian?[111] Similarly, since chili con carne and tamales were routinely mentioned in the same breath in the first decades of the twentieth century, why did mild, corn-based tamales stay foreign in the minds of Americans while rich, spicy chili did not?[112] Tracing the lineage of any kind of food is messy, and while it is usually impossible to identify precise reasons behind the ebbs and flows of food fashions, it is possible to describe broad changes in attitudes and practices.

Throughout the nineteenth century and into the twentieth, culinary discrimination had been virtually synonymous with culinary refinement, an association that built upon long-standing beliefs that people got more fastidious as they got more civilized and that those people with the greatest access to food resources could afford to be the choosiest. In 1906, for instance, one journalist had proudly described how some "extremely refined Americans" had left Italy immediately after watching Italians slurp up spaghetti.[113] But attitudes about pickiness and refinement were changing. Whereas turn-of-the-century journalists writing about foreign foods routinely sought to shock readers by describing the curious and repulsive things eaten elsewhere, by the 1920s, articles about foreign foods were much more likely to describe them as interesting, appealing, and chic. More and more, it was becoming fashionable to be an adventurous and experienced eater and unfashionable to be fussy or fastidious.

Foreign restaurants helped to effect some of these changes, as the historian Andrew Haley has described. In the mid-nineteenth century, restaurants owned by immigrants catered mainly to other immigrants. But starting in the 1880s and 1890s, they were increasingly frequented by white middle-class eaters more interested in novelty than nostalgia.[114] By the start of the twentieth century, diners in cities across the country could choose between western European restaurants—especially cheap French, German, and Italians ones—as well as, in many places, eastern European, South American, East Asian, and Middle Eastern restaurants. And as time went on they did not have to visit ethnic neighborhoods to find them, either, as foreign-born entrepreneurs opened more restaurants in middle-class neighborhoods and suburbs.[115] As it became more ordinary to eat at ethnic restaurants, middle-class city-dwellers pitted their increasingly wide-ranging culinary experiences against the narrow exclusivity of elites for whom culinary cosmopolitanism started and ended with French haute cuisine.[116]

Whether eaten in restaurants or cooked at home, spaghetti was probably the most common "foreign" food in the Progressive Era, and changing attitudes toward it were emblematic of changing attitudes toward foreign foods as a whole. Back in the mid-nineteenth century, most native-born Americans had known little about spaghetti except as a faintly unpleasant foreign curiosity. Pasta remained relatively exotic through the 1880s, although macaroni appeared with some regularity in nineteenth-century recipes as a vegetable side dish to be served by itself, as the base for cheese sauce, or sometimes as a starch to be used in sweet puddings.[117] In the 1890s and early 1900s, however, as Italian immigration surged and as Italian restaurants opened in cities around the country, spaghetti recipes started appearing in large numbers in American cookbooks, and pasta produced in U.S. factories was increasingly available on grocery shelves.[118] Spaghetti's long strands made its exoticism palpable, yet it was still a dish that people could make cheaply and easily at home, whether by cooking dried pasta in boiling water or, increasingly, by opening a can. Indeed, spaghetti entered mainstream American diets most vigorously by way of the can opener. By the early 1910s, brands like Franco-American, Van Camp, Purity Cross, and Heinz were all selling canned spaghetti to mass markets and meeting with remarkable success. Henry Heinz had originally been so skeptical about the public reaction to canned spaghetti that he had sent out a group of Italian chefs to tour grocery stores explaining what spaghetti was, but public demand turned out to be so high that Heinz quickly dropped the educational tour and expanded production facilities in order to meet it.[119] As early as 1911, the Van Camp Company affirmed that canned spaghetti was the most popular product it had ever made in its fifty-year existence.[120]

The fact that spaghetti was readily available in cans sold under trusted brand names accelerated its acceptance and gave it wide reach in markets where consumers might otherwise not have dared to cook dried pasta—still widely referred to as "Italian paste"—on their own.[121] Whereas nineteenth-century consumers had been rightfully dubious about the safety of canned goods and other industrially produced food, by the 1910s—in the wake of reliable mass production of cans and of the Pure Food and Drug Act of 1906—industrial processing increasingly stood for hygiene, safety, and consistency.[122] At the same time, canned spaghetti also meant familiar taste, so that consumers who first experienced pasta from a can would be unlikely to find its flavor off-puttingly peculiar. Van Camp, for example, loudly advertised the fact that the sauce it used in its canned spaghetti was the very same sauce it had long used in its pork and beans.[123]

This pasta-heavy version of Italian cuisine, already penetrating deeply into mainstream American diets by the 1910s, also got an enormous boost from the wartime food conservation campaign.[124] Italian dishes were considered ideal conservation foods since they tended to use large amounts of vegetables and grains and only small amounts of meat, and Italian American cookbook authors highlighted the cuisine's reliance on conservation foods like cheese, rice, cornmeal, and vegetable oils.[125] At conservation fairs, even women who were not Italian Americans themselves began to teach other women how to make risotto and polenta and other Italian dishes as conservation foods.[126] And while patriotic Americans otherwise minimized their wheat consumption during the war, they ate pasta because it was made with semolina flour, produced from high-protein durum wheat that food administrators considered inappropriate for bread making and thus did not prioritize for shipment to Europe. Some pasta boosters apparently believed many Americans would prefer to avoid eating pasta if they could, like one writer who said that eating more pasta and less white bread was a "stern dietetic reality" in wartime.[127] In general, however, Americans more and more reported that they *did* like pasta. In places like Oklahoma City and Cloverdale, Oregon, housewives testified that the new Italian recipes they were trying were "so frugal and so delicious" that they made food conservation easy.[128]

At the same time that the surging popularity of Italian cuisine was making pasta a widely acceptable food product, it also proved to be a vehicle for garlic's wider use. Amid general fears about the indigestibility of highly seasoned food and the addictive nature of strong flavors, middle-class Americans had long considered garlic to be noxiously overpowering. Yet Italian cuisine enthusiasts waged a gentle campaign to remove garlic's stigma. If "properly handled," used "in small quantities," and "thoroughly cooked," one cookbook author contended, garlic could be "inoffensive and wholesome."[129] Playing on lingering associations between race and the tolerance of strong tastes, an Italian American man joked that people with "Wop ancestry" should add garlic to their spaghetti sauce, while "pale people" could use onions. But he begged his flavor-phobic readers to "surely use one or the other."[130] Onions themselves were considered rather daring, too; as one 1922 cookbook writer typically put it, people could include onions in the recipe "if they have the courage."[131]

On the whole, American recipe writers tended to flaunt spaghetti's foreignness, not hide it, with recipes like Genuine Italian Spaghetti or Spaghetti—Italian Style.[132] But these nods to authenticity were halfhearted at best, and cooks generally sacrificed it when it suited them. For instance, one man who went out of his way to describe how he had personally collected his "real Italian" spaghetti recipe in Italy itself casually called for Eagle Chili Powder, a popular Mexican seasoning made in San Antonio.[133] In cookbooks, recipes for supposedly authentic Italian spaghetti recipes rubbed elbows with recipes like Creole Spaghetti, Spaghetti Rarebit, and Spaghetti à l'Americaine, which was spaghetti mixed with canned tomato paste and butter.[134] By the 1920s, spaghetti was widely known and widely loved, and recipes for it were ubiquitous in American cookbooks. When a cookbook editor in the early 1920s asked dozens of famous men for their favorite recipes, so many submitted recipes for spaghetti that the editor declared there must be "a decided male preference" for it.[135]

Even as spaghetti grew in popularity, however, some Americans remained unsold. Elongated pasta shapes seemed particularly foreign, and eating them was daunting for the uninitiated. One turn-of-the-century article had approvingly described an American tourist in Italy who resolutely cut his own pasta into "miniature strips" and was revolted by watching Italians forking up long, wormlike strands. The fact that poor Italians sometimes ate spaghetti with their hands was far worse.[136] Breaking or cutting pasta was one of the most obvious ways to make spaghetti seem less foreign, and recipes of the era routinely advised breaking it into pieces as small as an inch and a half, or even crushing it, before cooking.[137] Even when people cooked the strands whole, many continued to cut them into bits on their plates. Well into the twentieth century, many Americans remaining leery about the messiness and difficulty of eating long pasta shapes.[138]

Some also feared that spaghetti was inherently dirty, since Italians and Italian Americans regularly made pasta by hand and dried it in the sun, and reports circulated of racks of pasta drying outdoors as dogs and dirty children ran among them.[139] The great majority of the pasta Americans ate by the early twentieth century was not made by hand, however, but in factories. While it was normal for food companies at the time to tout the hygienic nature of their production practices, pasta companies went a step beyond, clearly responding to fears about foreign methods and of foreign hands themselves, proclaiming their pasta was "CLEANLY MADE BY AMERICANS" or "made the American way—by machines."[140] Even then, cookbook writers still regularly recommended that people wash pasta before cooking it.[141] In response to fears both about pasta's potential dirtiness and about its digestibility, Americans lavishly overcooked it, letting heat scour away germs and do some preliminary breaking down to lessen pasta's supposed burden on white American stomachs.[142] Hence advice that pasta could be digestible if it was boiled for half an hour—or an hour—then cooked again with sauce.[143] Yet as more and more Americans sampled pasta and liked it through the 1920s and 1930s, beliefs about its dirtiness, indigestibility, and essential foreignness faded, although they did not disappear.

As spaghetti's popularity rose, macaroni's soared, yet it did so increasingly as an American food, not as a foreign one. Macaroni's presence in nineteenth-century cookbooks had made it a familiar product, and when one 1915 writer said offhandedly that Americans "are all familiar with the regulation dish of macaroni and cheese," she was probably close to right.[144] Macaroni had become a very ordinary food by the 1910s, and that was true in virtually all sections of the country and among people from all income levels.[145] So domesticated was macaroni that by the mid-1910s a writer in the conservative *Boston Cooking-School Magazine* provided tricks that weary cooks could use to transform it *back* into a pleasingly exotic ethnic dish, such as boiling it in meat stock before adding sauce and scraps of meat.[146] But for the most part Americans decreasingly thought of macaroni as a particularly foreign food at all, serving up thoroughly Americanized dishes like Ham and Macaroni Scallop, Cheese and Macaroni Loaf, and Macaroni with Cottage Cheese.[147]

Besides Italian food, native-born Americans were also beginning to regularly discuss, and in some cases to cook and eat, "Oriental cookery."[148] In one of the first Asian cookbooks to be published in the United States, the 1914 *Chinese-Japanese Cook Book*, the authors claimed that Chinese cooking had become "very popular" in recent years, and no longer just among curiosity-seekers.[149] Indeed, while relatively few white Americans in the first decades of the twentieth century ate at Asian restaurants, Chinese restaurants and chop suey joints were gaining popularity among adventurous tourists and middle-class diners in big cities.[150] Yet many Americans clearly continued to think about Chinese cuisine as both mysterious and unpleasant. Some claimed that the act of eating Chinese food itself was naturally impossible for white Americans, who could never become adept at chopsticks even after years of practice.[151] During the war, jokes played on the conceit that no white person knew what went into Chinese food, and food administrators were supposedly forced to investigate "the secret art" of Chinese chefs as they verified restaurants' compliance with wheatless and meatless days.[152] Newspapers joked that when a Chinese American restaurant owner in Chicago asked local food administrators for help finding a meat substitute for meatless days, he had exposed the "mystery of chop suey" by revealing the fact that it usually contained meat.[153] Of course, an enduring irony of contemporary fears is that chop suey—the most popular "Chinese" dish of the era—did not actually come from China but rather was invented in the United States for American consumption, a recipe whose supposed foreignness began and ended with its nonsense name.

But even Americans who were enthusiastic about Asian cuisine tended to qualify their praise, and articles with titles like "Oriental Recipes that Are Worth the Making" clearly implied that many such recipes were not.[154] The authors of the *Chinese-Japanese Cook Book* argued that once people made Chinese and Japanese foods at home, they would "cease to feel that *natural repugnance* which assails one when about to taste a strange dish of a new and strange land."[155] Yet if some Americans did feel repugnance for Asian food, it was less common as time went on to assume that their revulsion *was* natural. "No one need be afraid of Chinese cooking," one American cookbook author assured readers in the early 1920s. She agreed that Chinese recipes for grubs or grasshoppers could sound alarming, but she noted, strikingly, that "no doubt, certain of our recipes must be to the Chinese," too.[156] In the 1920s and 1930s, more and more American cooks tried making nominally Asian dishes, although when such dishes did appear in American cookbooks and on American tables, they were often profoundly modified or even made up altogether, like chop suey itself. Sometimes recipes contained only the bare skeleton of supposedly Asian ingredients, like the recipe for Imperial Rice, which contained nothing but plain white rice and shredded chicken.[157] And sometimes ostensibly Asian recipes eagerly reintroduced familiar American staples, like Mabel Anderson's Chinese Puff, featuring grated cheese and white sauce, or Emilie Pfahl's Japanese Fritters, made with milk, crackers, and a sweet lemon cornstarch sauce.[158]

SLIGHTLY FOREIGN, JUST FOR FUN

Why did people have different eating habits in the first place? Despite the racial theories that had permeated explanations of varying food cultures in the early twentieth century, by the interwar period food scientists as well as popular food writers declared with confidence that food tastes were primarily cultural rather than biological, paralleling developments in the young field of cultural anthropology. Habit—not instinct, and not race—was "the most important factor in appetite," one writer in *Scientific Monthly* wrote in 1926, for instance. Yes, the "Irish like their potatoes; the Jews, their gefüllte fish; the Italians, their macaroni," but in all cases these were simply the foods to which these people had "been accustomed from early years."[159] The world contained an extraordinary diversity of food habits, but people were not *born* with these preferences. The wartime shifts in Americans' diets had contributed to the idea that food preferences were malleable, especially the insistence that a food prejudice was just that and that it was childish to cling to it instead of eating according to more rational criteria.[160] Increasingly it seemed that even very strong food prejudices could be reversed and new tastes could be acquired.

And acquire new tastes Americans did. Besides the slowly increasing use of garlic and garlic powder during the late 1910s, 1920s, and 1930s,

Americans also more regularly used a modest variety of other herbs, spices, and spice mixtures. A growing number of recipes made use of paprika by the 1920s, and its presence was enough to justify the use of "Hungarian" in any recipe title throughout the first half of the twentieth century. In the 1931 first edition of what would become the classic *Joy of Cooking*, Irma Rombauer described her delight at sampling a new rice dish and her shock to learn that its "delicious flavor" came from curry powder, which she had always avoided. She credited the success of this particular curry dish to the fact that it actually contained very little curry at all.[161] Tolerance of spices—even if the tolerance was sometimes very low by today's standards—was increasing even among people who had grown up believing that their discomfort with strong flavors was dictated by biology.

And a growing number of Americans throughout the interwar period did much more than simply tolerate foreign foods. They ate them in ethnic restaurants and at foreign-themed parties. They bought cookbooks crammed with recipes for them, made them at home, and served them at family meals and at formal dinners alike. They bragged about their experience with and knowledge of them. Self-consciously international cookbooks were popular, from books that focused on specific cuisines, like the 1928 *Mandarin Chop Suey Cook Book* or the 1929 *Ramona's Spanish-Mexican Cookery*, to more generally international cookbooks like the ever-popular *Settlement Cook Book* or the 1931 *Old World Foods for New World Families*.[162] Meanwhile, foreign recipes appeared not only in ethnic cookbooks but in virtually every cookbook, newspaper, and women's magazine. When the artist James Montgomery Flagg admitted sheepishly in the early 1920s that his favorite food was custard with wine jelly, he worried it sounded "ladieshomejournalish," since he well knew that a rougher or more exotic dish would sound more fashionable and more manly.[163] In fact, by the time Flagg wrote, popular women's magazines like the *Ladies' Home Journal* themselves rarely featured such delicate nineteenth-century dishes as custard with jelly, instead nonchalantly offering up hearty foreign-style dishes in every issue. Indeed, it became hard to find an American cookbook that did *not* include obviously foreign recipes, and more often than not dozens of them. Even books with titles like the 1922 *All-American Cook Book* overflowed with foreign recipes from Spanish Rice to Indian Curry, from Tamale Loaf to Chop Suey, from Pozole to Ravioli.[164]

Although the United States increasingly imported foods from around the world, the ingredients used in "foreign" recipes were rarely much different from those used in supposedly nonforeign foods. That overlap made the domestication of the recipes themselves easier.[165] Similarly, as foreign restaurants moved from immigrant neighborhoods to middle-class suburbs, they often changed their menus and their recipes, muting spiciness, cutting out garlic, and offering standard American options alongside ethnic dishes, even as they amplified the foreignness of the décor to appeal to diners looking for a novel experience.[166] At the same time, other ingredients that Americans had seen as distinctly foreign in the past were shedding those associations. For instance, through the early 1920s, broccoli had been rare in U.S. cookbooks, and when it appeared, it usually did so as an exotic Italian vegetable.[167] But broccoli roared to popularity in the mid-1920s, especially after the elegant Waldorf Astoria in New York started serving it in elevated pan-ethnic dishes like broccoli hollandaise and broccoli au gratin, with waiters instructed to inform patrons that it was related to cauliflower and "pronounced 'brok-kolee.'" By the end of the 1920s broccoli could be found on the menus of other restaurants and in ordinary grocery stores around the city and increasingly around the country, where housewives bought it eagerly.[168] Indeed, Americans adopted this "foreign" vegetable so quickly that many never thought of it as particularly foreign. Another food that made such a transformation was mayonnaise, which had seemed obviously and explicitly French early in the century but which became so widely adopted that it would come to seem like a wholly American condiment by the mid-twentieth century.

Generally, though, Americans in the 1920s and 1930s tended to play up—and play with—foods' international pedigrees. Sometimes they combined foods from different nationalities into new recipes and sometimes invented them altogether, creating crazy-quilt amalgams of ethnic, racial, and geographical culinary signifiers like Spanish Ragout, Chop Suey Spaghetti, or the pork chop dish named, improbably, Arabian Delight.[169] A dish called Japanese Suey was a drippy maple-syrup-and-marshmallow ice cream topping that appeared, of all places, in the southern-themed *Dixie Cook Book*, published by the Kansas City Business Woman's Club in 1921.[170] This sort of madcap culinary commingling is noteworthy not because it was exceptional but because it was so utterly commonplace in the interwar period, a time when playing with foreign foods showcased a shopper's command of a diverse range of products, a cook's familiarity with a world's worth of cooking styles and her creativity in melding them, and an eater's prerogative to subvert other people's definitions of identity in pursuit of pleasure. As the historian Kristin Hoganson writes, cooking and eating foreign foods helped "white, middle-class Americans define themselves as cosmopolitans in a world full of locals."[171]

By the 1920s and 1930s, foreign foods were both legion and increasingly mundane, comfortably sharing pages in cookbooks and magazines with tuna hot dishes and chicken pot pies—which of course were themselves mixed, foreign-influenced dishes that would have seemed coarse and distasteful by the standards of a turn-of-the-century food reformer. Indeed, many of those dishes that would come to seem most thoroughly all-American by the mid-twentieth century were first made acceptable by being presented *as* foreign, and thus as interesting and sophisticated. For instance, the 1922 recipe for Italian Delight was really a straightforward one-dish meal made by mixing spaghetti, ground beef, and canned soup.[172] And would Italian Delight really have tasted very different from the 1931 goulash recipe that called for spaghetti, ground beef, canned soup, and green peppers, or the 1936 chop suey recipe calling for spaghetti, ground beef, tomatoes, and bacon?[173] Just a few decades later, in fact, it is likely that any of those dishes would have simply been called a "hamburger casserole," a phrase whose increasing familiarity to American ears would obscure what would have seemed like the dish's own glaringly German and French origins earlier in the century.

Playing with foreign foods also showcased the glib rejection of staid rules from the recent past. Recipes like Japanese Suey were utterly at odds with prevailing advice in the first two decades of the twentieth century from nutritionists, who had generally frowned upon mixed foods, foreign foods, and frivolous foods alike. Even though some cookbook authors still deployed familiar values like nutrition and affordability when praising particular foreign recipes, people did not flock to these recipes just because of their vitamins. By the 1920s, foreign foods meant *pleasure* more than anything else. Bowls of noodles slicked with oil and suffused with garlic, hunks of meat falling apart into rich stews, spicy sauces flecked with chili and cheese: clearly, many of these foreign foods were delicious, and much of the pleasure Americans found in them came from their tastes, textures, and aromas. But it is also clear that some of the pleasure came from a sense of newness, and even of naughtiness. Eating foreign foods was a mild transgression, to be sure, but it was a transgression nonetheless, perhaps particularly so for people who had grown up during the high point of Progressive Era strictures against the threats foreign foods posed to digestion, health, and even identity.

By the mid-1920s, the sense of foreign foods' danger was contained enough to be exciting without being truly threatening. Companies selling products with an international flair worked to heighten, not dampen, their transgressive potential, like the ad for Dromedary brand shredded coconut that highlighted its Near East associations and promised it would give "an added thrill" to ordinary foods.[174] Heinz likewise advertized its canned spaghetti as "slightly foreign, just for fun."[175] But for many white, middle-class Americans during the interwar period, eating foreign foods made with mostly familiar ingredients—whether those foods were eaten at home or in restaurants patronized primarily by other diners like them— was more a temporary deviation from what they still thought of as their real eating habits than a concerted rejection of cultural or racial conventions.[176] Foreign foods let eaters deviate in small doses, meal by meal, without truly challenging their basic sense of order or of self.

Willingness to flirt with such boundaries, however, could signal an eater's bohemianism and modernity.[177] For instance, if most Americans still eagerly broke or cut spaghetti to make it easier to handle and less unapproachably foreign, eating it uncut was one of the surest ways to express comfort with this specific foreign food and with foreignness in general, and some vocally objected to cutting spaghetti as an affront to the dish's authenticity and to any hope of experiencing the dish in a meaningful way.[178] Some Italian Americans encouraged everyone to try eating long pasta shapes uncut, and one man provided sensual instructions to Americans to whirl the strands of spaghetti around their forks before tipping the whole "delectable mass" down their throats.[179] The Italian American writer John Moroso joked that spaghetti should be served alongside a revolver "so that the man who cuts his can be disposed of properly."[180] For non-Italians, eating their spaghetti uncut could testify to their experience with urban culture. For instance, one novelist in the early 1920s described the awkwardness of "a stanch American" knifing his spaghetti to bits at a restaurant, while the debonair man down the table—also an American, but a more cosmopolitan one—sucked his uncut spaghetti up through puckered lips while encouraging the beautiful woman next to him to do the same.[181] Willingness to seek out the foreign and to let themselves be changed by it lent eaters an air of the exoticism associated with foreign foods and foreign peoples themselves.

In other words, comfort with foreign foods was increasingly a sign of sophistication rather than its opposite.[182] When the cartoonist T. A. Dorgan reported in the early 1920s that chili con carne was his favorite food, he made clear that it was not because he was some country rube who did not know better, adding smugly, "I might have said Terrapin Maryland, or some other Ritzy dish."[183] Similarly, in 1931 the writer Harry Carr advised travelers that the "only right way is to 'eat native.' Meals that I shall never forget have been at cow camps with Indian vaqueros; with Chinese vegetable peddlers; with Mexican peons in the patios of adobe houses."[184] Carr was not writing in a handbook aimed at travelers on a shoestring budget but rather in the stylish *Fashions in Foods in Beverly Hills*, a compilation of recipes from movie stars and other wealthy Californians that brimmed with proudly internationalist recipes, with well over a third of its main dishes alluding to foreign origins, for instance.[185] And the book was absolutely typical of its times. The popularity of foreign foods in this era among the wealthiest and best-traveled Americans underlines their cachet, but ordinary cookbooks by single authors were similarly full of them.

Of course, by no means did all Americans embrace obviously foreign foods. Had they done so, in fact, foreign foods would not have seemed so thrilling and special to their devotees. When introducing particular foreign dishes, cookbook writers sometimes continued to acknowledge the fact that many people rejected "foreign foods" as a category and had little or no interest in trying them.[186] But as foreign foods became more stylish and more common throughout this era, rejecting them out of hand came to seem ever more provincial. By the 1920s and 1930s, it became much rarer for detractors to broadcast their aversions, as fussiness and culinary nativism came to look less like the purview of the highly refined and more like childish pickiness or uneducated ignorance.

TURNING THE MAH-JONGG TABLE INTO A
BISCUIT BOARD

Foreign food gained popularity amid the rapid and intense industrialization of the U.S. food supply. While the modern food industry has its roots in the 1860s, industrially processed food had reached Americans unevenly, getting its heaviest and most consistent patronage in the first two decades of the twentieth century from middle-class people in towns and cities. Through the 1910s, Americans still bought most of their foods unlabeled, in bulk.[187] By the interwar period, however, processed, mass-produced, and branded foods were increasingly available in cities, towns, and rural places, too. The basic structure of America's modern food industry was in place by the early 1920s and growing rapidly, including many of the brands and corporations that would dominate it throughout the century, such as Coca-Cola, General Foods, Del Monte, Heinz, Post, Dole, Quaker Oats, Standard Fruit, United Fruit, Campbell's, Borden, Kellogg, Kraft, the National Biscuit Company (later called Nabisco), Pepsi, Sunkist, and Armour, among many others.[188] As industrially produced food became more widely available, American consumers got more accustomed to it, and as it became more dependable, they became more dependent on it. By the end of the 1920s, the famed home economist Christine Frederick declared that canned goods had become so ingrained in the cooking and eating habits of middle-class families that housewives "would set up an instantaneous clamor" if deprived of them.[189] The pervasiveness of industrial food contributed to Americans' acceptance of foreign foods in one sense because foreign foods like canned spaghetti and canned chili were becoming widely available under trusted brand names. And industrial food's pervasiveness contributed in a different sense because some people welcomed the supposed authenticity and uniqueness of foreign foods as an antidote to the homogenizing effects of culinary mass production.

At the same time that the exoticism of foreign food was becoming not only acceptable but desirable, there was also a burst of interest in regional American cooking, fueled in part by the sense that distinct regional cuisines were in danger of extinction.[190] "Regional" foods had never stayed neatly in their regions, but their migrations and amalgamations were faster and more visible than ever in the 1920s and 1930s, thanks to increasingly centralized food production and the commodification of certain regional foods in industrialized forms, like canned New England clam chowder, southern biscuit mixes, packaged chili powder, and canned tamales.[191] At the same time, the unique climatic, geographical, and cultural features that had nourished regional diets and distinguished them from one another were being made irrelevant by modern transportation systems and food preservation technologies. The increasing omnipresence of such "regional" foods gave some the uneasy feeling that regional foods could not *stay* truly regional if cheap copies of them were to be had anywhere. As supposedly regional specialties became widely available in all corners of the country, people looked back nostalgically to times when, supposedly, southerners had lived on sweet potatoes, corn bread, and oysters by necessity and Yankees had subsisted on little but cod, clams, and cranberries.[192]

If regional cuisines were ailing, however, some thought they just needed to be nursed back to health. Responding to a New York writer who had claimed that old-fashioned southern food was disappearing, the author of a 1926 Atlanta editorial conceded that southern food was indeed threatened by scientific cookery, working women, and the South's own modernization. In "our strenuous efforts to wipe out sectionalism," he sighed, too many people had "converted the biscuit board into a mah-jong table." But he reassured readers that he still knew plenty of places where "an old 'Mammy cook'" was still producing "baked spareribs and candied yams, hoecake or waffles, creamed butterbeans and watermelon pickle in a cut-glass boat."[193]

In fact, it turned out that plenty of people all over the country were eager to put the mah-jongg table into biscuit-making service, not just the other way around. Interest in the foods of the Old South, in evidence since the end of the Civil War, exploded in the 1910s with a tremendous publishing boom of supposedly antebellum southern cookbooks, a boom that would last for decades.[194] While regular references to plantations and slave ownership in these antebellum revival cookbooks were shorthand for elite privilege, authors of many of the southern recipes that appeared in cookbooks, magazines, and newspapers clearly believed they also had a slumming appeal. Far from disguising their rural origins, recipes like "Near Possum"—in which pork was cooked to taste *like* possum—offered northerners the experience of eating like a poor southerner without having to contemplate hunting, skinning, and consuming a possum—or, for that matter, without actually having to interact with rural southerners.[195] Similarly, in "Hog Jowl and Turnip Greens," the recipe's editor noted with a wink that "beet greens could be used but they are not considered au fait, and to use spinach is an absolute faux pas," neatly signaling that he had the education to know all about high-class food, should he want it, but that he was also adventurousness enough to enjoy eating low, too.[196] By the end of the 1930s, the U.S. government would launch the America Eats program through the Works Progress Administration, sending some 200 writers and photographers around the country to document—and, administrators hoped, preserve—regional American eating practices.[197]

While worries over the homogenizing influences of industrial food helped sustain interest in regional cuisines, industrial food itself also shaped Americans' geographic and historical sense of what regional food meant in the first place. For example, references to "Boston Baked Beans" were rare in American cookbooks before the 1880s and almost nonexistent before the 1860s, when commercial canneries first started selling them as such. But by the late nineteenth century the popularity of canned "Boston Baked Beans" in grocers around the country cemented this formerly tenuous regional association.[198] At the same time, recipes for supposedly old-fashioned Boston Brown Bread often called for cooks to bake the bread in empty tin cans—items colonial Bostonians would hardly have had on hand.[199] Similarly, corn had been by far the most prevalent grain in the antebellum South, but in the early twentieth century, as improved milling processes and transportation networks made white midwestern flour cheap and widely available for the first time, white flour biscuits became the preeminent symbol of the cooking of the Old South.[200] And it was only in the 1910s and 1920s, as farmers in California and other western states invested heavily in pinto bean cultivation, that the beans' inclusion in the southwestern cuisine from the "old days" was codified.[201]

Moreover, the very line separating regional American food and foreign food was hazy on examination. In some cases, regional cuisines themselves were scarcely distinguishable from foreign cuisines, like the foods of the West and Southwest that were sometimes described as Spanish, sometimes as Mexican, and sometimes as regional American.[202] Meanwhile, supposedly foreign cookbooks, like the 1927 *Recipes from Many Lands*, compiled by North Dakota homemakers eager to produce foreign foods in their own kitchens, regularly included Chinese, Mexican, and various European recipes along with a wide selection of regional American ones.[203] Similarly, the Culinary Arts Press released a cookery series in the mid-1930s that included both international and regional cookbooks like *Chinese Cookery* and *'Round the World Cookery*, and books focusing on New England, southern, western, and Pennsylvania Dutch cooking.[204]

As categories of foreign food, national food, and regional food collided, the boundaries that for decades had defined acceptable foods, however uneasily, blurred.[205] Many of the foods that white, native-born Americans in 1900 had by and large rejected, and sometimes turned from in disgust, became components in a rapidly enlarging national repertoire of unembarrassedly regional and foreign dishes and cooking styles, less a canonized cuisine than a proudly polyglot and eagerly acquisitive approach to eating. As Christine Frederick boasted in the late 1920s, "Many, many countries have contributed foods until the present day American bill-of-fare can be truly said to be the most cosmopolitan in the world."[206] If anything, describing oneself as admirably adventurous when it came to food was a new way of describing oneself as discriminating.[207]

FOR MANY AMERICANS in the first decades of the twentieth century, the thought of foreign foods and foreign ways of eating conjured foul-smelling tenements and the weird, insalubrious foods of the poor. By these lights, the inscrutability of mixed, foreign foods was closely tied to their supposed dirtiness and indigestibility. Food became a major target of Americanization efforts as reformers sought to convince immigrants— along with everyone else—to conform to the supposedly historical American practices of eating plain, unadorned foods with few constituent ingredients.

But even at its height in the late 1910s, Americanization was changing course. One of the most glaring signs of the redirection of the original campaign to Americanize immigrant eating practices is that the meaning of "Americanization" itself changed in the decades that followed.[208] Instead of primarily describing immigrants becoming like native-born Americans, "Americanized" increasingly described foreign products or dishes that were appropriate for American consumption. Recipe titles from the 1930s like Americanized Cuban Pan Tamale, Americanized Chop Suey, or Americanized Smörgåsbord would have signaled to readers that these dishes had foreign influences but ultimately domestic personalities, that they had been stripped of potentially threatening ingredients, and that they could be easily reproduced in American kitchens.[209]

Similarly, the term "melting pot" first came into use in 1909 as a term to describe the United States and its panethnic identity, and it is telling that throughout this era, melting—in the sense of melding or mixing together—became a more popular metaphor for immigrants' incorporation into American culture than wholesale transformation.[210] Indeed, whether Americanization reformers liked it or not, the United States was a place where diverse people had always mixed and melded, a process disrupted but hardly eliminated by the restrictions set by the Immigration Act of 1924. It is also noteworthy that this metaphor of culinary melding caught on just as mixed foods themselves were starting to become more broadly acceptable, and more recognizably American.

A singular irony is that as food reformers in the first two decades of the century worked hard to articulate a vision of American cuisine that was wholesome, authentic, and unchanging, American diets were in reality becoming more homogenous in important ways. While individual Americans were eating relatively more varied diets throughout the first four decades of the twentieth century, other factors were also working to unify ideas about what Americans ate, from improved transportation to the growth of industrial food to the explosion of the advertising industry to the rise of national brands and national grocery chains. Even the emerging discipline of statistics itself, combined with the use of the calorie to measure food's energy, helped to structure ideas about what Americans ate simply because such things could finally be calculated.[211] The burgeoning of printed cookbooks helped to promote notions of normal eating, too, and more Americans than ever were using phrases like "national dish," "our national diet," and "the American diet."[212] Food reformers had led this reevaluation of the national diet early in the century, with their narrow notion of American food as pure, plain, and sparsely seasoned, but ideas about American diets became less exclusionary as time went on. Increasingly, indeed, many said that their diet was defined and enriched by its very diversity—a diversity premised upon their own admirable adventurousness and their country's wealth and international reach.[213] Indeed, as Americans rethought what it meant to eat like an American, inclusion was coming to seem like a *uniquely* American trait, with culinary diversity one more manifestation of American abundance.

7

THE TRIUMPH OF THE WILL

The Progressive Body and the Thin Ideal

Lay your double chin on the altar of liberty!
—*Hackensack Record*, 1917

The woman fades out as the double chin fades in.
—*Washington Post*, 1925

Sometime in the 1910s, a woman named Nina Putnam decided to go on a diet. She had been slim as a young bride, and for a few years she had stayed that way by cleaning her own house and doing all her marketing on foot. But as her husband's salary increased, they acquired new things: a vacuum cleaner, an automobile, an apartment in a building with an elevator, and a maid to do the housework. Putnam grew much less active and much less slim, eventually coming to feel like a "hippopotamus" and worrying she was in danger of becoming a "mere wife, instead of a sort of standardized best girl as heretofore." After finally deciding to lose weight, she saw ads for weight loss products everywhere and tried scheme after scheme, from a reducing corset to an electric massaging roller to special mail-order wheat buns to a dance regimen that involved wearing little but a small towel and a large rubber band. Eventually, seeing that nothing was getting smaller except her bank account, Putnam had a revelation. All those dieting companies were selling, she realized, was "nothing in the world but my own strength of mind" and "a visualization of the courage necessary to diet carefully." Putnam decided to diet relying on nothing but willpower, and it was then that she really began to lose weight. She restricted herself severely, eating no potatoes, bread, pasta, cake, pie, pastries, ice cream, cheese, mayonnaise, nuts, olives, grapes, or bananas, and allowing herself only extremely small amounts of soup, sauces, milk, butter, cream, bacon, and sugar. She was always a little hungry, and she considered that a mark of her success.[1]

Nina Putnam eventually lost fifty pounds and was so delighted with the triumph of her will that she wrote a book about it. *Tomorrow We Diet* was published in 1922, and in it Putnam shared the secrets of her success, detailing her list of forbidden foods and stressing that readers could *never* have a lapse in dieting, any more than they could have a lapse "in ethics or true religion." To get thin and stay that way, self-control was needed at every turn, at almost every moment. "You can get as slim as you want to," Putnam wrote, but "two things are required of you—two little eenty weenty things. Self-control and intelligence." Of course, she fully realized that there was nothing tiny about either, and she related her own desperate struggles with her appetites: "There have been times when the sight of a potato ... has brought tears of longing to my eyes! Times, too, when I have reached out a trembling hand and surreptitiously patted the soft cheek of a Parker House Roll." Her willpower won out over her passing desires, however, and she stressed that all her suffering was nothing compared to "the subsequent heavenly, sublime joy" of changing her body, feeling youthful and energetic, and throwing out old clothes that were too big.[2]

Putnam's weight loss narrative touched upon many of the themes underlying Americans' changing ideas about bodies and bodily mastery in the 1910s through the 1930s: the open deprecation of the overweight, the difficulties of dieting and the preeminent importance of willpower in doing so successfully, the joy in being thin, and the centrality of thinness to sex appeal and marital happiness, particularly for women. Weight loss testimonies were not new. They had appeared in the mid-nineteenth century in a few tracts aimed at men, most famously in William Banting's popular *Letter on Corpulence*, first published in 1863 and then many times thereafter.[3] But it was only starting in the 1910s, as thinness became the dominant beauty ideal for both men and women, that weight loss narratives saw their full flowering as a popular new kind of success story, a kind of success obtainable by almost anybody, in theory. In these narratives, those people with enough determination not only changed their bodies for the better, but they transformed their entire lives. Weight loss supposedly led to greater beauty and personal appeal, prolonged youthfulness and improved health, more energy and efficiency, heightened intelligence and ambition, and subsequent benefits like success in business and pleasure in marriage.[4]

While the Great War had lasted, pronouncements about self-discipline and sacrifice as ends in themselves had been nearly ubiquitous. In fact, such pronouncements had been so commonplace and so potent that they nearly muffled associations between food conservation, weight loss, and a growing conviction that thinness was the physical ideal. Yet these associations existed, and they were gaining enormous cultural power during the era. The notion that wartime food restrictions might result in Americans becoming desirably thin was an idea unthinkable during Civil War food shortages. Its attractiveness in the 1910s shows how the idealization of thinness that surged into popularity at the end of the Great War, and that came to overwhelm American conceptions of beauty in the twentieth century, was profoundly compatible with Progressive ideals of self-control, moral righteousness, and asceticism.

A variety of factors contributed to the explosion of weight loss culture during and after the Great War, and one especially potent factor was the creep of metrics into daily life. The application of calories to food in the late nineteenth century and the emerging discipline of statistics resulted in well-publicized comparisons of food consumption and body weights between individuals and across populations.[5] At the same time, life insurance statistics were revealing new correlations between excess weight and chronic disease. More and more Americans, meanwhile, were purchasing newly affordable home scales and buying their clothing ready-made, and thus increasingly thinking of their bodies in terms of numbers and sizes instead of, say, just making clothes to fit their individual bodies.[6] Moreover, metrics grew more prevalent in daily life just as the motion picture industry was taking off and as a visually oriented print media continued to expand.[7] Handed the tools to make physical comparisons, Americans eagerly made them. The growing ease of numerical and visual comparisons contributed directly to the valorization of thinness. But what accounts for the moral stigma that leeched onto the idea of being overweight? The answer lies at the heart of the Progressive ideology of self-control, a value that transcended the Progressive Era itself, both supporting and thriving within the enduring associations between thinness, willpower, and beauty.

IF YOU ARE DOING YOUR BIT, DO NOT FEAR FOR YOUR FIGURE

Today, the food conservation diet suggested for Americans in World War I sounds an awful lot like a weight loss diet. Government administrators urged Americans to eat less red meat, white flour, butter, and sugar, and to eat more lean meat, whole grains, fruits, and vegetables. The reasons for these recommendations had nothing to do with losing weight, of course, since administrators simply wanted to send dense, high-calorie commodities to Europe. Although the reasons for these changes were not to make Americans thinner or healthier, however, Americans during the war increasingly believed—and hoped—that they might.[8] For the first time during the 1910s, slenderness and attractiveness were becoming nearly inseparable as mainstream aesthetic ideals, and middle-class Americans who had been eating more and exercising less in previous years celebrated the idea that wartime food conservation might also improve their "health and physical appearance."[9] Columns appeared suggesting that young women "desirous of having a slender, sylphlike form and graceful carriage" or "all adipose ladies and gentlemen who wish to preserve their figures and serve the nation" had special incentive to eat less in wartime.[10] It was no coincidence that when Dr. Lulu Hunt Peters first published her fantastically popular *Diet and Health, with Key to Calories* in 1918—a book that would become one of the best-selling diet books in American history—she dedicated it to Herbert Hoover.[11]

Fat was not universally reviled in this era, however. Americans had long associated thinness with malnutrition and poverty, and in the 1910s they still regularly used *fat* to describe beauty and good health. Mothers of soldiers in the Great War were happy to hear their sons were "growing fat and strong" in army camps, for example, and some people reported happily that they had "gained considerably in weight as well as in health" even while following food conservation rules.[12] People in the 1910s often *wanted* to be fatter than they were, and advice columns in U.S. magazines and newspapers regularly featured queries about how best to gain weight. Skinniness—or looking like "an animated walking stick"—was wholly undesirable aesthetically.[13] Many were proud of Americans' reputation for having "robust physique[s]" and of statistics demonstrating that they ate more on average than people anywhere else in the world.[14] Indeed, the idea that the United States was "the fat nation of the earth" was central in appeals to Americans to spare some of their abundance for hungry Europeans.[15] Immigrants often came to the United States in order to escape situations of true deprivation and prolonged hunger, and for many recent immigrants and poor Americans, full figures for men and women remained positive symbols of security and success.[16]

Moreover, until the early twentieth century, thinness and self-control had not necessarily seemed to be allied concepts. Yes, many believed that the obese were sinfully self-indulgent, but at the turn of the century most people who were very thin were so because of poverty, regular physical labor, or illness—not because of willpower. According to most nutritionists at the time, in fact, endocrinal problems were generally more to blame for extra fat than overeating.[17] Before the application of calories to food energy and a thorough understanding of the workings of metabolism, people had not even necessarily believed that eating too much *caused* someone to become overweight, since according to casual observation, an active person might eat abundantly and not gain weight, while someone else might gain weight even while eating sparingly, especially if they ate mainly high-calorie foods.[18] And even when calories *were* applied to food, many people thought about food's energy in a completely positive light. For example, today a nutritionist might conceptualize calories by saying that someone would have to walk an extra mile to burn off the energy in three teaspoons of sugar. But in the early twentieth century, Americans more often thought of three sugar lumps as helpfully providing enough energy that they *could* walk an extra mile.[19]

For a brief time in the 1910s, public opinion was fairly balanced on the question of overweight and underweight.[20] Indeed, those words had only come into existence at all in 1899, premised on the novel concept that there was an ideal and supposedly *normal* weight to compare them against.[21] In the first decade and a half of the twentieth century, diet specialists were as likely to help people gain weight as they were to help them lose it.[22] But the scales of public opinion were tipping fast. For one thing, underweight actually *was* less and less of a public health issue. The growing popularization of automobiles and other automated forms of transport, combined with increasing urbanization and the expansion of a sedentary, white-collar workforce, resulted in fewer Americans regularly performing physical activities.[23] At the same time, improvements in food distribution and preservation systems had resulted in a more stable and abundant food supply in all seasons, and rising U.S. wages in previous decades had allowed a broader swath of people to buy adequate amounts of it, steep price increases in the early twentieth century notwithstanding.

As underweight receded as a public health concern, worries about overweight took its place. Some blamed industrial food for Americans' rising weights.[24] One food reformer, for example, said that new foods, concentrated foods, and out-of-season foods tempted Americans at every turn, confusing them into spending too much, eating too much, and choosing foods based on what tasted good rather than what *was* good.[25] And of course, at the high point of the temperance movement, commentators also drew connections between the intemperance of drinking alcohol and the intemperance of overeating.[26] If anything, food was more insidious than alcohol because opportunities to abuse it were everywhere.[27] And like excessive alcohol, excessive food was increasingly thought to be not just morally corrosive but also physically harmful.[28]

Indeed, another important factor in fat's vilification was rapidly accumulating evidence that fat was unhealthful, even deadly. In the recent past, U.S. doctors had generally agreed that the greatest danger regarding food was too little of it, since being underweight could indicate malnutrition and predisposed people to tuberculosis, pneumonia, and other diseases.[29] In 1912, for instance, one dieter had said it was uncomfortable to be fat but scoffed at the idea that fat was actually harmful.[30] Attitudes were changing, however. Most damningly, new mortality studies sponsored by life insurance companies revealed that after the age of thirty-five, death rates increased steadily and predictably the more people weighed.[31] In fact, they showed that people actually lived longest when they weighed ten pounds less than average.[32] As study after study revealed the thin outliving the fat, life insurance companies contracted their range of acceptable weights and considered weight as they calculated risk.[33] Dietitians were becoming important contributors to the field of medicine in this era, while doctors were beginning to pay serious attention to their patients' eating habits.[34]

Another startling change in the late 1910s was that chronic diseases like heart disease, cancer, and diabetes for the first time surpassed epidemic diseases as the leading cause of death among Americans. And experts tended to attribute chronic diseases to living habits—increasingly defined as bad habits—like drinking too much or smoking, getting insufficient exercise, worrying excessively, and especially overeating.[35] The weight loss authority Lulu Hunt Peters informed readers in 1918 that they should either diet or prepare to die: "no joke; you can't tell how near you are to it if you are much overweight."[36] As doctors and nutritionists stated with growing confidence that being thin was actually healthy, people who had previously considered themselves problematically underweight more and more heard that their "problem" was in fact no such thing. For example, when women in 1918 wrote to *Good Housekeeping* magazine complaining that they were "extremely thin," the food expert Harvey Wiley informed them that unless their low weight was caused by tuberculosis or a parasite, they should rejoice at being thin.[37]

The wartime food conservation campaign both reflected and magnified rising concerns about body fat. Far from worrying that overzealous housewives might damagingly underfeed their families, people started worrying that food conservation had not gone far enough in mitigating "excessive personal tubbiness."[38] Some claimed that the health of Europeans who were eating less because of war conditions was improving, and one doctor began a study based on that premise at the Carnegie Nutrition Institute laboratories in 1917, aiming to prove that Americans would be healthier by eating 10 to 20 percent less.[39] Doctors argued that "Self-Martyrizers" who fervently followed food conservation directives were not martyrs at all, because eating less would actually do their bodies good.[40] So obvious were the benefits of eating less that one journalist in a small-town Wisconsin paper felt the need to reassure readers that nothing was detracted from the moral act of going without food "either as a religious or a patriotic exercise by the knowledge that it is a health exercise as well."[41] Wartime weight-loss clubs formed, like the "Fatless League," which encouraged Americans to order food by calories instead of simply ordering different dishes, and the "180 Club" in Los Angeles, which aimed to reduce the weight of any "fat men" who weighed more than 180 pounds.[42]

As part of the personality cult around Herbert Hoover, physical descriptions often cast him as strong and trim. Hoover was certainly trimmer in the war years than when he entered the White House a decade later, but he was never particularly slender, and the starched collar fashionable for men in the 1910s only accentuated his ponderous jowls and tendency toward a double chin. Still, one journalist described Hoover as "slight of build," and another author claimed that he "thinks himself thin," and that his "rather spare figure" resulted from his "abstemious personal habits" as well as from his intensive brainwork.[43] Others described him as "angular," physically "Herculean," or "Samsonlike," and people wrote that in contrast to average "flabby invertebrates," Hoover radiated strength.[44] One journalist said Hoover was the model of the sort of "he-men" the country needed, and another wrote that Hoover "gives at once an impression of force. His limbs look hard; his smooth face is strong."[45] This was not simply a case of changing ideas about what constituted a lean or a heavy person. If anything, the changing standards for men go in quite the opposite direction; after all, Hoover himself—who weighed between 180 and 190 pounds—would have qualified as a "fat man" according to the standards of the 180 Club.[46] In an age when photographs were still a relatively expensive luxury in print media, detailed physical descriptions were common fare in journalism, but the almost phrenological assessments of Hoover hint at an expectation that if those who shirked food conservation were the "fat and disloyal," then food conservation personified was righteously hard and lean.[47]

Indeed, popular political imagery throughout the war relied on visual disparities between the patriotically lean and the treacherously fat, as Americans readily connected the "greed" of food speculators with the "greed" of overeaters. Given rising food prices and fears that European food shortages might soon extend to the United States, some people secretly stockpiled nonperishable food during the war, hoping to resell the food at a profit after prices rose higher. The government actively denounced such profiteering as wicked and unpatriotic, and Americans used the language of fat to describe it: the "Greedy Few Must Not Fatten on Nation's Sufferings."[48] Political cartoonists imagined food speculators as hogs, gorging in ravaged market baskets, and they pitted a gaunt and virile Uncle Sam against bloated profiteers.[49] In one cartoon, Uncle Sam enters a butcher shop carrying a bat labeled "Price Regulation" to confront a hugely fat "Profiteering Butcher."[50] In another, a bony Uncle Sam wrests the reins from an obese profiteer who has been recklessly driving a carriage piled high with the nation's food.[51] Many also associated the reviled high cost of living—which had ballooned in the previous two decades due largely to rising food costs—with fat. One wartime cartoon portrayed Herbert Hoover as a doctor dispensing his "Celebrated Reducing Tonic" to an overweight, middle-aged woman representing the swollen "Cost of Living."[52]

Not only did Americans use the language of fat to describe hoarding, but even more tellingly, they also used the language of hoarding to describe excess body weight. People's pantries might be laudably sparse, but their bodies could still be "hoarding food in the shape of fat."[53] Indeed, Americans increasingly articulated the idea that there were other ways to waste food besides throwing it in the kitchen garbage pail, and one of the most common was by *eating it* when they did not need to. While the patriotic scrimped and even fasted, fat people had "vast amounts" of extra food "stored away in their own anatomy."[54] Writers demanded, "Are You a Fat Hoarder?" and "How dare you hoard fat when your nation needs it?"[55] By the calculations of *Popular Science Monthly* magazine, the excess weight on all Americans was the equivalent of almost 700 million loaves of bread, or enough to feed an army of 3 million men for two months. At a time of international food shortages, some Americans looked at fat people as wasted "loaves of bread perambulating throughout the country."[56]

Because patriotic food conservation supposedly resulted quite naturally in a healthfully trim weight, patriotism was visible in a way it had never been before. "If you are doing your bit, do not fear for your figure," the writer of one Department of Agriculture pamphlet warned.[57] Similarly, a New Jersey paper published the slogan, "Lay your double chin on the altar of liberty!"[58] People who did lose weight during the war sometimes described their accomplishment in patriotic terms, like one formerly obese

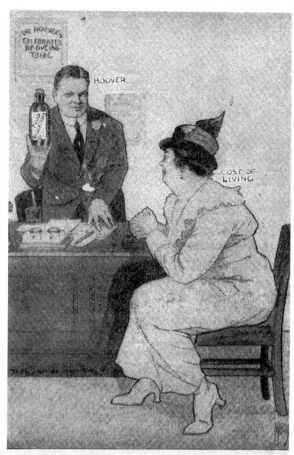

"OH, DOCTOR, WILL IT MAKE ME NORMAL AGAIN?"

In this cartoon, the high cost of living personified is an overweight woman. Fortunately, "Dr. Hoover" is on hand to dispense a weight-loss tonic in the form of food regulations. Literary Digest, *1 September 1917, 13*

Texas man who boasted that his diet was helping to win the war.[59] Extending this argument, however, meant that anyone who was not either thin or actively losing weight was disloyal. Journalists declared that a person "cannot be fat and be patriotic" and that attempts to be both at once smacked of hypocrisy.[60] For instance, one writer sneered that those "stout persons who sit around listening to war lectures and imagining they are doing their bit" were treacherously deluded, because the "one way a fat person can help the government is to lose weight and quickly."[61] So grave did the problem of excess weight seem in the context of international food shortages that some called for scales in state buildings and said that everyone should be weighed in public once a month.[62] Others suggested quite seriously that obesity be declared a misdemeanor, and that fat men and women be arrested.[63] People were not just watching their own weights. They were keeping an eye on their neighbors' weights, too.

By the end of World War I, Americans' longtime appreciation of fat was fading and a new idealization of thinness was taking firm hold. Americans increasingly associated slimness with admirable self-control and excess fat as a uniquely visible expression of moral weakness. When Americans thought about the consequences of eating too much, their perceptions themselves were changing. By the late 1910s, most Americans no longer saw a few extra pounds on someone as an admirable sign of success and well-being, a physical margin of error between their possessor and hard times. Instead, they envisioned excess fat as the sum of all the extra food these overweight people had needlessly, and greedily, consumed.

VICTORY OVER SELF

Americans had condemned fat as immoral in the context of wartime food shortages, but condemnation of fat survived the war. In fact, it thrived in the decades that followed, and dieting culture roared into popularity in the 1920s and 1930s as the idealization of thinness seeped into mainstream conceptions of beauty. Associations between good health and wise eating, combined with widespread new desires to be thin, profoundly affected Americans' food choices. By the late 1920s, the popular home economist and consumption expert Christine Frederick proudly asked, "Where else do women think so much before they eat?" And where besides America would women "sit down to a rare lamb chop and a slice of pineapple"—a popular weight loss diet of the day—"while all the time craving chicken salad and mayonnaise, a slice of cocoanut cake and a cup of chocolate with whipped cream?" For all her enthusiasm about weight loss in the abstract, however, Frederick struggled with her own "reducing agonies."[64] She once joked darkly that her status as a consumption expert felt ironic at those times when she was twenty pounds overweight.[65] By 1930, a *New York Times* journalist doubted whether there was anyone in the country—and especially any woman—who was capable of eating a meal without thinking about her figure.[66]

The idealization of thinness was so powerful in the post–World War I years that dieting maintained a tenacious hold on American culture even during the Great Depression. Some in the early 1930s had anticipated that widespread economic woes would be an adequate check on overeating all by themselves, like the newspaper columnist who speculated, "During these trying times I don't think many of us will have to diet or reduce."[67]

In fact, however, dieting culture hardly budged during the decade, and for all but the poorest Americans, concerns about slimness stayed keen even while budgets tightened. Economic austerity and the idealization of thinness were even potentially complementary. For example, in the first edition of *The Joy of Cooking*, published in 1931, Irma Rombauer wrote that she compiled the books' recipes "with one eye on the family purse and the other on the bathroom scale."[68]

During this era, some of the most open deprecation of fat came from people who had once been overweight themselves. One man said that for twenty years he had been "disgustingly fat," with "all the bodily characteristics of a bale of hay."[69] Nina Putnam called herself a "hippopotamus," while Dr. Luella Axtell, who later became a specialist on obesity, recalled the "nausea of abhorrent self-loathing" that had surged through her after she had caught sight of her arm quivering and shaking "with its burden of fat. How hideous! How loathsome!"[70] Lulu Hunt Peters remembered her days as an overweight bride, sighing, "Never can I tell pathetically 'when I was married I weighed only one hundred eighteen, and look at me now.' No, I was a delicate slip of one hundred and sixty-five when I was taken."[71] In all cases, of course, deprecating their former selves was a way of elevating their present ones. If they were once disgusting, now they were not; if Peters could not sigh that she had gone from a slim bride to a hefty matron, all the better to smile that she had gone from hefty to slim. And because they were talking about *themselves*, after all, anti-fat rhetoric from the lips of the formerly fat passed as self-deprecation rather than bigotry.

For many successful dieters, however, the most dramatic transformation was not a transformation of their bodies but a transformation of their wills. Willpower was the central theme of dieting advice in this era, and again and again dieters credited their wills for their success. A man named Samuel Blythe described his epic struggles with his own powers of self-control and attributed his eventual weight loss to "the triumph of the will over the appetite." For months after he first radically cut back on food, Blythe was hungry all the time, and sometimes he had to leave the table to gain control of himself or grip the sides of his chair to keep from reaching out for more food. It was the hardest struggle of his life, he said, because no fat person simply *lost* weight; the weight was "fought off, beaten off . . . a grueling combat to the finish, a task that appalls and usually repels."[72] Of course, the fact that the combat did not repel *him* in the end—that his will eventually triumphed—made the triumph all the greater. Luella Axtell proudly reported how she had woken her husband out of a sound sleep by declaring out loud in the middle of the night that she would no longer be fat, after having a midnight revelation that she possessed the "power of victory over self."[73] "Self control!" another diet author exulted. "That is the base of it all."[74]

Dieting writers in the 1920s and 1930s generally told reducers to stick to their diets no matter what and warned them that any lapse at all meant self-defeat.[75] Sylvia Ullback, a Norwegian-born dieting guru who billed herself as "Sylvia of Hollywood," had dieted down to less than a hundred pounds herself and doled out uncompromising weight loss advice to dozens of film stars and, later, to readers of her popular books.[76] Dieters had "to have gumption!" Sylvia thundered. "You've got to have courage and will power! You've got to shake yourself rid of *laziness* and work as you've never worked before!"[77] Sylvia demanded an intense regimen involving colonic irrigations, vigorous scrubbing under cold showers, no alcohol, and most importantly, very little food.[78] To "chaste[n]" their stomachs and show them that they were "master," Lulu Hunt Peters advised dieters to fast for at least one day at the start of a diet.[79] And dieters in this era did chasten their bodies. For instance, as a teenager in the mid-1920s, a girl named Yvonne Blue—who later married the behaviorist B. F. Skinner—wrote giddily in her diary about staying up late with a friend one spring night making grilled cheese and eating "the lovely soggy, melt-in-your-mouthy-buttery sandwitches."[80] But only a few months later she declared she was tired of "being fat" and vowed to lose thirty pounds and "get slim and sylphy-like" before going back to school in the fall.[81] Sometimes fasting for days at a time, Yvonne filled her diary with descriptions of the lemonade, cakes, and cookies she denied herself, writing that whenever she was tempted she repeated to herself, "I have a will!"[82] Likewise, the young opera star Marion Talley lost more than twenty-five pounds in two months after signing a contract with the film company MGM, relying on nothing but "will power" as she subsisted on coffee, skim milk, and salads dressed with indigestible—and thus calorie-free—mineral oil.[83]

The daily menus recommended by dieting books of the era were often miserly, and some popular fad diets consisted of little but bananas and milk, or spinach and pineapple, or pineapple and lamb, echoing in their monotony some of the fad diets popular at the turn of the century.[84] One of the best-selling American dieting books in the 1930s was Victor Lindlahr's *7-DAY Reducing Diet*, which promoted a painfully austere, albeit temporary, diet of only about 650 calories a day.[85] The problem, of course, was that temporary diets rarely effected lasting change. Indeed, most weight loss authors stressed that returning to old habits meant returning to the old body, and reducers could not relax their willpower even after they had reduced their weights. For instance, one author warned dieters that they could never slacken their vigilance as long as they lived, never even casually stealing "a few grapes for yourself while arranging the dish of fruit."[86] Lulu Hunt Peters hated it when people asked if they would *always* have to count calories. "Yes!" she seethed. "You will always have to keep up dieting, just as you always have to keep up other things in life that make it worth living—being neat, being kind, being tender; reading, studying, loving." Dieting was like having a bath—it was not enough to simply do it once.[87] Willpower had to become a part of who they were.[88]

As Americans more and more saw excess fat as both harmful and avoidable by those who exercised their willpower, they reinterpreted plumpness as a mark of laziness or gluttony rather than the natural result of heredity, glands, or aging, the prevailing explanations for weight gain in earlier decades. For example, one man who lost fifty-five pounds looked back on the slow weight gain of his youth as "legitimate enough. I put it on myself. There was no hereditary nonsense about it."[89] There was a joke in the 1910s about an overweight woman who was sure heredity was to blame for her fat: the one time she dieted she gained weight, even though she "didn't eat a thing but what the doctor ordered, besides [her] regular meals."[90] Perhaps the most important change in popular beliefs about the biological nature of body weight was that people increasingly said it was unnecessary to gain weight as one aged, an idea that contrasted sharply with nineteenth-century beliefs that most people naturally grew stout as they grew old, and that fat offered warming and protective properties desirable for the elderly.[91] By the 1920s and 1930s, observers increasingly concluded that people gained weight when they consumed more calories than they used, and that was that.[92] Anyone who claimed to be an exception to that rule was probably lying.[93]

Refuting biological justifications for fat meant that anyone could potentially become thin, as long as they had the will.[94] The problem, many feared, was that overweight people by definition did not possess much willpower at all. Fat people might claim to be eager to do whatever was necessary to lose weight, but that eagerness usually lasted only until the next meal, when "their appetites refuse to be bridled."[95] Thin people, by contrast, were *willing* to bridle themselves—it was why they were thin in the first place. Even worse, once a body was coated with excess fat, it was widely believed, the fat itself physically affected the body and the mind, sapping energy and dulling intelligence and self-discipline. As Lulu Hunt Peters wrote, "[W]ill power with a layer of fat on it gets feeble."[96] Yet, increasingly, people suggested that those who did not already possess a steely will could learn how to cultivate one. The term "will-power" was only coined in the 1870s, but it was a powerful concept that had entered mainstream vocabularies very quickly.[97] Starting around the turn of the century, a new genre of self-help books dedicated to developing and strengthening willpower had rocketed into success on both sides of the Atlantic, including hugely popular works like Jules Payot's *The Education of the Will*, first published in 1895 and republished dozens of times afterward in French and English, and Frank Haddock's spectacularly successful 1907 *Power of Will*.[98] Moreover, one of the best ways to "train the flabby will" was the act of dieting itself.[99] In other words, those who managed to follow a strict diet not only could shrink their will-sapping fat, but they could strengthen their self-control by exercising it.[100]

Increasingly, physical exercise seemed to be a vital complement to diet in the battle to lose weight.[101] Interest in exercise had been expanding since the mid-nineteenth century. While health reformers in the early nineteenth century had promoted sexual and dietary restraint as the bases of physical health, by the second half of the century reformers were turning to exercise as another important tool.[102] Starting in the 1870s, the first formal physical education programs in the United States had come into being under the auspices of universities and secondary schools, with advocates harkening back to the rigorous physical training undertaken by the Ancient Greeks.[103] By the turn of the twentieth century, more than 270 U.S. universities and even more city school systems had started physical education programs, and that number grew rapidly in the following years, eventually including virtually every school in the country.[104]

It was no accident that physical education rose to national prominence just as members of the expanding American middle class were doing less physical labor as part of their daily lives, or that reducing diets as well as exercise regimens targeted middle-class Americans rather than farmers, servants, or other manual laborers. Twentieth-century Americans as a whole were less likely to require as much food energy as previous generations due to technological changes in everything from transportation to home appliances to farm equipment, but the difference in calorie needs was most acute in the middle classes. In the nineteenth century, middle-class Americans had emphasized their ability to afford relatively sedentary lives as an important distinction between themselves and poorer people. But by the early twentieth century, they were rethinking and even romanticizing physical labor as an invigorating form of exertion and a means to attain health and beauty. "If you want to eat like an ogre and get thin," one dieting author wrote, "become a farmer!" It was little wonder that city men were growing "heavy and flabby and lazy and always wish something else would happen to them."[105] In earlier times, when most Americans had done hard manual work all day, it was logical that they had breakfasted on meat, beans, hot cakes, and pie, while now a commuter with a city job could barely stomach an egg with toast.[106] Indeed, one of the sharpest changes in American eating habits in the early twentieth century was the transition from large, hot breakfasts heavy on meats to lighter breakfasts centered around toast or cereal, a change that reflected Americans' decreasing levels of physical activity as well as the growing availability of industrially produced breakfast cereals. Indeed, American meals were shrinking in general, and by the 1920s contemporary studies reported that Americans ate less food per capita than they had in previous decades.[107]

Just as white-collar office workers were unlikely to toil physically as part of their jobs and more likely to ride a train or drive an automobile between suburban homes and urban workplaces, some worried that women were getting fat because they were not doing enough housework. The health and beauty expert Susanna Cocroft advised wealthy patients trying to lose weight to scrub their own floors, and the columnist Dorothy Dix argued that wealthy women essentially paid other women to do their exercise for them.[108] "Many a rich woman," Dix claimed, "envies her maid the hipless figure, her small waist, her firm, exquisitely modeled arms," and it was "strange that she has not realized that she, too, could attain these attractions in the same school of physical development."[109] Yet not all servants were thrilled with their own figures, like one African American maid in Houston who wrote to a newspaper advice column because she was desperate to get rid of the fat under her arms and at the back of her neck.[110] Indeed, even for women who did it full time, housework simply required less physical exertion than it had for previous generations, as labor-saving devices like vacuums, gas stoves, and modern plumbing became features of more and more homes.[111] As one beauty writer grumbled in 1927, "Civilization and prosperity have made women slothful. We don't even sweep since vacuum cleaners have been invented."[112]

In the first three decades of the twentieth century, as engines, appliances, and other technological aids made daily life less physically taxing than ever before, middle-class Americans increasingly took up exercise as a formal pursuit outside the realm of ordinary activities. Exercise was at once a form of recreation, a means of attaining vigor and beauty, and an emblem of self-discipline, and large numbers of those men and women who had the time and money to do so pursued activities like golf, tennis, skating, horseback riding, hiking, and recreational walking.[113] Though potentially fun, these activities also had a moral dimension since they required discipline, exertion, and sometimes training—and because doctors and physical educators so vocally touted their contributions to health and longevity as well as to a fashionable figure. By the 1920s, exercise was taking on the hybrid identity it would have throughout the twentieth century: an activity that was not work and yet was not simply leisure, either.

Not all the era's dieting material focused on self-denial, by any means. Dozens of books and hundreds of small companies capitalized on people's fears of hunger and discomfort, hocking products that promised to take off weight with little emotional or physical duress.[114] Some of the era's most popular dieting methods were steam baths, diet pills, and laxative chewing gums.[115] Companies produced dieting cookbooks describing products like Knox Gelatin or Kellogg's All Bran cereal as painless substitutes for fattier foods.[116] Reducing salts, added to bath water or swallowed all by themselves, were another weight loss fad, and devices like electrical massagers and "Shimmey Chairs" promised to jiggle away weight.[117] Meanwhile, special "Reducing Soap" supposedly melted away fat on any part of the body where people scrubbed themselves.[118]

These painless weight loss methods rarely lasted long, however. The soaps and salts and Shimmey Chairs simply did not work, while laxatives led to intestinal ills, and diet pills could be dangerous. The popular diet drug dinitrophenol, for example, caused so many deaths that it was outlawed by the late 1930s.[119] Despite the fads for effortless weight loss, the majority of advice in the interwar period came back to the basic formula that would stay consistent in the decades that followed: to lose weight you had to eat fewer calories than your body required, and for most people this meant a struggle with their desires, day after day after day. In the long run, however, the well-publicized difficulties of losing weight only added to the prestige of having done so. Willpower remained the defining motif of dieting advice from the 1910s through the 1930s, and it was not simply because a strong will was the most effective way to become thin. In popular imaginations, willpower remained a vital component of thinness itself, part of the ends as well as the means. Thin was beautiful precisely because it was a physical manifestation of self-control.

AS THE BODY IS, SO THE SOUL IS!

Visual media took on profound new power throughout the first four decades of the twentieth century. Advertising ballooned, doubling in the

1920s alone, and more ads than ever contained graphics and pictures.[120] Books, fashion magazines, and newspapers all contained more images, too, with many specializing in photographs of young female models and actresses. Indeed, popular forms of entertainment often explicitly encouraged appraisals of and comparisons between women's bodies. In the Miss America Pageant, for example, which started in Atlantic City in 1921 and drew hundreds of thousands of spectators within a few years, judges went out of their way to select contestants with unbobbed hair who did not resemble flappers, but they still expected them to be as slender as the latest film stars: the women were evaluated while wearing swimming costumes and their waists were measured.[121] Americans were looking more at other people throughout the 1920s and 1930s, and they were also looking more at themselves. There were more mirrors inside American homes, appearing especially in places like bathrooms, where self-scrutiny could accompany daily weighing on newly purchased home scales.[122] Dieters sometimes described how their own reflections motivated them. As she lost weight, for instance, Nina Putnam said that she fought off the temptation to devour a pan of frying bacon by looking in a mirror.[123] Others used the mirror as confirmation that they were on the right track, like one successful dieter who described the satisfaction he found in looking in a full-length mirror: "I am confronted by the reflection of a slight man, slim-waisted, with narrow, beautiful legs."[124]

One of the most striking changes in the postwar world was that bodies were more visible than ever before, as fashions in the 1920s quite suddenly became tighter, lighter, and more revealing. For women, heels became higher, skirts and hair drastically shorter, and arms, legs, and necks were all more visible.[125] Men's suits were more tightly tailored. Bodies were increasingly on display, and for many, this meant that "bodily defects"— sometimes newly conceived of as such—were shamefully revealed.[126] One 1920s writer commented that while the full dresses popular in decades past had only suggested the bodies underneath, in clothing "where the material is drawn closely about the figure, it is the reality which counts."[127] And skimpiness was not the only change. Ready-made clothing was becoming ubiquitous, and weight loss authors encouraged people to judge themselves by the standards of standardized clothing. Sylvia Ullback demanded, for instance, "[H]ow do your clothes fit? Can you walk into a good shop, ask for your size fourteen or whatever it is, and have your garment fit? Or must the hip seams be let out, the shoulders narrowed? This test will give you a pretty good idea of just where you're wrong if you can't see it yourself."[128] One African American fashion commentator described overweight women "trailing from shop to shop, trying on 'stylish stouts,'" and "sobbing with disappointment." But she laughed that the new fashion for slimness was not going away, so heavy women should either lose weight or go back to wearing bonnets and shawls.[129]

The growing popularity of motion pictures further promoted and valorized thinness. Overweight women had no business in show business, one African American man wrote in the *Chicago Defender*, saying that if it were up to the audience the only fat women would be "in the side shows."[130] One diet advertisement informed readers matter-of-factly that the movies required "slender figures" because "almost everybody dislikes fat."[131] Film companies in the 1920s also began including weight limits in the contracts they signed with actresses. In one, for instance, a company reserved the right to "terminate the contract at any time after the weight of the artist shall exceed 130 pounds."[132] The president of First National Pictures boasted about his company's strict weight limits and claimed they were good for the actresses as well as good for the company. Yet the one actress quoted in a news story about the company's weight limits, Doris Kenyon, was less than enthusiastic as she described how hard it was "to keep such a constant watch over your weight and food" and how "disconcerting to be a hostess and adhere to a diet while my friends are enjoying their favorite dishes."[133] Other stars of the era also discussed their struggles to conform to increasingly severe expectations. Before filming a new movie, the silent film star Theda Bara reported eating nothing but two baked potatoes a day with milk. Another film star, Myrtle Stedman, confided that she was so sick of dieting that "the ambition of her life" had become "to retire and eat a breakfast of ham and eggs and hot biscuits."[134] Constraining as Hollywood actresses felt such expectations to be, women across the country emulated them. The "Hollywood 18-Day Diet," enormously popular in the late 1920s and 1930s, promised followers they could lose a pound a day by living off little but grapefruit.[135] In New York, one article reported, women of all backgrounds—from stenographers to debutants to housewives—were subsisting on grapefruit in the hopes of gaining movie star proportions.[136]

As visual media came to dominate popular culture, physical appearance was more and more taken as an indicator of character and personality. "As the body is, so the soul is!" the authors of one 1918 cookbook wrote, and they meant it.[137] Indeed, while excess weight on someone pointed to all the overeating he or she had done, that fat also supposedly revealed a host of other character traits: fat people were sad; they lacked ambition; they were dimwitted and slow; they were followers rather than leaders.

Americans had long drawn associations between the inner and outer selves, from obsession with racial taxonomy to interest in phrenology, and in many ways twentieth-century attempts to read into fat were one more expression of this long-standing interest. In the nineteenth century, popular culture had regularly suggested that overweight people were jolly and easygoing, and books of collected jokes encouraged readers to "Laugh and Grow Fat."[138] By the 1910s, however, people increasingly suggested that overweight people were not jolly at all, but rather aimless, anxious, or sad.[139] Vance Thompson, the author of one of the best-selling weight loss books of the 1910s, wrote that no fat person was truly happy. "No; the fat man may clown and slap himself and wag a droll forefinger, but he is not merry at all; and if one should sink a shaft down to his heart—or drive a tunnel through to it—one would discover that it is a sad heart, black with melancholy."[140] Many also described the fat as inherently lazy, like one poor Michigan woman who had reported her "fat and lazy" neighbor to the government during the war for sitting around eating ice cream all day.[141] Some said that people became fat because they lacked a sense of purpose, and that the state of being fat further drained ambition. "Get a purpose in life," Susanna Cocroft told clients, "and then you will get a waist line!"[142]

Intellectually as well as morally, fat people were held to be inferior to their slimmer counterparts, and some people advanced physiological arguments to explain the difference. A glutton "possesses a fat mind, and thinks clumsily," according to a journalist in an Alabama paper, whereas a light eater supposedly had "room enough in his mind for the big impulses and blood enough in his body to feed all the tissues of it—including the brain."[143] Some said that fat blanketed the nerves, making the overweight calmer and slower, less alert and less efficient.[144] For example, Lulu Hunt Peters had worked as a hospital superintendent when she was at her heaviest, and after losing seventy pounds years later, she proclaimed that she felt like refunding the salary she got at that time because "efficiency decreases in direct proportion as excess weight increases. Everybody knows it."[145] Others said that constantly having so much food in the body caused blood to rush away from the brain and to the stomach, and that the "foggy feeling" that plagued overeaters could be "dispelled by simply eating less."[146] Fat men were rarely great men, purportedly, because they lacked the drive and ambition that would give them a singular purpose in life. For instance, a doctor in the 1920s joked that fat men's "footprints on the sands of time would be quite noticeable—if they made any. But as a rule they do not."[147] Another diet author noted smugly that William Taft—who had weighed upwards of

300 pounds during his presidency—had not been competent enough to earn a second term.[148] Thinness, by contrast, was both the result of ambition and the source of new energy and drive. With their supposedly more sensitive nervous systems and freely flowing blood, thin people were described as sharp, energetic, and highly keyed.[149] The body building enthusiast and physical culture pioneer Bernarr McFadden claimed in 1923 that "many of the worlds' greatest thinkers are light eaters and attribute their superior mental efficiency, in part at least, to their abstemious diet."[150] It was the thin who were the world's natural leaders and thinkers, the thin who got things done.[151]

As a result of the toll that fat allegedly took on intellect and energy, people who did manage to lose weight supposedly underwent a stunning mental alteration in the process. Dieting transformed one "tub of a man" into "a greyhound type, keen and alert instead of heavy-footed and sluggish."[152] Another dieter claimed that he became "mentally and physically" stronger after losing thirty-five pounds.[153] One man's business "took a decided up-hill trend" after he went on a diet, "as his brains grew less fuddled with food and his body more willing and active."[154] And because it would supposedly result in sharper intellect and greater ambition, authors swore that weight loss boosted earning power.[155] In the year following significant weight loss, one writer promised dieters, they would make more money and "be more successful, no matter what your profession or vocation."[156] When women fretted that losing weight would cause their faces to become wrinkled, Lulu Hunt Peters shot back that weight loss would cause more wrinkles in their brains, and that was what mattered.[157]

NOBODY LOVES A FAT GIRL

Dieting in the first two decades of the twentieth century had by no means been a starkly gendered activity. In fact, dieting had been a primarily masculine activity throughout the second half of the nineteenth century, when most Americans had seen dieting and fasting—and the rigorous physical self-control they entailed—as practices appropriate only for men.[158] When women in large numbers did start to diet in the early twentieth century, it was one important way that they asserted modern women's capacity for physical activity, in a conscious departure from nineteenth-century beliefs that women could not and should not endure stern bodily trials.[159] As thinness became a truly mainstream ideal starting in the late 1910s, dieting culture still did not exclusively target women. New fashions emphasized dramatically slimmer figures for both sexes, and columnists cautioned,

"Mr. Man, beware!" as fashionable male waistlines shrank.[160] Writers coolly repeated the old saying, "Nobody loves a fat man."[161]

But by the 1920s, they were going further. "Nobody loves a fat man," Nina Putnam sighed, "but the subject doesn't even come up about a fat girl."[162] Although the contraction of stylish silhouettes affected physical expectations for men, women had become the primary targets of dieting discourse by the 1920s. Putnam resigned herself to the idea that "men get by with more pounds and less hair than any woman would dare attempt, even if the money were mostly hers."[163] But misogyny, and not just resignation, laced through much of the era's dieting advice. One beauty writer said overweight women "should be spanked," and Sylvia Ullback wished she were in Congress so she could "try to get a law passed that sloppy fat women should be arrested."[164] Some suggested that women not only lacked *character*, in the form of willpower and resolve, but they lacked *personhood* itself, that women did not meaningfully exist when they gained weight. A male author in the mid-1910s had written that some of the women he had loved had "drowned" and "vanished" in an ocean of fat, and nine years later a different journalist agreed, writing that the "woman fades out as the double chin fades in."[165] Another male diet author said a fat face had no capacity "for mirroring the soul."[166] At the same time, even as women were increasingly expected to diet rigorously, they were also criticized for losing too much weight, or losing it in the wrong places, or in the wrong way.[167] Tony Gaudio, a Hollywood camera man who worked with some of the biggest film stars of the era, insisted that women be thin but complained that stars' dieting made their faces, necks, and shoulders look "scrawny" and "grotesque." He did not suggest how women might lose weight on some parts of their bodies but not on others, but he was sure a doctor would know.[168] Others criticized women for showing any signs of the stress caused by chronic hunger, complaining that nothing made women dull and cranky like strict dieting.[169]

To be taken seriously—even to be noticed—it seemed crucial to many women by the 1920s to be thin. It was at once particularly hard to be thin in the modern age, due to sedentary habits and industrializing food supplies, and particularly *important* to be so. Indeed, thinness was a prerequisite for *being* modern. Bodies had to be sleek and streamlined to achieve "up-to-date lines," one writer declared; they had to be thin to "fit into our civilization."[170] Another cookbook author wrote in 1934 that there was "no room for the fat woman in this age."[171] Even as she privately struggled with her own weight, Christine Frederick celebrated women's dieting know-how as a preeminent sign of their modernity. While grandmother might have resigned herself to "the 'middle-aged spread' of the hips which made her fat, fair and forty," Frederick wrote, the modern woman "at once watches her weight, buys an electric exerciser, eats less, and in many cases counts her calories daily."[172] New expectations about thinness brought related new pressure on women to, somehow, stay young.[173] Indeed, in the booming youth culture of the 1920s, nothing was so modern as being young and energetic. Modern fashions were "built around youthful curves," and observers praised the "childlike figure[s]" of extremely thin women.[174] Anti-aging sentiments were embedded in advice that women should *keep* their beauty and health by dieting.[175] One woman who signed herself "Dorothy" asked an advice columnist in 1928 how she could possibly be expected to diet and keep looking young when she was already exhausted by taking care of her child and home and husband. The columnist responded scathingly that she knew a vivacious woman with five children who wore the same dress size as her teenage daughter. With only one child to look after, she said, Dorothy "ought to look like a flapper and act like one."[176]

Commentators also increasingly described thinness as crucial to both women's general attractiveness and their marital happiness.[177] Like Nina Putnam, who thought her excess weight had put her in danger of becoming a "mere wife," many women lost weight—or were told that they should—because it would supposedly improve their marriages.[178] For instance, one young woman wrote to a newspaper advice column because she weighed more than 200 pounds and her slender husband made fun of her and no longer took her out. Even if she was overweight, she wrote, "I have a heart the same as if I only weighed 110, and I don't enjoy doing all of the lovemaking." While the columnist responded that she personally thought the nicest wives were women "who love good food and set a good table, who get a little heftier and a little sweeter as the years go by," she still informed the woman that if her husband had started comparing her to flappers, she had better start counting calories.[179] When a different woman wrote to Lulu Hunt Peters for advice because her husband "hates me to be fat," Peters said she was glad there was at least one husband who did not pretend not to prefer slender women.[180] Sylvia Ullback scolded women for expecting to be loved simply for being warm mothers, agreeable companions, and good housekeepers, saying those accomplishments did not "excuse a woman from being a pleasant eyeful as well."[181] At age fifty-one, Ullback herself had divorced her longtime husband and married a thirty-year-old movie star.[182] But not all women wanted to lose weight in order to please the men in their lives, and some even dieted in spite of protests from their husbands and boyfriends. For example, one African

American woman who described herself as "stout" aimed to lose at least thirty pounds even though her husband "'likes 'em plenty heavy.'"[183] Likewise, a woman named Elaine wrote to Egypsy Ann, the advice columnist in the *New York Amsterdam News*, complaining that although she wanted to lose weight, her boyfriend "prefers them with curves."[184]

While some African Americans clearly rejected mainstream glorifications of thinness, many others embraced the increasingly rigid associations between thinness and beauty. Articles about dieting and ads about weight loss products and services filled African American newspapers in the 1910s, 1920s, and 1930s, like the electric weight reducing treatments a woman calling herself "Madame Lococo" offered in Harlem.[185] Women regularly wrote to advice columns in the black press to ask about losing weight, and journalists described the importance of self-denial and willpower in achieving thinness.[186] In 1932, a young middle-class black woman living in Atlanta wrote that she felt "entirely too fat" at five feet three and 150 pounds. She had "lost all of [her] beaux" because of her weight, she said, and it seemed that she was losing her slender "girl pals," too. Despite what she described as her desirably "light brown skin" and the fact that she had finished college, she believed her fat was ruining her happiness.[187] Indeed, the stakes of dieting for African American women were heightened precisely because the rise of dieting culture took place in the midst of nostalgic white celebrations of imagined Mammy figures, contented slaves whose pleasure-seeking nature and physical laxity were expressed for all the world to see in their invariably rotund bodies.[188]

DURING AND AFTER THE GREAT WAR, growing hostility to fat found its most virulent expression in aesthetics, but the idealization of thinness was not built on the shifting sands of the fashion world. Rather, the thin ideal arose from bedrock intellectual and moral convictions at the dead center of Progressive ideas about social order, especially the increasingly steadfast conviction that physical self-control indicated a capacity for moral and political self-government. These ideals found their public apogee in the Progressive Era, but they survived in the private weight loss struggles of individual Americans throughout the century that followed. The endurance of the Progressive idealization of thinness points to the stability of its intellectual and moral foundations.

The conviction that dieting was more than vanity fueled the explosion of dieting after the war. Thinness came to seem indispensable to beauty in the postwar years, but a thin body also contributed to health, success, and happiness. As chronic disease rates rose, doctors broadcast the message that weight loss improved health and added years to life expectancy. Sloughing off weight also supposedly boosted efficiency and intelligence, since excess weight was thought to pad nerves and slow blood flow to the brain. Weight loss made people look younger by restoring youthful figures, but it also increased energy, making people feel younger, too. Moreover, by increasing attractiveness and sex appeal, thinness improved marital prospects or strengthened marriages already in place. Simply put, it increasingly seemed that thinness made people happy, and it came to seem hard for any person—and especially for any woman—to be authentically happy if she was fat.

Men were not exempt from hardening associations between outer thinness and inner righteousness. But starting in the 1920s, just as women were gaining unprecedented political, social, and sexual freedom, they bore the full force of morally charged inducements to be thin. Sylvia Ullback not only swore that fat women "can't be happy," but she said they "might as well be dead."[189] This sort of cruelty was only socially possible because of the conviction, breathtakingly common by the 1920s and 1930s, that at a very basic level fat people *chose* to be fat. Excess weight did not result from glands or parentage or any other biological predisposition, medical authorities concluded. Instead, it resulted from repeated failures of the will, from spineless capitulations, day after day, to pleasure and appetite. If they could only summon the will to rein in their animal desires, thinness was supposedly anyone's for the taking.

MORAL FOOD AND MODERN FOOD

Be a Little Hungry!—*Erie Herald*, 1918

In the late 1910s, Americans sent soldiers abroad to fight in what many believed was actually a *great* war, one they hoped would forever vanquish a Prussian system of government that represented autocratic control by the few and the slavish submission of everyone else. In this morally electric context, an unprecedented foreign food aid project turned cooking and eating into intensely political activities on the American home front, and reformers ushered in a new era of scientific food by stressing the moral importance of approaching food rationally. Food reform generally and food aid specifically were quintessentially Progressive projects, bolstered by scientific expertise and by moralistic efforts to make daily life more rational. By looking at the modernization of American food, which took place at a time of national transformation and international crisis, this book has considered America's transition to modernity, a process that continues to shape the nation and the world.

Nowhere is this clearer than in the birth of international food aid itself, the firing line of the Progressive quest for rational food. The federal government gained extraordinary influence over eating habits and food production in the United States during World War I, as food administrators encouraged Americans to exercise self-discipline instead of relying on a formal rationing program. Yet such calls to arms from the government were only possible because a remarkable number of individual Americans at the same time were expressing the idea that when people disciplined themselves around food, prioritizing the needs of the state or of science or of the collective good over their personal desires, they demonstrated their fitness for political citizenship itself. In conjunction with Progressive debates over the meaning of democracy, Americans in large numbers boldly associated the capacities for physical and political self-government. The fervency of patriotic food control helped fuel a quasi-religious asceticism that transcended the demands of the war itself, giving rise to an enduring brand of popular self-denial premised on physical and moral mastery of the self.

Few Americans would have conserved food without a strong positive motivation to do so. European hunger became a tool of mass mobilization on the U.S. home front, with food administrators claiming that Americans' food choices would decide the fates of Allied civilians and the course of the war itself. It was a good argument, and Americans voluntarily conserved food so that people elsewhere might eat with a level of commitment they would never equal again. For many Americans, daily food conservation was the most direct and meaningful way they experienced the war, and it inspired an elevated vision of America's place in the world. The focus on needy Europeans underlined American abundance and power, both widening Americans' consciousness of the world outside their borders and deepening their confidence in the role they might play in it. In part because of the resounding success of the World War I program, food aid would become a hallmark of U.S. foreign policy in the twentieth century, both as a demonstration of American abundance and as a powerful strategic tool.

The war also made basic nutrition literacy a distinguishing feature of American middle-class identity. A decade after the war, in the late 1920s, the leading home economist Christine Frederick looked back at the recent leaps in popular nutrition knowledge and gave the war much of the credit. Wartime nutrition education had pushed Americans' knowledge forward by ten or even twenty years, she estimated, noting that the wartime appeal to save butter and sugar "was the first time that many a housewife knew that there *were* distinctions between fats or sugars, or that eating a potato was not the same thing as eating a tomato." After the war, nutrition education had continued through public schools, newspapers, advertisements, and food exhibits, she noted, and it had become hard to find any women's magazine that did not carry "page after page of material and articles on foods." The average reader might still not understand just how vitamins worked, but she understood that her family needed them, and she went out of her way to buy foods like oranges, spinach, bran, and liver. Frederick knew that many of the war's lessons had been forgotten, and she smiled that a 1920s housewife was "no longer interested in making an eggless-butterless-cake," but she nevertheless saw the war's lasting mark in Americans' unusually high interest in and engagement with nutrition.[1]

Indeed, by the time Frederick wrote, scientific eating had moved from the domain of a few nutritionists and food faddists at the turn of the century to become an extraordinarily mainstream interest. By 1930, the doctor and syndicated columnist William Brady declared that the "dumbest layman is more or less hot and bothered about his diet nowadays."[2] Another journalist that same year pointed to the recent sevenfold increase in demand for lettuce as proof that Americans in large numbers had come to accept the importance of green vegetables.[3] Yet things were not quite so simple. American diets did change markedly during the first half of the century: between 1910 and 1950, Americans on average bought fewer grain products and more milk, fruits and vegetables, beans, nuts, and frozen fish and meat.[4] But there were many reasons for these changes. For one thing, it is likely that some of those purchases supplanted foods that Americans in earlier years had grown—or caught—themselves. For another, electric refrigeration became more common in homes, industry, and transportation starting in the 1910s, radically extending the distance perishable foods could travel and the time that could elapse before they perished.[5] New knowledge about nutrition might have spurred a 1920s housewife to buy lettuce, in other words, but in most places she only had the option of doing so in the first place because of changes in technology.[6] Meanwhile, the continuing growth of the canning industry further contributed to mounting meat, dairy, and produce consumption. These and other industrial and commercial changes, including rapidly industrializing agriculture and the growth of national grocery chains, gave Americans unprecedented access to a variety of foods year-round, while rising standards of living meant that people could afford to buy more of the foods on offer.[7]

Still, all the refrigerated lettuce and frozen spinach and canned green beans in the world would not have transformed eating habits on their own if Americans had not simultaneously embraced the idea that these foods were important and desirable. The cascade of nutrition education during World War I was a watershed moment that had long-range effects on American diets. It was during the war that nutrition truly became a *popular* science, one whose basic precepts a remarkable number of Americans applied to their daily lives.

Moreover, the World War I food aid program also lent nutrition a sense of *moral* urgency, and this proved to have equally long-lasting effects on American eating. Since the turn of the century, reformers of all stripes had been urging Americans to set aside taste and tradition when they stood in the way of eating according to more rational criteria. The wartime campaign to send American staples to Europe provided a megaphone for those arguments. Reformers believed, of course, that by showing the backwardness of pleasure they were opening the way for superior culinary rules based on science and reason. Yet reformers' own basic culture blindness hobbled rational food. Although science would play a major role in industrializing the American food supply in the century that followed, by the early twenty-first century "industrial food" had become shorthand for intensely flavored, fattening food with little nutritive value: seemingly the very opposite of Progressive ideals.[8]

Meanwhile, the American women whose labor underwrote World War I food aid drew support from the home economics movement, which was infusing cooking and housework with scientific legitimacy and social prestige. In large part because of home economics' expansive influence, white, middle-class women throughout the first decades of the twentieth century increasingly performed full-time housework in their own homes without the aid of servants. As molded by home economics, the modern housewife was a fundamentally limited role, one whose claims to professionalism and political relevance remained largely rhetorical. But at the time, that rhetoric was enormously important. It gave weight to the idea that women could be competent citizens and voters, and it placed broad new emphasis on voluntarism, which would characterize postwar cooperative activities. And the exaltation of cooking as scientific and prestigious helped make housewifery a fashionable choice for middle-class women for at least four decades after the war, while also contributing to the growing social acceptability of men's cooking throughout the century.[9]

As cooking got more scientific for whites in the early twentieth century, they went out of their way to emphasize that it had never been scientific for anyone else. Southern black cooking, in particular, came to symbolize African Americans' supposedly instinctive relationship with food at the same time it threw into relief whites' supposedly more detached and rational approach to diet. One of the most significant results of these racialized views of food was the rise of euthenics, a new discipline that united the concerns of eugenics with those of home economics by arguing that environmental factors—food preeminent among them—affected racial development. Diet's alleged influence on racial fitness heightened the urgency of the quest for rational food, as both black and white reformers sought to improve race by improving diet. Although the discipline of euthenics vanished from public consciousness soon after the war, its basic principles continued to affect American thinking about diet. In fact, euthenics' underlying premise, that dietary choices and other environmental factors profoundly affect mental and physical development, remained at the very center of mainstream understandings of health throughout the twentieth century and beyond, gaining new strength by the early twenty-first century through the emerging field of epigenetics.

Even as Progressive nutritionists searched for food's effects on race, modern nutrition science itself was slowly eroding old boundaries between foreign, national, and regional diets. World War I saw the height of efforts to Americanize immigrants by bringing their daily habits into line with American practices, including the supposedly time-honored tradition of eating plain, unmixed, lightly seasoned food. Despite such reform enthusiasm, however, in reality more and more Americans of all backgrounds were increasingly thinking of selected foreign and immigrant dishes— albeit watered-down versions of these dishes—as important parts of the American diet itself. Interest in self-consciously foreign foods expanded steadily in the century after Americanization's peak, helping to make the diversity of American diets one of their most singular characteristics and to make culinary cosmopolitanism an increasingly valuable form of cultural currency.

In fact, a new word—"foodie"—has emerged recently to describe modern culinary sophisticates, people who are eager to relish the many pleasures food has to offer and to deploy their knowledge about it and expand their skills in producing it. Just as sophisticated eating by the Progressive Era was no longer confined to four-star restaurants, self-described foodies today are anti-elitist in certain contexts, even aggressively so. They enthusiastically cross class and cultural borders in the name of eating well, praising the offerings of holes-in-the-wall or small farms, peasants' food production techniques, and the supposedly customary specialties to be found in small towns. There are real reasons to enjoy such food, of course, starting with taste. Moreover, in a food world dominated by industrial production, bypassing the tracks laid by Big Food and Big Ag can be an important way of preserving cultural diversity, reviving dying recipes or ingredients, minimizing an eater's toll on the environment, or supporting alternative food networks and businesses. Foodies sometimes fight for food justice, and the same people who care passionately about what they eat are at times the same people fighting against hunger, malnutrition, and unequal access to food resources.

But being a foodie hardly guarantees activist bona fides.[10] Just as middle-class Americans in the early twentieth century used nutrition knowledge as a badge of their own education, modernity, and privilege, the foodie movement serves social purposes, too—perhaps even primarily. Crossing both literal and figural boundaries in order to eat more deliciously advertises an eater's familiarity with a range of different foods and his or her boldness in seeking them out, just as it did for foreign and regional food enthusiasts in the Progressive Era. Today, as conspicuous consumption takes on ever more literal meaning, foodies' embrace of the far-flung and the low can actually elevate their social status. Self-proclaimed foodies find pleasure in foods from a conspicuously wide array of cultures and social levels. But their very willingness to eat widely—and their ability to discern which of the many foods at their disposal are the most pleasing and the most interesting—becomes a steep new boundary in its own right, effectively separating their own informed, appreciative, and wide-ranging food choices from the presumably nonspecial way that everyone else eats.[11] For instance, the subtitle of *Saveur*, a popular cooking magazine with highbrow pretensions, instructs readers to "Savor a World of Authentic Cuisine," a phrase that both celebrates diversity and implies access to a rarefied world of global encounter. It is telling that *Saveur* also bills itself as a travel magazine, because possessing the resources to sample "authentic" cuisines at their source, at least occasionally, is an important part of being a foodie. The foodie movement is founded upon attitudes that are direct descendents of ideas that first gained mass popularity in the Progressive Era, especially the belief that knowledge about food and cooking could denote education and social standing rather than their opposites, and the stance that true cosmopolitans are culinary adventurers rather than picky discriminators.

Yet of all the changes in American food culture forged in the era of the Great War, perhaps the most extreme and lasting is in Americans' attitudes toward their bodies. To a degree unprecedented in the whole of human history, large numbers of Americans in the Progressive Era began to consider fat to be both physically unattractive and morally repugnant. At the same time, of course, thinness became an aesthetic and moral ideal, a sign of inner strength and self-control, and the necessary precondition of beauty. Even as Americans in the century since the Progressive Era have grown bigger and heavier, the glorification of extreme thinness remains a form of both individual and collective homage to the moralization of self-control, one that each generation has replicated, with stunningly little variation, ever since.

Indeed, in recent decades the moralization of self-control around food has only intensified as it has become a pillar of arguments condemning obesity as a personal choice and a personal failure. Especially since the turn of the twenty-first century, the so-called obesity epidemic has become a source of both national anxiety and national fascination, with stories about Americans' growing weights appearing in national media outlets with remarkable regularity. There are some concrete reasons for the interest, not least of which is the perception that obesity and overweight contribute to declining national health and rising health care costs, seemingly matters of shared concern. But this alone hardly explains the fixation. Other factors also affect Americans' health and medical spending, from epidemic diseases to environmental toxins to climate change, but no other threat to public health can match obesity's hold on the public imagination.

Indeed, there is a special fervor reserved for obesity, with the non-obese typically leading the charge. If it is no longer socially possible to run headlines quite like the 1915 *Washington Post* article "Number of Fat Women Is Appalling!," it is acceptable to decry other people's fat in the name of their physical health, like the 2008 *Washington Post* feature, "How Obesity Harms a Child's Body."[12] Likewise, newspapers might no longer declare "Cannot Be Fat and Be Patriotic," as the *Boston Post* did in 1918, but concern about obesity's effects on national security have only sharpened since the U.S. surgeon general equated the dangers it posed with the threat from terrorism in 2006.[13] For people who are not obese themselves, deploring others' apparent vulnerability to the so-called epidemic draws attention to their own unique resistance. In fact, while environmental explanations for obesity seem superficially less vitriolic than condemning it as a personal failure, they are far from neutral. The geographer Julie Guthman points out that environmental explanations imply that "if junk food is everywhere and people are all naturally drawn to it, those who resist it must have heightened powers."[14] As a result, contemplating others' obesity can be both satisfying and socially rewarding for the non-obese; when succumbing to an "epidemic" becomes tantamount to succumbing to temptation, successfully avoiding obesity becomes a visible and ever more meaningful sign of self-control. In this context, indeed, self-control has become more of a moral virtue than ever, as obesity's ostensible threats legitimize its moral condemnation.[15]

In many ways, attitudes toward food that were forged in the Progressive Era have shaped Americans' understandings of their dietary choices and the food systems that support them ever since. The specific contexts have changed, but current debates over everything from industrial food, sustainability, and poverty to obesity and self-control have been animated by the same fundamental conviction, articulated with passionate certainty by Americans a century earlier, that food is a moral issue.

NOTES

INTRODUCTION

1. The chemist Wilbur Atwater was surprised when his own data demonstrated that poor people's food was sometimes more nutritious than what rich people ate. Levenstein, *Revolution at the Table*, 47.

2. Letter from Harvey Wiley, D.C., to Honorable Murray Hulbert, D.C., 22 June 1917, folder "1917," box 124, Harvey Wiley Papers, LOC.

3. For more on Progressivism, see Gilmore, *Who Were the Progressives?*; Rodgers, *Atlantic Crossings*; Gilmore, *Gender and Jim Crow*; Sanders, *Roots of Reform*; Crunden, *Ministers of Reform*; Stears, *Progressives, Pluralists*; Link, *Paradox of Southern Progressivism*; and Wiebe, *Search for Order*.

4. Robert Crunden likewise argues that Progressivism was more of a "climate" of thought than an organized social movement. Crunden, *Ministers of Reform*, ix.

5. Gabaccia, *We Are What We Eat*, 60.

6. Ray Wilbur, speech at Memorial Church, no location given, 4 April 1918, folder "Dr. Wilbur. Speeches. Articles. Statements. Notes. II-1918," box 2, series 5H, USFA Collection, Hoover Institution.

7. The word "overweight" was coined in 1899. *Oxford English Dictionary Online*, s.v. "overweight, adj."

8. Coveney argues that nutrition has always been imbued with moral judgments and advice, and it is precisely those elements that make nutrition "so compelling, so engaging, so judgemental, and so strangely popular" (*Food, Morals and Meaning*, viii).

9. Some of the boxes of general correspondence in the National Archives' Food Administration collection had not been re-catalogued since they were originally filed shortly after the end of World War I. In those boxes, the folders holding the letters were crumbling away to dust. When I could not read the name of a folder as a result, I have indicated "folder illegible" in the endnotes.

10. For materials in the Press Clipping section, the original archivist placed the clippings in folders labeled with the name of the newspaper from which they came, writing either "News" or "Edit" after each newspaper title to indicate whether the clipping came from the news or the editorial section of the paper. However, since many newspaper titles themselves end with the word "News," such as the *Birmingham News*, the resulting folder name in those cases contains the phrase "News News," as in the "Birmingham News News (AL)" folder. This is not a typo.

CHAPTER ONE

1. Ration card, n.d., folder "New York—Rationing," box 18, series 6H, USFA Collection, Hoover Institution.

2. USFA press release no. 619, 29 January 1918, folder "New York—Rationing," box 18, series 6H, States Division, USFA Collection, Hoover Institution.

3. Ibid.

4. "N.O. Women Pledge Food Rationing: Here's Hoover Limit for Each Weekly," 31 January 1918, folder "New Orleans Item News (LA)," box 556, RG 4, NARA.

5. "Wealthy Women to Go on War Diet," 10 February 1918, folder "Baltimore News News (MD)," box 556, RG 4, NARA.

6. "Women Ask for Rationing Plan," 6 April 1918, folder "Altoona Tribune News (PA)," box 568, RG 4, NARA.

7. "United States Food Administration, 'Chronological Sketch with Directory of Members, May 1917–June 1919,'" March 1920, New York, folder 40, box 17, NYSCHER;

"Organizer's Manual," National Family Pledge Card Campaign, For Guidance of State, County, City, Town and Township Chairmen, October 21–28, 1917, USFA Conservation Division, folder "Home Card Campaign, Aug–Nov 1917," box 3, series 5H, USFA Collection, Hoover Institution.

8. Bonzon and Davis, "Feeding the Cities," 310. Germans suffered as a result of the Allied blockade, with government rations often hovering around 1,400 calories a day, though a thriving black market supplemented this paltry amount. Offer, *First World War*, 29–30.

9. Offer, *First World War*, 66.

10. Hoover, *American Epic*. Remaining in London when the Great War broke out in the summer of 1914, Hoover had immediately started working to repatriate Americans stranded in Europe. Within a few weeks, the U.S. ambassador to Britain, Walter Hines Page, asked Hoover if he would also undertake the task of organizing relief to civilians in areas of Belgium and northeastern France occupied by Germans troops. Brand Whitlock, "How American Relief First Came to Starving Belgium," *Washington Post*, 21 June 1918, SM5, PQHN. For more on the Commission for Relief in Belgium, see Nash, *Life of Herbert Hoover: The Humanitarian*.

11. Because of the occupation, French wheat and oat production fell by more than a third and sugar beet production plunged by almost 70 percent. Bonzon and Davis, "Feeding the Cities," 310; "Acreage of Important Crops in France for 1913, 1916, 1917," bulletin no. 58, 23 July 1917, Food Administration Statistical Department Information Service, folder "FA I-A/Statistical Department Information Service, Bulletins #1–400, 1917 Incomplete," box 3, USFA Collection, Hoover Library; Offer, *First World War*, 62–63. Although contemporary reports of German atrocities were sometimes overstated or invented for Allied propaganda, the German occupation of Belgium was one of brutality and "routine terror," as Larry Zuckerman puts it. Zuckerman argues that the occupation of Belgium was "a forerunner of Nazi Europe." Zuckerman, *Rape of Belgium*, 1–2. See also Vernon Kellogg, "The Authentic Story of Belgian Relief: Americans to the Rescue," June 1917, *World's Work*, folder "June 1917, The Authentic Story of Belgian Relief," box 12, USFA Collection, Hoover Library.

12. The commission bought its own foodstuffs and imported them on a fleet of cargo ships that sailed under a special commission flag. It operated railway cars, factories, mills, and warehouses, and every month volunteers distributed 220 million pounds of bread, 20 million pounds of bacon, and tons of beans, sugar, powdered milk, and other commodities and canned goods. Local committees stored food in warehouses and distributed it according to ration tickets, which civilians either bought or received for free, if they were deemed to be destitute. "America's Obligations in Belgian Relief–Address before the Chamber of Commerce in the State of New York," 1 February 1917, 5–8, bound folder "Addresses, Letters, Magazine Articles, Press Statements, Etc. Inclusive Dates: February 1, 1917–April 6, 1918," box 93, vol. I, part 1, Hoover Collection, Hoover Institution. Commission volunteers could only deliver foodstuffs up to the border of Belgium or occupied France, where distribution was taken over by Belgian and French organizations. "Belgian Relief Commission Food and Clothing Program Announced for Coming Year," Official Statement of the United States Food Administration, no. 5, 1 October 1918, Washington, D.C., folder "FA I-A/Official Statements #1–18, 1918–1919," box

2, USFA Collection, Hoover Library. Soup was the ideal vehicle for absorbing the motley and unpredictable food donations, and soup kitchens staffed by local women were the most common method for distributing food on the ground. Hoover, *American Epic*, 28.

13. Vernon Kellogg, "Herbert Hoover, as Individual and Type," *Atlantic*, March 1918, folder "Writings about Hoover," box 219, Hoover Collection, Hoover Institution.

14. Of the 50,000 volunteers working with the commission by then, the majority were local French and Belgians, but the most prominent leaders were Americans. "The Man Who Fed Belgium," 17 July 1917, folder "Pomona Bulletin Edit (CA)," box 530, RG 4, NARA; "Mr. Hoover in Retrospect," clipping from the *Evening Post*, New York, 23 October 1918, folder "Tom Ellis, Congressional and Legislative Resume," box 39, series 12H, USFA Collection, Hoover Institution.

15. Pasta made an acceptable bread substitute because it was usually made with durum wheat, which was considered inappropriate for bread making.

16. At the end of the nineteenth century, new gold discoveries had dispelled nineteenth-century fears of deflation and sparked, instead, rampant inflation. See Jacobs, *Pocketbook Politics*; Macleod, "Food Prices"; and Rauchway, "High Cost of Living."

17. Jacobs, *Pocketbook Politics*, 15.

18. Macleod, "Food Prices," 375; Levenstein, *Revolution at the Table*, 109–10.

19. Jacobs, *Pocketbook Politics*, 53–55; Levenstein, *Revolution at the Table*, 109–10; Frank, "Housewives," 257.

20. Margueritte Wilkinson, "The Food Riots," May 1917, reprinted in Van Wienen, "Poetics of the Frugal Housewife," 64.

21. Spelling original. Address from Sallie Bardette, Prudence, W.V., to "The President or Congressman or Senitors," 25 July 1917, folder illegible, box 288, RG 4, NARA.

22. Mullendore, *History of the United States Food Administration*, 53–54.

23. "Autocracy in Democracy," 10 August 1917, folder "San Diego Union Edit (CA)," box 531, RG 4, NARA.

24. Lever Act, no. 41, 65th Congress, H.R. 4961, folder "FA I-A—Press Clippings, 1917–1918," box 2, USFA Collection, Hoover Library.

25. Letter from Mr. C. Williams, Rusk County, Tex., to USFA, September 1917, folder "Propaganda, German," box 159, USFA Collection, Hoover Institution.

26. Pledge card campaign canvassers reported encountering such fears of government food confiscation from Arkansas, Connecticut, Delaware, Georgia, Kansas, Kentucky, Illinois, Indiana, Iowa, Maine, Michigan, Minnesota, Mississippi, New Hampshire, New Jersey, New York, North Carolina, Ohio, Pennsylvania, South Dakota, Tennessee, Texas, Virginia, West Virginia, and Wisconsin. Home Conservation Division, Correspondence and Data, RG 4, NARA; May Ayres Burgess and Florence Ball, "How the People of the Country Criticize the Policies of the Food Administration," memorandum to Dr. Wilbur, 14 September 1917, folder "How the People of the Country Criticize the Policies of the Food Administration," box 3, series 5H, USFA Collection, Hoover Institution; USFA Intensive Food Campaign, transcript of meeting, 12 September 1917, folder "Home Card Campaign, Aug–Nov 1917," box 3, series 5H, USFA Collection, Hoover Institution.

27. Letter from Miss Amelia Worthington, Birmingham, Ala., to USFA, 17 September 1917, folder "Propaganda, German," box 159, USFA Collection, Hoover Institution.

28. The act already made it illegal to import distilled spirits into the United States. Lever Act, no. 41, 65th Congress, H.R. 4961, folder "FA I-A—Press Clippings, 1917–1918," box 2, USFA Collection, Hoover Library.

29. See Hall, "Wilson and the Food Crisis."

30. Lever Act, no. 41, 65th Congress, H.R. 4961, folder "FA I-A—Press Clippings, 1917–1918," box 2, USFA Collection, Hoover Library. Conversion into contemporary money is based on the commodity price index figures in McCusker, *How Much Is That in Real Money?*, 57.

31. The Lever Act guaranteed the price of wheat for the next eighteen months, or until May 1919, an attempt to boost production by assuring a profit for farmers for every grain of wheat they could grow. The price was originally set at $2.00 a bushel, later raised to $2.20 for the 1918 crop. If imported wheat was selling at cheaper prices than U.S. wheat, the Lever Act allowed for tariffs to equalize the prices. Lever Act, no. 41, 65th Congress, H.R. 4961, folder "FA I-A—Press Clippings, 1917–1918," box 2, USFA Collection, Hoover Library. Legislators prioritized wheat production in large part because western Europeans got more than half their calories in the form of wheat. Dickson, *Food Front in World War I*.

32. Mullendore, *History of the United States Food Administration*, 61–62.

33. As soon as he signed the Lever Bill into law on August 10, 1917, President Wilson created the Food Administration by executive order, effectively transferring the full powers granted him by the act to Hoover as chief food administrator.

34. These "normal" prices were based on wholesale prices plus what administrators deemed acceptable profit margins. Jacobs, *Pocketbook Politics*, 61.

35. While individual food conservation remained voluntary, the compliance of businesses and restaurants was not, with those that violated the Lever Act subject to fines of up to $5,000. Especially early in the war, punishments tended to be relatively minor; one of the most common was to force a restaurant or store that had violated food regulations to "advertise its disgrace" by putting up signs to that effect in its windows. Sometimes restaurant owners or merchants who had hoarded or profiteered were forced to close for a few days or to give "donations," usually between $10 and $100, to war charities. But both food regulations and the punishments for violating them got stricter as the war progressed. In October 1918, the Food Administration released a strict new list of foods that could not be served in restaurants on certain days, and the increasingly stringent regulations excited little public protest, which commentators attributed largely to Hoover's popularity. See "Sugar Questions," USFA bulletin, August 1918, folder "Publications," box 5, series 5H, USFA Collection, Hoover Institution; "A Badge of Shame," excerpt from *New York Tribune*, 30 July 1918, folder "New York—Enforcement," box 16, series 6H, States Division, Hoover Institution; "Penalties Imposed by the Food Administration in Texas for the Month of November," *Texas Federal Food Administration Bulletin* 1, no. 7, December 1918, folder "Texas," box 30, Hoover Institution; "Michigan Federal Food Bulletin," no number, n.d., folder "Michigan," box 14, series 6H, Hoover Institution; and "Restaurants to Close Next Tuesday: Violators of Meatless Day Rule Punished by Food Administration," typed document, 21 March 1918, folder "New York—Enforcement," box 16, series 6H, States Division, Hoover Institution. The first criminal prosecution for hoarding did not take place until September 1918,

when two German American café owners who had been hoarding sugar were fined the maximum $5,000. Letter from USFA to all Federal Food Administrators, 27 September 1918, folder "Regulations," box 74, series 43H, Hoover Institution. More often by the fall of 1918, if farmers refused to sell their wheat, the food administration seized their crops. For example, when two German American brothers in New Mexico refused to sell wheat at the legally established price, the Food Administration seized all their stores of wheat. "Ways in Which Women Can Help Win," Agricultural Speaker Service bulletin no. 11, 8 April 1918, folder "FA-II/Agricultural Speaker Service Bulletins #1–26. Information for Speakers," box 7, USFA Collection, Hoover Library; "Mr. Hoover in Retrospect," *Evening Post*, New York, 23 October 1918, folder "Tom Ellis, Congressional and Legislative Resume," box 39, series 12H, USFA Collection, Hoover Institution.

36. Woodrow Wilson, speech, 19 May 1917, excerpted in "United States Food Administration, 'Chronological Sketch with Directory of Members, May 1917–June 1919,'" March 1920, New York, folder 40, box 17, NYSCHER.

37. Koistinen, *Mobilizing for Modern War*, 255–56.

38. The Food Administration received hundreds of admiring letters addressing Hoover by these titles. Home Conservation Division, General Correspondence, USFA Collection, RG 4, NARA. Even articles with seemingly sarcastic titles like "Hail, Hoover, Dictator," were wholly praising and enthusiastic. "Hail, Hoover, Dictator," 16 August 1917, folder "West Palm Beach Post Edit (FL)," box 533, RG 4, NARA.

39. Consumption levels either decreased absolutely or decreased in relationship to population. The discipline of statistics was central to this food conservation enterprise. It was only in the 1910s that statisticians were able to determine with any level of accuracy food consumption in the United States. Previously, scientists could hazard "only the roughest guesses as to the total domestic consumption of all but a few items," specifically the wheat and sugar crops, whose levels government officials had tracked for several decades. During the war, food administrators regularly received what Raymond Pearl, the chief U.S. government statistician, called "the naive and simple question" of how much of which foods Americans ate each year. Before 1920, statisticians had few accurate answers to give. Pearl, *Nation's Food*, 243–44, 209.

40. Ibid., 243–44.

41. These export figures are compared to those of the immediate prewar years. "Annual Report of The United States Food Administration for the year 1918," folder "FA I-A/Annual Report, 1918; Report to Feb. 1918; Food Program for 1919," box 1, USFA Collection, Hoover Library; Jacobs, *Pocketbook Politics*, 54; Koistinen, *Mobilizing for Modern War*, 262–67; Frank, "Housewives," 257.

42. USFA Home Card, folder 56, box 17, NYSCHER; Hoover, introduction to Mullendore, *History of the United States Food Administration*, 12.

43. Administrators donated the fines to the Red Cross. "Organize State Food Police," 20 September 1918, folder "Philadelphia Bulletin News (PA)," box 568, RG 4, NARA. All forty-eight states, as well as Alaska, Hawaii, Puerto Rico, and the greater metropolitan areas of Washington, D.C., New York, Philadelphia, and St. Louis, had a federally appointed state food administrator.

44. May Stranathan, "Scale-Carrying Bread Sleuth Creates Panic in Restaurants," 9 February 1918, folder "Pittsburg Dispatch News (PA)," box 569, RG 4, NARA.

45. "Every Loyal Lady in Lorain a Police-Woman," 28 January 1918, folder "Lorain News Edit (OH)," box 567, RG 4, NARA.

46. Helen Dare, "Don't Be a Kicker—Be Your Own Policeman!," 21 October 1918, no. 424, folder "Press Releases, States Section, Educational Division #400–470," box 10, USFA Collection, Hoover Library. They should also learn to be their "own drillmaster." "Master or Slave," 15 March 1918, folder "Santa Ana Register News (CA)," box 551, RG 4, NARA.

47. Ray Wilbur, typed text of article for *Ladies' Home Journal*, untitled, 4(?) June 1917, folder "Dr. Wilbur. Speeches. Articles. Statements. Notes. I-1917," box 2, series 5H, USFA Collection, Hoover Institution.

48. Governor [Thomas] Bickett, "Saturnalia of Extravagance," 2 November 1917, folder "Raleigh State Journal Edit (NC)," box 544, RG 4, NARA; "Dr. Wiley Predicts German Race of Weaklings While Americans Become Strong," n.d., folder "Washington Herald News No. 2 (DC)," box 552, RG 4, NARA; "Wheat Saving Program for the Household," USFA brochure, Washington, D.C., April 1918, folder 50, box 17, NYSCHER.

49. Helen Belknap, "A New Adventure—Helping a World Cause by Thrift," The War Time Pastor in Town and Country, bulletin no. 3, The Presbyterian Board of Home Missions, New York City, folder illegible, box 288, RG 4, NARA.

50. Untitled blurb, 1 March 1918, folder "Tulsa World News (OK)," box 570, RG 4, NARA; H. E. Barnard, "War Restoring Kitchen to Its Pioneer Place as Center of Home," 16 January [?] 1918, folder "Chagrin Express News (OH)," box 566, RG 4, NARA; "B'klyn Women to Incorporate Frugality Ass'n," 21 June 1917, folder "Brooklyn Daily Times (NY)," box 288, RG 4, NARA; "Vice of Overfeeding," 14 July 1917, folder "Salt Lake City Herald Edit (UT)," box 548, RG 4, NARA.

51. "Curtailing of Waste," 4 June 1917, folder "Long Beach Press Edit (CA)," box 530, RG 4, NARA; "Wheat-Mixing and Food Conservation," 1 February 1918, folder "Medina Gazette Edit (OH)," box 567, RG 4, NARA.

52. Untitled blurb, 17 October 1917, folder "Medford Sun Edit (OR)," box 546, RG 4, NARA.

53. Bennett, *World's Food*, 242–43.

54. Cullather, "Foreign Policy of the Calorie," par. 4.

55. "How We Americans Eat," 4 February 1918, folder "Montgomery Advertiser Edit (AL)," box 549, RG 4, NARA; "National Food Chief Coming to Columbus," [?] October 1918, folder "Columbus Citizen News (OH)," box 567, RG 4, NARA.

56. "Candy," 1 September 1918, folder "Erie Dispatch Edit (PA)," box 568, RG 4, NARA.

57. "Miss Blow's Letters to a Mother," *American Kitchen Magazine* 14, no. 4 (1901): 224; Cocroft, *Self-Sufficiency*, 61.

58. Ray Wilbur, "The Sugar Ration," n.d., folder "Dr. Wilbur. Speeches. Articles. Statements. Notes. I-1917," box 2, series 5H, USFA Collection, Hoover Institution; Hoover, "The World's Food Shortage—Address Delivered at the Smithsonian Institution, Washington, D.C. (U.S. Food Administration. Bull. 7)," bound folder "Addresses, Letters, Magazine Articles, Press Statements, Etc. Inclusive Dates: February 1, 1917–April 6, 1918," box 93, Hoover Collection, Hoover Institution.

59. W. W. Stanley, untitled piece in the *Christian Sun*, 20 June 1917, folder "Elon College, Christian Sun Edit (NC)," box 544, RG 4, NARA; photograph of Home Economics Exhibit by Fort Worth, Texas, W.C.T.U., *Union Signal*, 24 May 1917, 1.

60. Letter from USFA to Greenhut Co., N.Y., 22 November 1917, folder "USFA papers concerning letter G," box 118, USFA Collection, Hoover Institution.

61. John Nicholls, "Life-Sustaining Food vs. Life-Destroying Drink," *Union Signal*, 17 May 1917, 5; cover, *Union Signal*, 31 May 1917.

62. "Conservation of Grain the Crying Need of the Hour," *Union Signal*, 7 June 1917, 5.

63. Edwin Ellis, "American-German and Pro-German Traitors," handwritten essay, May 1918, folder "Prohibition Letters," box 405, RG 4, NARA.

64. Letter from C. J. Boppell, St. Maries, Idaho, to Hoover, 30 June 1917, folder illegible, box 288, RG 4, NARA.

65. Emphasis original. Abstract of letter from Mrs. Charles William Towne, Waukon, Iowa, to USFA, 22 July 1917, folder "How the People of the Country Criticize the Policies of the Food Administration," box 3, series 5H, USFA Collection, Hoover Institution.

66. "Answers to Questions," n.d., folder 9, box 1, series 5H, USFA Collection, Hoover Institution.

67. "Output of Brewers in 1917," USFA Statistical Bulletin no. 1341, 27 July 1918, folder "FA I-A/Statistical Department Information Service, Bulletins #1335–1419, 1918 Incomplete," box 5, USFA Collection, Hoover Library.

68. For more on the temperance movement, see Tyrrell, *Woman's World*; Bordin, *Woman and Temperance*; and Szymanski, *Pathways to Prohibition*.

69. Hoover was embarrassed when the press discovered his house-building plans, and he ended up delaying construction until just after the war. Allen, *Independent Woman*, 72–73, 80; Hoover, quoted in originally anonymous interview in Irwin, "First Aid to America: How Civilians Must Get Together and Get Behind Strong Leaders," *Saturday Evening Post*, 24 March 1917, 18–19, bound folder "Addresses, Letters, Magazine Articles, Press Statements, Etc. Inclusive Dates: February 1, 1917–April 6, 1918," vol. I, part 1, box 93, Hoover Collection, Hoover Institution. Irwin later wrote, "In the SATURDAY EVENING POST of March twenty-fourth I published an interview with an eminent American, under the title First Aid to America. The victim was Hoover" (Irwin, "The Autocrat of the Dinner Table," *Saturday Evening Post*, 23 June 1917, folder "Writings about Hoover," box 219, Hoover Collection, Hoover Institution).

70. Quote from Hoover, "The European Food Position, draft of speech," 10 May 1917, folder "Speeches and Writings," box 149, Hoover Collection, Hoover Institution.

71. Alma Whitaker, "Sumptuous Waste," 15 March 1918, folder "Los Angeles Times News (CA)," box 551, RG 4, NARA; Vernon Kellogg, "Patriotism and Sacrifice," USFA bulletin, (Washington, D.C.: GPO, June 1918), folder "Dr. Vernon Kellogg 4 (1)," box 58, series 27H, USFA Collection, Hoover Institution.

72. Typed transcript of meeting, n.d., folder "New York," box 15, series 6H, States Division, USFA Collection, Hoover Institution.

73. Atwater, "Guide to the Nation's Dietary Needs." Helen Atwater was the daughter of Wilbur Atwater, who first used calories to measure food energy.

74. Bollet, *Plagues and Poxes*, 153–72.

75. Clipping from unnamed paper, 14[?] December 1917, folder "J-K 356 Oct. 1," box 321, RG 4, NARA.

76. Mabel Kittridge, "The Way Some East Side Women Are Managing Their Budgets," n.d., typed document, folder "New York," box 15, series 6H, USFA Collection, Hoover Institution.

77. "Address by Alonzo Taylor," USFA, 20 May 1918, folder "Address. Taylor, Dr.," box 22, USFA Collection, Hoover Institution.

78. Spelling original. Letter from Gust Stohlberg, Grand Rapids, Mich., to Hoover, folder "F-G 354 Feb. 1," box 321, RG 4, NARA.

79. Abstract of letter from Mrs. Fannie T. Farris, Medon, Tenn., to USFA, 12 July 1917, folder illegible, box 296, RG 4, NARA.

80. Typed transcript of meeting, folder "New York," box 15, series 6H, States Division, USFA Collection, Hoover Institution.

81. "Where the Food Campaign Fails to Get Across," 28 January 1918, folder "Where the Food Campaign Fails to Get Across," box 3, series 5H, USFA Collection, Hoover Institution.

82. "To Workers," USFA Campaign, no. 4, October 1917, no folder, box 15, series 6H, USFA Collection, Hoover Institution; abstract of anonymous letter from Boston to USFA, 6 July 1917, folder "How the People of the Country Criticize the Policies of the Food Administration," box 3, series 5H, USFA Collection, Hoover Institution.

83. Typed abstract of letter written from "Farmer's Daughter," no location given, to Hoover, 27 September 1917, box 328, RG 4, NARA.

84. "Short Rations!," 1 February 1918, folder "Savannah News Edit (GA)," box 553, RG 4, NARA.

85. Abstract of letter from John Donahue, Pittsburgh, to USFA, 11 July 1917, folder "How the People of the Country Criticize the Policies of the Food Administration," box 3, series 5H, USFA Collection, Hoover Institution.

86. Hoover, "Food and the War," *The Day's Food in War and Peace*, 11, bound folder "Addresses, Letters, Magazine Articles, Press Statements, Etc. Inclusive Dates: February 1, 1917–April 6, 1918," vol. 1, part 1, box 93, Hoover Collection, Hoover Institution.

87. "Civil War Food Shortage," 2 February 1918, folder "Mansfield News News (OH)," box 567, RG 4, NARA.

88. Spelling, grammar, and emphasis original. Letter from Miss Ida P. Beale, Cherrydale, Va., to Hoover, 1 June 1917, folder illegible, box 288, RG 4, NARA; "Sacrifices Today and in the '60s," 26 October 1917, folder "Columbia State News (SC)," box 547, RG 4, NARA.

89. Letter from Ernest G. Baldwin, Memphis, Tenn., to Hoover, 21 June 1917, folder illegible, box 288, RG 4, NARA; letter from J. W. Bachman, Chattanooga, Tenn., to Hoover, 22 June 1917, folder illegible, box 288, RG 4, NARA; "To My Comrades Everywhere/Whether They Wore the Blue or the Gray," farm recruitment poster, Phoebus, Va., folder illegible, box 288, RG 4, NARA; letter from Annie Booth McKinney, Knoxville, Tenn., to Hoover, 24 June 1917, folder "NS 238," box 293, RG 4, NARA.

90. David Blight argues that in the fifty years after the Civil War, desires for sectional reunion evaded and repressed descriptions of the war as a fight spurred and sustained by divisions over slavery. By the 1910s, what Blight calls reconciliationist visions,

grounded in white supremacy, had soundly triumphed over emancipationist visions in popular American memories of the war. Blight, *Race and Reunion*.

91. For more on antimodernism as a rebellion against—and a way of coping with—industrial capitalism at the turn of the century, see Lears, *No Place of Grace*.

92. Richards and Norton, *Cost of Food*, 8.

93. Dickson, *Food Front in World War I*, 24.

94. Such suggestions were part of a larger interest in the revival of colonial food, which started in the nineteenth century. Carroll, "Forefathers' Day Dinners"; "Simple Life Desirable," 21 September 1917, folder "Manhattan Mercury Edit (KS)," box 535, RG 4, NARA; letter from Margaret H. J. Lampe, Bloomington, Ill., to Hoover, 6 August 1917, folder "LM—217," box 292, RG 4, NARA.

95. "The Simple Life for 1918," 2 January 1918, folder "Philadelphia Inquirer Edit (PA)," box 568, RG 4, NARA; "Corn," USFA leaflet, December 1917, folder "FA-II/Home Cards," box 8, USFA Collection, Hoover Library; "Did Lincoln Hooverize? Read His Menu from 1818," 28 December 1917, folder "Cleveland Press News (OH)," box 567, RG 4, NARA; "Benjamin Franklin Knew Value of Food Saving," 23 February 1917, folder "Chambersburg Opinion News (PA)," box 568, RG 4, NARA.

96. "United States Food Administration, 'Chronological Sketch with Directory of Members, May 1917–June 1919,'" March 1920, New York, folder 40, box 17, NYSCHER.

97. Bradley, *Cook Book*, 51; Edith Gooding, "Hooveritis," reprinted from B.R.P Railway Employes' [*sic*] Magazine, *Food and the War: Federal Food Administration for South Dakota* 1, no. 3, 15 February 1918, folder "South Dakota," box 30, USFA Collection, Hoover Institution.

98. Offer, *First World War*, 67.

99. Ray Wilbur, typed text of article for *Ladies' Home Journal*, untitled, 4[?] June 1917, folder "Dr. Wilbur. Speeches. Articles. Statements. Notes. I-1917," box 2, series 5H, USFA Collection, Hoover Institution.

100. Hoover, "Food Conservation and the War," *American Journal of Public Health*, November 1917, bound folder "Addresses, Letters, Magazine Articles, Press Statements, Etc. Inclusive Dates: February 1, 1917–April 6, 1918," vol. I, part 1, box 93, Hoover Collection, Hoover Institution.

101. *Oxford English Dictionary Online*, s.vv. "undernourished, adj.," "malnourished, adj.,".

102. Griffith, *Born Again Bodies*.

103. Letter from Horace Fletcher, Copenhagen, to Vernon Kellogg, 11 June 1918, folder "Fletcher, Horace," box 127, USFA Collection, Hoover Institution.

104. Stearns, *Fat History*, 42.

105. Ray Wilbur, notes on his speech at unnamed conference, 17 August 1918, folder "Dr. Wilbur. Speeches. Articles. Statements. Notes. II-1918," box 2, series 5H, USFA Collection, Hoover Institution.

106. Interoffice memo from Vernon Kellogg to W. A. Dupee, 28 June 1918, folder "W. A. Dupee," box 11, series 6H, USFA Collection, Hoover Institution.

107. Untitled blurb, 1 March 1918, folder "Tulsa World News (OK)," box 570, RG 4, NARA. As one home economist wrote in 1914, "Modern science has disproved the ancient maxim that whatever pleases the palate nourishes" (Austin, *Domestic Science*, 69).

See also Goudiss and Goudiss, *Foods That Will Win the War*, 83. Distrust of taste had a long history. Fifty years earlier, for instance, two cookbook authors wrote that "it by no means follows that food which gives the greatest delight in the mouth, will be equally agreeable when swallowed" (Lyman and Lyman, *Philosophy of House-Keeping*, 24).

108. Reformers had long preached the importance of teaching children "the subjugation of appetite," but if subjugation could be learned, that meant adults could learn it, too. Snyder, *Practical Hygienic Preparation of Foods*, 14; letter from Mrs. B. C. Anthony, El Paso, Tex., to Hoover, 22 June 1917, folder 11, box 288, RG 4, NARA.

109. Emphasis original. Rose, *Everyday Foods in War Time*, 49.

110. Letter from Marie Broomfield, Providence, R.I., to USFA, folder "C 52 Nov. 1," box 299, RG 4, NARA.

111. "Satisfying Hoover," 25 May 1918, folder "Salem Herald Edit (OH)," box 567, RG 4, NARA.

112. Spelling original. Edward Arps, "Conservation of Food: What It Means and What It Will Unfold," typed circular, folder illegible, box 288, RG 4, NARA.

113. *Bulletin for the Clergy* 1, no. 1 (November 1917), folder "Cooperating Organizations. Religious, Fraternal, Patriotic, Labor, Agricultural, Commercial, etc.," box 3, series 5H, USFA Collection, Hoover Institution.

114. Crunden, *Ministers of Reform*. Griffith also examines the Protestant fervor that ran through questions of physical self-control around the turn of the twentieth century, particularly for men. Griffith, *Born Again Bodies*.

115. "Billy Sunday's Sermon Yesterday: 'Present Your Bodies,'" 28 March 1918, folder, "Chicago Herald News," box 554, RG 4, NARA.

116. "Food Administration Invites Every Woman to Register and Sign Pledge," June 1917, folder 9, box 1, series 5H, USFA Collection, Hoover Institution; "Resume of Letters Sent to All Federal Food Administrators, August 10, 1917 to February 1, 1918," folder "FA I-A/Annual Report, 1918; Report to Feb. 1918; Food Program for 1919," box 1, USFA Collection, Hoover Library.

117. "Lenten Fasts to Aid Nation in Saving Food," February 1918, folder "Cleveland Plaindealer News (OH)," box 567, RG 4, NARA; "Wasting Fats," 21 November 1918, folder "Cleveland Plaindealer News (OH)," box 567, RG 4, NARA.

118. Hoover, quoted in "Report of the Library and Exhibits Section of the Educational Division," September 1918, folder "Library and Exhibits Section. Edith Guerrier," box 42, series 12H, USFA Collection, Hoover Institution.

119. "It Does Us Good," 31 October 1917, folder "Wichita Eagle Edit (KS)," box 535, RG 4, NARA.

120. Letter from H. L. Bailey, Piqua, Ohio, to Hoover, 21 June 1917, folder illegible, box 288, RG 4, NARA; "Conserve Food to Save Yourselves," 27 May 1918, folder "Salem News News (OH)," box 567, RG 4, NARA. Despite general enthusiasm, some religious figures refused to cooperate, usually citing either reluctance to ask their congregations to go without wheat while beer production continued, or simply refusing to "prostitute the pulpit" for secular concerns (letter from D. S. Pickett, Vera, Okla., to Hoover, 25 June 1917, folder illegible, box 294, RG 4, NARA).

121. "Resolutions adopted at a conference of bishops, secretaries and editors of the Methodist Episcopal Church," 1 August 1917, folder "Methodist Episcopal," box 401,

RG 4, NARA; "Science Church Takes Hoover Food Pledge," 22 October 1917, folder "Christian Science Church," box 401, RG 4, NARA; William Chambers Covert, Letter to Pastors and Committees, in Bulletin for the National Service Commission of the Presbyterian Church in the U.S.A., 10 August 1917, folder "Cooperating Organizations. Religious, Fraternal, Patriotic, Labor, Agricultural, Commercial, etc.," box 3, series 5H, USFA Collection, Hoover Institution.

122. Dr. G. H. Herald and L. A. Hansen, "S.D. Adventists and the Food Administration," 14 September 1917, folder "Adventist Church," box 401, RG 4, NARA.

123. Joseph Krauskopf and Sidney Goldstein, "Open Letter to the Jewish Summer Hotels and Boarding Houses," n.d., folder "Methodist Church (North) [sic]," box 401, RG 4, NARA.

124. Reverend Dr. Joseph Krauskopf was in charge of food conservation propaganda aimed at Jewish people. Subcommittees were sometimes formed to carry out food conservation propaganda within individual religious organizations. Letter from Hoover to M. Angelo Elias, 9 August 1917, folder illegible, box 290, RG 4, NARA; Augustin M'Nally, "The Conversion of the Rosenblooms," *Keep Old Glory Waving*, no. 6, n.d., folder "New York," box 15, series 6H, USFA Collection, Hoover Institution; Joseph Krauskopf and Sidney Goldstein, "Open Letter to the Jewish Summer Hotels and Boarding Houses," n.d., folder "Methodist Church (North) [sic]," box 401, RG 4, NARA.

125. Letter from William Anthony Aery, Hampton Institute, Hampton, Va., to Hoover, 7 July 1917, folder illegible, box 291, RG 4, NARA; letter from Bertha Harris Arnold, Takoma Park, Md., to Lou Henry Hoover, 17 November 1917, box 298, RG 4, NARA.

126. A. U. Craig, "List of Colored Men to Aid the Food Campaign," 30 June 1917, folder illegible, box 289, RG 4, NARA.

127. Letter from A. U. Craig, D.C., to W. A. McKenzie, D.C.(?), 11 September 1917, folder "Colored Organizations," box 401, RG 4, NARA.

128. "How the Negro Can Help Make Food Win the War," USFA bulletin, April 1918, 6–7, folder "FA-II/Food Conservation, General," box 8, USFA Collection, Hoover Library.

129. For example, letter from W. H. Mixon, Birmingham, Ala., to Hoover, 2 August 1917, folder "TZ-249," box 293, RG 4, NARA; letter from Reverend C. H. Groover, Blitchton, Ga., to Hoover, 17 June 918, folder "D," box 405, RG 4, NARA.

130. Spelling original. Conservation Campaign, USFA Memorandum on Publicity Agencies Available to Assist Home Card Distribution, October 1918, folder "FA-II/Food Conservation, General," box 8, USFA Collection, Hoover Library.

131. Some of the many proposals for fasting were "National Fast Day Proposed," 13 February 1918, folder "Mansfield Shield News (OH)," box 567, RG 4, NARA; letter from Rev. Richard C. Jones, Cambridge City, Ind., to Hoover, 23 June 1917, folder "NS—198," box 292, RG 4, NARA; and letter from Milton M. Bales, Dade City, Fla., to Hoover, 25 June 1917, folder illegible, box 288, RG 4, NARA.

132. See Flake, *Politics of American Religious Identity*.

133. Kirby, "Sermons before the Commons," 528–48. Fasting had also been an American commemorative device at various points in the eighteenth and nineteenth centuries. During the Civil War, Abraham Lincoln set aside a national fast day after a series

of Union defeats in April 1863. Jefferson Davis, president of the Confederacy, called on southerners to fast on at least four different days during the war. Earlier, President John Adams had appointed a day of national fasting in 1798 because of the troubles brewing with France. "As to a National Fast Day," 4 March 1918, folder "Providence Journal News (RI)," box 570, RG 4, NARA; "A Chance for Mr. Hoover," 23 January 1918, folder "Beaver Springs Weekly Herald News (PA)," box 568, RG 4, NARA.

134. "Here's a Thought for Days of Lent," 13 February 1918, folder "Columbus State Journal News (OH)," box 567, RG 4, NARA; "Lenten Fasts to Aid Nation in Saving Food," February 1918, folder "Cleveland Plaindealer News (OH)," box 567, RG 4, NARA.

135. Letter from USFA to Mr. Ira J. Anderson, Sapulpa, Okla., 6 February 1918, folder "H-I 25 Nov. 1," box 298, RG 4, NARA; letter from Cyrus V. Berger, N.Y.C., to Hoover, 29 January 1918, folder "C 42 Nov. 1," box 299, RG 4, NARA.

136. Letter from Mr. Ira J. Anderson, Sapulpa, Okla., to Hoover, 28 January 1918, folder "H-I 25 Nov. 1," box 298, RG 4, NARA.

137. "Hooverizing," 1 March 1918, folder "Columbus State Journal Edit (OH)," box 567, RG 4, NARA.

138. "Spiritual Issue at Bottom," *Bulletin for the Clergy* 1, no. 2 (January 1918), folder "Cooperating Organizations. Religious, Fraternal, Patriotic, Labor, Agricultural, Commercial, etc.," box 3, series 5H, USFA Collection, Hoover Institution.

139. Hoover, "United States Food Administration—Letter to all Representatives of the Food Administration," 12 November 1918, bound folder "Addresses, Letters, Magazine Articles, Press Statements, Etc.," vol. I, part 2, box 93, Hoover Collection, Hoover Institution.

140. Everitt Brown, "The Food Administration: A Test of American Democracy," *The Historical Outlook: A Journal for Readers, Students and Teachers of History* 10, no. 5 (May 1919), Philadelphia, folder "Writings about Hoover," box 219, Hoover Collection, Hoover Institution.

141. Amy Bentley sees the same phenomenon affecting notions of sacrifice during World War II. Bentley, *Eating for Victory.*

142. Letter from Mary Bradford Shockley, Palo Alto, Calif., to Vernon Kellogg, D.C., 28 January 1918, folder "California," box 12, series 6H, USFA Collection, Hoover Institution; letter from unsigned woman, 11 January 1918, folder 41, box 17, NYSCHER; Martha Van Rensselaer [?], untitled report on trip to Pennsylvania Food Administration, folder 42, box 17, NYSCHER; abstract of letter from O. G. Small, Portland, Oreg., to Hoover, 24 January 1918, folder 41, box 17, NYSCHER.

143. Capozzola, *Uncle Sam Wants You*; Capozzola, "Only Badge Needed."

144. For example, in Flint Hill, Virginia, Mr. Towson Smith wrote to Hoover to report that a neighbor girl helped herself to a slice of cornbread but only ate half of it. When the girl told him defensively that children in her school always wasted food, he proceeded to extract the names of all the children from her and mailed the list in his letter to Hoover, hoping the government would make such a strong example of them that others would be scared into economy. Letter from Mr. Towson E. Smith, Flint Hill, Va., to Hoover, 16 November 1917, folder "TZ 349 Jan 1," box 320, RG 4, NARA.

145. Tristan Scott, "UM Students Seeking Pardons for Those Convicted of Sedition 85 Years Ago," *The Missoulian*, 9 April 2006, 3, accessed online.

146. Letter from Annie Irving Keeler, Jacksonville, Fla., to USFA, n.d, folder 41, box 17, NYSCHER.

147. Abstract of letter from Mrs. J. A. Tillotson, Nowata, Okla., to USFA, 16 November 1917, folder "T 36," box 328, RG 4, NARA.

148. Mrs. C. D. Anthony in New York City was one of hundreds of women who wrote Hoover to say she was tired of "wrestl[ing] with the servants" over food conservation, and she believed under rationing "servants would have to co-operate" (abstract of letter from Mrs. C. D. Anthony, N.Y.C., to USFA, folder "A 1, 2," box 327, RG 4, NARA).

149. Typed summary of "Confidential Meeting on the Food Needs of the Poor," 5 February 1918, N.Y.C., folder 60, box 17, NYSCHER.

150. Letter from Helen Moore, Milwaukee, Wisc., to USFA, 25 January 1918, folder 41, box 17, NYSCHER; *Food and the War: Federal Food Administration for South Dakota* 1, no. 18 (1 December 1918), folder "South Dakota," box 30, USFA Collection, Hoover Institution.

151. Letter from Marie Broomfield, Providence, R.I., to USFA, folder "C 52 Nov. 1," box 299, RG 4, NARA.

152. "Befo' de' Wa' Bread Is With Us Again," 13 November 1918, folder "Baltimore Star News (MD)," box 556, RG 4, NARA.

153. Coe originally typed "many of us, are not yet." Letter from Rev. H. Gertrude Coe, Waterbury, Conn., to Hoover, 8 June 1918, folder "C," box 405, RG 4, NARA.

154. Ray Wilbur, "Food Conservation for 1918–19," typed essay, n.d., apparently published in the *Journal of the American Medical Association*, folder "American Medical Association," box 325, RG 4, NARA.

155. Cocroft, *Self-Sufficiency*, 61.

156. "The Food of Other Days," 20 March 1918, folder "Oklahoma City Times Edit (OK)," box 570, RG 4, NARA.

157. Ray Wilbur, "Food Conservation for 1918–19," typed essay, n.d., apparently published in the *Journal of the American Medical Association*, folder "American Medical Association," box 325, RG 4, NARA; 1880 U.S. Census, *Boonesboro, Boone, Iowa*, Roll: T9_328, Family History Film: 1254328, Page: 121.1000, Enumeration District: 8, Image: 0326, Ancestry Library Edition database, accessed online.

158. Nash, *Life of Herbert Hoover: Master of Emergencies*, 229.

159. S. A. Mitchell and H. Alexander Smith, "A Perspective of [*sic*] the British Food Rationing System," July 1918, folder "R 93–97 Great Britain," box 115, USFA Collection, Hoover Institution.

160. Ray Wilbur, "Food and the War," speech at public meeting, Memorial Hall, Columbus, Ohio, 3 December 1917, folder "Dr. Wilbur. Speeches. Articles. Statements. Notes. I-1917," box 2, series 5H, USFA Collection, Hoover Institution.

161. Wilbur was the president of the American Medical Association in 1923 and 1924, and he served as the secretary of the interior under Hoover from 1929 to 1932, all while maintaining his job as president of Stanford. He was president from 1916 until 1943, the longest presidential tenure in Stanford's history. Swain, "Ray Lyman Wilbur."

162. "Ray Lyman Wilbur," n.d., folder "Dr. Wilbur. Speeches. Articles. Statements. Notes. I-1917," box 2, series 5H, USFA Collection, Hoover Institution.

163. Ray Wilbur, "Outline of a Statement," April 1918[?], folder "Dr. Wilbur. Speeches, Articles. Statements. Notes. II-1918," box 2, series 5H, USFA Collection, Hoover Institution; "Biographic Sketch of Ray Lyman Wilbur, Secretary of the Interior," March 1929, folder "Press Releases, Wilbur Biography," box 26, Ray Wilbur Collection, Hoover Library.

164. Ray Wilbur, notes on speech at unnamed conference, 17 August 1918, folder "Dr. Wilbur. Speeches, Articles. Statements. Notes. II-1918," box 2, series 5H, USFA Collection, Hoover Institution.

165. "Vital Issues after the War," summary of address by Ray Wilbur to National Security League, Chicago, 22 February 1918, folder "Dr. Wilbur. Speeches, Articles. Statements. Notes. II-1918," box 2, series 5H, USFA Collection, Hoover Institution.

166. "A Little Talk to the Food Hoarder," 17 January 1918, folder "Oklahoma City News (OK)," box 570, RG 4, NARA.

167. Letter from Hoover to Educational Institutions with Women Students, 25 January 1918, folder illegible, box 296, RG 4, NARA.

168. "Vital Issues after the War," summary of address by Ray Wilbur to National Security League, Chicago, 22 February 1918, folder "Dr. Wilbur. Speeches, Articles. Statements. Notes. II-1918," box 2, series 5H, USFA Collection, Hoover Institution.

169. Wilbur spoke in reverent terms of the utterly "autocratic position" Hoover had occupied as head of the Commission for Relief of Belgium (Wilbur, "Address at Conference of County Food Committees of Ohio," Columbus, Ohio, 3 December 1917, folder "Dr. Wilbur. Speeches. Articles. Statements. Notes. I-1917," box 2, series 5H, USFA Collection, Hoover Institution).

170. This sort of name recognition contributed to Hoover's early political success, although similar monikers haunted him by the time of the Depression's "Hoovervilles."

171. "Food Administrator Would Welcome Visit from Mice," 18 February 1918, folder "Pittsburgh Post News (PA)," box 569, RG 4, NARA.

172. For example, letter from Mrs. Emma West, St. Albans, W.V., to Hoover, 4 June 1917, folder illegible, box 296, RG 4, NARA; and letter from Mrs. M. E. Ruffin, Mobile, Ala., to Hoover, 6 July 1917, folder illegible, box 291, RG 4, NARA.

173. Harris Dickson, "Save and Serve with Hoover: What Will Feed Three Will Feed Four," *Collier's: The National Weekly*, ed. Mark Sullivan, 11 August 1917, folder "Writings about Hoover," box 219, Hoover Collection, Hoover Institution; Gooding, "Hooveritis," *Food and the War: Federal Food Administration for South Dakota* 1, no. 3, 15 February 1918, folder "South Dakota," box 30, USFA Collection, Hoover Institution; Mable I. Clapp, "Hoover's Goin' to Get You," *Ladies' Home Journal*, November 1917, folder "Writings about Hoover," box 219, Hoover Collection, Hoover Institution; "Hoover—that's all" poem, quoted in Morgan, *Reds*, 91, original source not cited; letter from Horace Fletcher, Copenhagen, to Vernon Kellogg, 11 June 1918, folder "Fletcher, Horace," box 127, USFA Collection, Hoover Institution.

174. Letter from Mrs. Elizabeth N. Bousall, Clifton Heights, Pa., to Hoover, 17 March 1918, folder "D-F 43 Feb. 1," box 299, RG 4, NARA.

175. Emma F. Way, San Diego, Calif., to Hoover, 4 November 1918, folder 50, box 17, NYSCHER; abstract of letter from Mrs. W. C. Mendenhall, Richmond, Va., to Hoover, 14 November 1917, folder "M 23, 24, 25," box 328, NARA.

176. Grammar and punctuation original. Ray Wilbur, memo to USFA staff, 21 July 1917, folder 8, box 1, series 5H, USFA Collection, Hoover Institution.

177. Interoffice memo from H. G. Andrews to H. J. Hill, 8 November 1917, folder "25 Andrews, Mr. H. G.," box 298, RG 4, NARA.

178. Hoover, quoted in an originally anonymous interview. Irwin, "First Aid to America: How Civilians Must Get Together and Get Behind Strong Leaders," *Saturday Evening Post*, 24 March 1917, 18–19, bound folder "Addresses, Letters, Magazine Articles, Press Statements, Etc. Inclusive Dates: February 1, 1917–April 6, 1918," vol. I, part 1, box 93, Hoover Collection, Hoover Institution.

179. Emphasis added. "The Man Who Fed Belgium," 17 July 1917, folder "Pomona Bulletin Edit (CA)," box 530, RG 4, NARA.

180. The second title alludes to Oliver Wendell Holmes Sr.'s popular 1858 book, *The Autocrat of the Breakfast Table*. Irwin, "The Autocrat of the Dinner Table," *Saturday Evening Post*, 23 June 1917, folder "Writings about Hoover," box 219, Hoover Collection, Hoover Institution; Louis Magid, "In Favor of Autocratic Food Control," *Evening Post: New York*, 21 December 1917, folder "Mag-May Correspondence," box 147, USFA Collection, Hoover Institution; "Supreme Food Dictator," [month illegible] 1918, folder "Oklahoma City Oklahoman Edit (OK)," box 570, RG 4, NARA; untitled article, 10 August 1917, folder "Los Angeles Graphic Edit (CA)," box 530, RG 4, NARA.

181. "National Will Power," 7 August 1917, folder "Brockton Times Edit (MA)," box 537, RG 4, NARA.

182. "Vital Issues After the War," summary of address by Ray Wilbur to National Security League, Chicago, 22 February 1918, folder "Dr. Wilbur. Speeches. Articles. Statements. Notes. II-1918," box 2, series 5H, USFA Collection, Hoover Institution.

183. "Master or Slave," 15 March 1918, folder "Santa Ana Register News (CA)," box 551, RG 4, NARA; Governor [Thomas] Bickett, "Saturnalia of Extravagance," 2 November 1917, folder "Raleigh State Journal Edit (NC)," box 544, RG 4, NARA; "Simple Life Desirable," 21 September 1917, folder "Manhattan Mercury Edit (KS)," box 535, RG 4, NARA.

184. "Autocracy, But Not Prussian," 30 May 1917, folder "Philadelphia Public Ledger Edit (PA)," box 546, RG 4, NARA.

185. The historian Charlotte Biltekoff argues that "self-control was central to the meaning of a good diet and eating right" throughout the twentieth century. Biltekoff, *Hidden Hunger*, 9.

186. Wilson, "Labor Must Be Free," 12 November 1917, address to the American Federation of Labor Convention, Buffalo, N.Y., John T. Woolley and Gerhard Peters, eds., American Presidency Project online, http://www.presidency.ucsb.edu/ws/?pid=65402.

187. "Self-Control," 13 November 1917, folder "Leadville Democrat Edit (CO)," box 532, RG 4, NARA.

188. "United States Food Administration, 'Chronological Sketch with Directory of Members, May 1917—June 1919,'" March 1920, New York, folder 40, box 17, NYSCHER.

189. Hoover, "Food Administration in Relation to the Farmer—Address before Conference of Editors and Publishers of Farm Papers, Chicago," 25 August 1917, bound folder "Addresses, Letters, Magazine Articles, Press Statements, Etc. Inclusive Dates:

February 1, 1917–April 6, 1918," vol. I, part 1, box 93, Hoover Collection, Hoover Institution.

190. "United States Food Administration, 'Chronological Sketch with Directory of Members, May 1917—June 1919,'" March 1920, New York, folder 40, box 17, NYSCHER.

191. "Until Next Harvest," USFA pamphlet, April 1918, folder 6, box 18, NYSCHER. This slogan also appeared in other administration literature, including on the widely disseminated 1918 pledge card.

192. Edward Arps, "Conservation of Food: What It Means and What It Will Unfold," typed circular, folder illegible, box 288, RG 4, NARA.

CHAPTER TWO

1. "Cat Meat May Soon Appear on Bill of Fare," 19 February 1918, folder "Urbana Citizen News (OH)," box 567, RG 4, NARA.

2. "Host Feeds Cat Meat to Trusting Guests: Possible Item Added to War Menu, but Some are Doubters," *Los Angeles Times*, 17 February 1918, 15, PQHN; "Cat Meat May Soon Appear on Bill of Fare," 19 February 1918, folder "Urbana Citizen News (OH)," box 567, RG 4, NARA.

3. He got the job when his eldest brother, the prominent eugenicist Paul Popenoe, took a leave from the journal to work with the war effort. Herbert Popenoe, World War I Draft Registration Form C, 4-4-24, 12 September 1918, Los Angeles County, California, Roll: 1531198, Draft Board: 6, Ancestry Library Edition database, accessed online.

4. Wiley had been chief chemist at the Department of Agriculture since 1883. Letter from Wiley to Mrs. Charity Dye, Indianapolis, 26 January 1917, folder "1917," box 124, Harvey Wiley Papers, LOC.

5. "Quit Waste, Eat Dog and Cat, Says Wiley," 27 March 1918, folder "Philadelphia Bulletin News (PA)," box 568, RG 4, NARA.

6. Rabinbach, *Human Motor*, 262.

7. Hoover, "Some Phases of the War Food Problem," *American Medicine*, June 1918, bound folder "Addresses, Letters, Magazine Articles, Press Statements, Etc. Inclusive Dates: April 30, 1918–September 16, 1919," box 93, Hoover Collection, Hoover Institution; "Food Control," 10 March 1917, *New Republic*, folder "March 10, 1917 Food Control," box 11, Hoover Library. "Carbohydrate" dates from the late 1860s, and "protein" dates from the 1840s. "Cholesterol" was coined in 1894, though it did not become a byword for another fifty years. *Oxford English Dictionary Online*, s.v. "cholesterol."

8. Levenstein, *Revolution at the Table*, 86.

9. "What the Nation Is Eating and Drinking," *New York Times*, 20 February 1910, SM6, PQHN.

10. Books like Jacques Buttner's *A Fleshless Diet* made explicit connections between vegetarianism and rationality. Luff, *Gout*, 248.

11. Wiley, *Not by Bread Alone*, 305–6.

12. Wallace, *Rumford Complete Cook Book*.

13. Food Administration literature worked to convince Americans that corn was as readily digestible as wheat. Katherine Blunt, Frances L. Swain, and Florence

Powdermaker, *Food Guide for War Service at Home*, Collegiate Section of the USFA (New York: Charles Scribner's Sons, 1918), folder "FA-II/Food Saving & Sharing, Food Guide . . . (booklets)," box 8, USFA Collection, Hoover Library; Alonzo Taylor, reprinted speech, Hotel Astor, New York, 8 February 1918, printed pamphlet (Roanoke, Va.: Union Printing & Manufacturing Co., 1918), 8–9, folder "FA-II/Addresses by Grew, Merrill, Pearl, Smith, Taylor, Wilbur," box 7, USFA Collection, Hoover Library.

14. For instance, when the influenza epidemic broke out in 1918, food administrators urged state representatives to make sure flu victims got extra sugar to boost their energy. USFA press release no. 1275, 30 October 1918, Public Information Division, folder "Press Releases, #1200–1299," box 12, USFA Collection, Hoover Library; Goudiss and Goudiss, *Foods that Will Win the War*, 58–60; letter from Zadia M. Olmstead, Duluth, Minn., to USFA, 7 September 1918, folder 60, box 17, NYSCHER; letter from J. W. Barnes, Bridgeport, Conn., to USFA, 12 September 1918, folder 60, box 17, NYSCHER; typed document about Cocoa, n.d., folder "Beverages," box 89, USFA Collection, Hoover Institution; Eleanor Franklin Egan, "The Modern Samaritan: How Charity Pays Its Way in Belgium," *Saturday Evening Post*, 21 October 1916, box 219, Hoover Collection, Hoover Institution; Wallace, *Rumford Complete Cook Book*, 29; Rose, *Everyday Foods in War Time*, 18.

15. Bryce, *Modern Theories of Diet*, 235.

16. Letter from H. L. Atkinson, San Francisco, to Julius Kahn, House of Representatives, 25 June 1917, folder illegible, box 288, RG 4, NARA; Pietkiewicz, "La Mastication," 179.

17. "Butter Camouflage," press release for farm journals, 2 March 1918, folder "Farm Journals Sections. Press Releases. 1918," box 41, series 12H, USFA Collection, Hoover Institution; Luff, *Gout*, 253.

18. Luff, *Gout*, 254–55.

19. Letter from Mark Barrett, Eau Claire, Wisc., to Hoover, 15 July 1917, folder illegible, box 288, RG 4, NARA.

20. Carrington, *Vitality, Fasting and Nutrition*, vii–ix.

21. Bryce, *Modern Theories of Diet*, 295.

22. Stearns, *Fat History*, 38.

23. Langworthy and Milner, *Investigations on the Nutrition of Man*, 18. Cookbook authors also increasingly provided the estimated cost of each dish along with the recipe, and they calculated the maximum calories available for ten cents. See Bradley, *Cook Book*, 11; Behnke and Henslowe, *Broadlands Cookery-Book*, 74–75; McCollum, "Some Essentials to a Safe Diet"; Murray, *Economy of Food*; and Richards and Norton, *Cost of Food*.

24. "Your Fuel Need," typed document, 2, n.d., folder 8, "Dr. Ray Lyman Wilbur. 17 May–24 November 1917," box 1, series 5H, USFA Collection, Hoover Institution.

25. Typed document about Cocoa, n.d., folder "Beverages," box 89, USFA Collection, Hoover Institution; Cummings, *American and His Food*, 139; "The Food Value of Milk," USFA bulletin no. 13, March 1918, folder "FA-II/Bulletins, #1–17," box 7, USFA Collection, Hoover Library.

26. Bradley, *Cook Book*, 11; Behnke and Henslowe, *Broadlands Cookery-Book*, 74–75; "Potatoes," advertisement sponsored by Wholesale Grocery Brokers' Association

of Kansas City, *Kansas City Star*, 30 April 1918, folder "Kansas," box 13, series 6H, USFA Collection, Hoover Institution.

27. Edna Noble White, "Meat and Meat Substitutes," *Agricultural College Extension Bulletin* 10, no. 4, December 1914, folder "Home Demonstration Agents," AAFCSR, #6578, DRMC.

28. Behnke and Henslowe, *Broadlands Cookery-Book*, 13; "Food Which Will Provide the Most Protein at Smallest Cost," 8 January 1918, folder "Guthrie Leader News (OK)," box 570, RG 4, NARA.

29. "Cost of Food in Relation to their Body-Building and Energy-Producing Values," bulletin no. 425, 24 November 1917, folder "FA I-A/Statistical Department Information Service, Bulletins #1–400, 1917 incomplete," box 3, USFA Collection, Hoover Library.

30. The Food Administration announced that peanut butter "has attained an important dietary place, especially as a nutritive article of food for the working man" (unnumbered press release, 8 July 1917, folder "Press Releases, #1–99," box 10, USFA Collection, Hoover Library). See also "Some Data on the Value of the Peanut as a Food Crop," Statistical Division bulletin no. 38, 9 July 1917, folder "Peanuts and Peanut Products," box 156, USFA Collection, Hoover Institution; and letter from Sam Blum, New Orleans, to USFA, 9 April 1918, folder "Nuts," box 154, USFA Collection, Hoover Institution.

31. McCollum, "Some Essentials to a Safe Diet," 95; "Your Fuel Need," typed document, n.d., folder 8, "Dr. Ray Lyman Wilbur. 17 May–24 November 1917," box 1, series 5H, USFA Collection, Hoover Institution; Cullather, "Foreign Policy of the Calorie," par. 13; Levenstein, *Revolution at the Table*, 110.

32. Harvey Wiley, "The Chemistry, Nutritive Value and Economy of Foods," Lecture IV, Westbrook Free Lectureship, Philadelphia, March 1918, folder "1918," box 126, Harvey Wiley Papers, LOC.

33. Levenstein, *Revolution at the Table*, 45.

34. McCollum, "Some Essentials to a Safe Diet," 99–100; letter from Eula McClary, N.Y.C., to Hoover, 7 May 1917, folder "DE–223," box 292, RG 4, NARA.

35. "Margin of Food," 6 August 1917, folder "Utica Globe Edit (NY)," box 544, RG 4, NARA.

36. Benton, *Gala-Day Luncheons*, 154; Sangster, *Good Manners for All Occasions*; Benton, "Poverty Luncheon Club"; Kingsland, "If You Are Well Bred"; Hall, *Handbook of Hospitality*, 269; Kingsland, *In and Out Door Games*, 382.

37. See Fitzgerald, *Every Farm a Factory*.

38. Gabaccia, *We Are What We Eat*, 55–58; Petrick, "Feeding the Masses," 29. See also Cronon, *Nature's Metropolis*; Levenstein, *Revolution at the Table*; and Jacobs, *Pocketbook Politics*.

39. "Value of commodities destined for domestic consumption, by type: 1869–1919," table Cd378–410, in Carter et al., Historical Statistics.

40. "Modern Miracle," advertisement for Kraft Cheese Loaf, *Chicago Daily News*, 20 November 1921, 23, PQHN.

41. "Standardize Your Table to Standardize the Nation," 22 March 1918, folder "Columbus Dispatch News," box 567, RG 4, NARA.

42. Wiley, *Not by Bread Alone*.

43. Levenstein, *Revolution at the Table*; Stearns, *Fat History*, 28. See also Cravens, "Establishing the Science of Nutrition."

44. Cummings, *American and His Food*.

45. "Food for Your Children," U.S. Food Leaflet no. 7, 1917, 104, folder "Publications," box 5, series 5H, USFA Collection, Hoover Institution; letter from Alonzo Taylor to Miss Stephenson, no place or first name given, duplicate, 25 May 1918, folder "Medical Questions," box 150, USFA Collection, Hoover Institution; "Food," *Crisis*, July 1918, 165; Luff, *Gout*, 253; Lorand, *Health through Rational Diet*, iii.

46. Charles Cristadoro, "Macaroni the Oldest National Joke," 9, typed article, folder "Macaroni," box 149, USFA Collection, Hoover Institution.

47. Letter from Carson Cook, Stockton, Calif., to Secretary of Agriculture, 4 September 1917, folder "Peanuts and Peanut Products," box 156, USFA Collection, Hoover Institution.

48. Rose, *Everyday Foods in War Time*, 4.

49. Cullather, "Foreign Policy of the Calorie," par. 4.

50. Cooper, *New Cookery*.

51. Press release no. 59, 14 January 1918, States Publicity Section, USFA Public Information Division, folder "Press Releases, States Section, Educational Division #1–99," box 9, USFA Collection, Hoover Library.

52. Antoinette Donnelly, "Watch Your Weight! Says Lulu Hunt Peters, A.B., M.D.," *Chicago Daily Tribune*, 15 September 1915, B4, PQHN.

53. Brewster and Brewster, *Nutrition of a Household*, 3–4; Carrington, *Vitality, Fasting and Nutrition*, vii–ix.

54. For example, one food reformer in the mid-1910s proclaimed that overeating could cause emaciation if digestion was faulty. Christian, "Emaciation, Its Cause and Cure," 2; Greer, *Food*, 177; "Good News for the Fat," 2 June 1918, folder "Pittsburg Dispatch News," box 569, RG 4, NARA; "Eat and Grow Thin—Fast and Fatten," 26 March 1918, folder "Bridgeport Post News (CT)," box 550, RG 4, NARA.

55. *Food Questions Answered*, USFA bulletin, March 1918, 7, folder "Publications," box 5, series 5H, USFA Collection, Hoover Institution.

56. "What Is Calorie [*sic*]?," 14 June 1918, folder "Erie Times News (PA)," box 568, RG 4, NARA.

57. Landis, "Dietary Habits and their Improvement."

58. Brewster and Brewster, *Nutrition of a Household*, 5, 8–9. See also Rabinbach, *Human Motor*; Pietkiewicz, "La mastication," 174; DuPuis, *Nature's Perfect Food*; "What Is Calorie [*sic*],?" 14 June 1918, folder "Erie Times News (PA)," box 568, RG 4, NARA; Wood and Hopkins, *Food Economy in War Time*, 3; Cocroft, *Let's Be Healthy*, 10; letter from Horace Fletcher, Copenhagen, to Vernon Kellogg, 11 June 1918, folder "Fletcher, Horace," box 127, USFA Collection, Hoover Institution; and W. H. Crawford, "Men Who are Winning the War," *Leslie's Weekly* 125, no. 3226, folder "July 5, 1917. Men Who are Winning the War," box 12, Hoover Library.

59. Levenstein argues that vitamin research created the next stage in nutrition research, beyond the calorie-centric reasoning of the "New Nutrition" and into what he calls the "Newer Nutrition" of the 1920s and beyond. Levenstein, *Revolution at the Table*, 147–60.

60. For example, an 1860 nutrition table defined grains as the most nutritious food and vegetables as the least nutritious. Cambell, *Practical Cook Book*, 9; Gratzer, *Terrors of the Table*, 143–48.

61. Dewey, *New Era for Woman*.

62. Cummings, *American and His Food*, 131.

63. Gratzer, *Terrors of the Table*, 163.

64. Ibid., 163–64.

65. Ibid., 166; McCollum, *Newer Knowledge of Nutrition*; Levenstein, *Revolution at the Table*, 147–60.

66. Gratzer, *Terrors of the Table*, 162–69.

67. Katherine Blunt, Frances L. Swain, and Florence Powdermaker, *Food Guide for War Service at Home*, Collegiate Section of the USFA (New York: Charles Scribner's Sons, 1918), 11, folder "FA-II/Food Saving & Sharing, Food Guide . . . (booklets)," box 8, USFA Collection, Hoover Library; Flora Rose, "Points in Selecting Meals," 2 November 1917, folder "Abby L. Marlatt: Isabel Bevier: F. W. Van Sicklin: Flora Rose," box 2, series 5H, USFA Collection, Hoover Institution; Rose, *Everyday Foods in War Time*, 47.

68. "Get the 'Scientific' Slant," 1 March 1918, folder "Augusta Journal News (ME)," box 556, RG 4, NARA; "Hundred-Calorie Exhibit Draws Women to Window," 21 May 1918, folder "Philadelphia Public Ledger No. 1 (PA)," box 569, RG 4, NARA; letter from Fred Lawrence Foster, San Jose, Calif., to USFA, 10 January 1918, folder 41, box 17, NYSCHER; "After Hoover What?," 20 November 1918, folder, "Greensburg Tribune Editorial (PA)," box 568, RG 4, NARA.

69. Letter from Bessie Dixon, Norfolk, Va., to Hoover, 8 August 1917, folder illegible, box 290, RG 4, NARA.

70. Gilman, "Housekeeper and the Food Problem."

71. Brewster and Brewster, *Nutrition of a Household*, 3–4; Hitchcock, "Relation of the Housewife to the Food Problem"; "What I Would Like Women to Do," *Ladies' Home Journal*, August 1917, bound folder "Addresses, Letters, Magazine Articles, Press Statements, Etc. Inclusive Dates: February 1, 1917–April 6, 1918," box 93, vol. I, part 1, Hoover Collection, Hoover Institution.

72. Spelling and grammar original. Abstract of letter from Mary O. Gallery, Chicago, to Food Administration, 3 July 1917, folder "NS—348," box 295, RG 4, NARA; letter from Mrs. Kathleen M. Heide, Fitzgerald, Ga., to Hoover, 1 March 1918, folder "87 Congress of Mothers & Parent-Teachers Ass'n., National," box 301, RG 4, NARA.

73. For more on nutrition knowledge as a mark of middle-class identity in this era, see Biltekoff, "Hidden Hunger."

74. "Am I a Good Cook," February 1918, folder "Cedar Rapids Modern Brotherhood Edit (IA)," box 556, RG 4, NARA.

75. For example, on a rare occasion when wealthy Chicago ladies attended a wartime food conservation show in 1918, they brought their kitchen servants with them, since, after all, it was the servants who would be doing the shopping and cooking. "Society Folk as Conservators," 24 January 1918, folder "Dayton Journal News (OH)," box 567, RG 4, NARA.

76. "Hoover's Disciple on Calories' Trail," [?] February 1918, folder "Cleveland Plaindealer News (OH)," box 567, RG 4, NARA.

77. Cream of Wheat advertisement, painted by Edward V. Brewer for Cream of Wheat Co., 26 January 1922, 56, *The Youth's Companion*, American Periodicals.

78. "Food Conservation in Relation to Social Service and Charity Work," typed document, no author, folder "348 Social Service Worker," box 320, RG 4, NARA.

79. Wiley, *Not by Bread Alone*, 305–6.

80. Ibid.

81. Love and Davenport, *Defects Found in Drafted Men*, 27, 28–29.

82. Harvey Wiley, "Importance of Food in the National Defense," typed speech, 3 June 1917, folder "1917," box 125, Harvey Wiley Papers, LOC. Some of the books that explicitly applied rationality to eating and cooking were Buttner, *Fleshless Diet*; François Xavier Gouraud, *What Shall I Eat? A Manual of Rational Feeding* (New York: Rebman Company, 1911); Susannah Usher, *Some Points to Be Considered in the Planning of a Rational Diet*, 2d ed. (Urbana: University of Illinois, 1912, 1914); Isaac Thompson Cook, *Health through Rational Living* (Saint Louis, 1913); Lorand, *Health through Rational Diet*; Harry Finkel, *Health via Nature: The Health Book for the Layman, including a Rational System* (New York: Society for Public Health Education, 1925).

83. See Levenstein, *Revolution at the Table*, 72–146.

84. Goudiss and Goudiss, *Foods That Will Win the War*, 83. One home economics stricture that entered food conservation wisdom was the importance of accepting any food that was served "without question or comment." "Care of Children," Home Demonstration in Care and Feeding of a Normally Well Child, no. 276, Department of Home Economics, Cornell University, 1919[?], folder 2, box 18, NYSCHER.

85. Hoover, "Some Phases of the War Food Problem," *American Medicine*, June 1918, bound folder "Addresses, Letters, Magazine Articles, Press Statements, Etc. Inclusive Dates: April 30, 1918—September 16, 1919," box 93, Hoover Collection, Hoover Institution.

86. "Examiner News Editorials," 12 December 1917, folder "Yuma Examiner Edit (AZ)," box 529, RG 4, NARA.

87. Harvey Wiley, "Importance of Food in the National Defense," typed speech, 3 June 1917, folder "1917," box 125, Wiley Papers, LOC.

88. Even nutritionists at the time were not convinced that the substitute diet was more healthful, although they were starting to lean in that direction. It is noteworthy that food conservation rules also encouraged Americans to eat foods like peanut oil, cheese, chicken fat, and a variety of other foods that might strike a twenty-first-century reader as less than ideally healthful.

89. Ray Wilbur, typed article for Labor Press, n.d., folder "Dr. Wilbur. Speeches. Articles. Statements. Notes. I-1917," box 2, series 5H, USFA Collection, Hoover Institution; "Food Values," 11 January 1918, folder "Columbus Dispatch News (OH)," box 567, RG 4, NARA; "Food Economy for the Housewife," Home Economics Series, bulletin no. 1, July 1917, State College of Washington library, 4.

90. Letter from Carson Cook, Stockton, Calif., to Secretary of Agriculture, 4 September 1917, folder "Peanuts and Peanut Products," box 156, USFA Collection, Hoover Institution; Allen, *Mrs. Allen's Book of Sugar Substitutes*, 80.

91. In contrast, in the early 1920s the French writer M. Marguey took issue with overly mechanical descriptions of digestion. Lost in the emphasis on science, math,

and hygiene, he said, was the simple fact that people should enjoy eating. Marguey, Introduction to *La cuisine et la table moderne*, iii–iv.

92. Goudiss and Goudiss, *Foods That Will Win the War*, 26, 42, 63.

93. "Home Economics Teaching under Present Economic Conditions," 5 September 1917, Department of the Interior, Bureau of Education leaflet, folder "Dept. Interior," AAFCSR, #6578, DRMC.

94. Prof. Stoughton Holburn, "The Kitchen in England," 28 February 1918, folder "East Stroudsburg Press News (PA)," box 568, RG 4, NARA.

95. Letter from Alonzo Taylor, Philadelphia, to Hoover, 15 July 1917, folder illegible, box 293, RG 4, NARA.

96. Harvey Wiley, "Food Conservation," typed essay or speech, undated, folder "1917," box 125, Harvey Wiley Papers, LOC.

97. Harvey Wiley, "The Chemistry, Nutritive Value and Economy of Foods," 21, Lecture I, Westbrook Free Lectureship, Philadelphia, March 1918, folder "1918," box 126, Harvey Wiley Papers, LOC.

98. "Meat Recipes," n.d., folder 47, box 17, NYSCHER.

99. Jean Prescott Adams, "Military Life Influences Food Habits," from "The Business of Being a Housewife," 6 September 1918, printed leaflet produced by Armour & Co., folder "22 Armour & Co. Feb. 1," box 298, RG 4, NARA; "Meat Recipes," n.d., folder 47, box 17, NYSCHER; Food Conservation Notes, no. 22, 24 August 1918, folder "FA-II/ Food Conservation Notes," box 8, USFA Collection, Hoover Library. See also McWilliams, *Revolution in Eating*.

100. Food Conservation Notes, no. 24, 7 September 1918, folder "FA-II/Food Conservation Notes," box 8, USFA Collection, Hoover Library; "Food Administration Activities," press release for farm journals for week ending 15 June 1918, folder "Farm Journals Sections. Press Releases. 1918," box 41, series 12H, USFA Collection, Hoover Institution; "Food from the Forest," press release for farm journals for week ending 22 October 1918, folder "Farm Journals Sections. Press Releases. 1918," box 41, series 12H, USFA Collection, Hoover Institution; "The Marsh Rabbits," January or February 1918, folder "Lima Times-Democrat Edit (OH)," box 567, RG 4, NARA; Food Conservation Notes, no. 25, 14 September 1918, folder "FA-II/Food Conservation Notes," box 8, USFA Collection, Hoover Library.

101. Food Conservation Notes, no. 22, 24 August 1918, folder "FA-II/Food Conservation Notes," box 8, USFA Collection, Hoover Library.

102. "Win the War with Snails," 3 February 1918, folder "Dayton News Edit (OH)," box 567, RG 4, NARA; "Help Win War by Raising Frogs," 22 November 1917, folder "Anaheim Gazette News (CA)," box 530, RG 4, NARA.

103. "Eating Horse Meat," *Chicago Daily Tribune*, 28 May 1917, 8, PQHN.

104. "Eats Horse Meat: Says It Is Fine," *Chicago Defender*, 14 April 1917, 1, PQHN.

105. "Resume of Important Rulings and Letters Sent to Federal Food Administrators," August 1st to August 15th, folder "FA I-A/Resume of Important Rulings, for district & county Administrators, April–Aug. 1918," box 3, USFA Collection, Hoover Library; Ritvo, *Platypus and the Mermaid*, 204–5.

106. "Heard in Corridors of Washington Hotels," *Washington Post*, 10 May 1918, 6, PQHN; and "Horseflesh Control in England," press release for farm journals for week

ending 5 November 1918, folder "Farm Journals Sections. Press Releases. 1918," box 41, series 12H, USFA Collection, Hoover Institution.

107. Lévi-Strauss, *Totemism*, 89.

108. "Dogs and Cats as Food," 30 March 1918, folder "Wilkesbarre Record Edit (PA)," box 568, RG 4, NARA.

109. Letter from Harvey Wiley to Mr. J. A. Burkhardt, Kansas City, Mo., 28 May 1917, folder "1917," box 124, Harvey Wiley Papers, LOC.

110. "Eat Cutlets—Scientist Offers Hoover New Food Item after Dining on Feline Meat," *Chicago Daily Tribune*, 16 February 1918, 7, PQHN.

111. "Cat Meat May Soon Appear on Bill of Fare," 19 February 1918, folder "Urbana Citizen News (OH)," box 567, RG 4, NARA.

112. "Host Feeds Cat Meat to Trusting Guests: Possible Item Added to War Menu, but Some Are Doubters," *Los Angeles Times*, 17 February 1918, 15, PQHN.

113. Grier, *Pets in America*, 288.

114. "Dogs or Babies?," 9 June 1918, *Selma Times*, folder "Georgia Miscellaneous," box 553, RG 4, NARA; "Campaign Pledge Press Statement No. 16," n.d., folder "Campaign Pledge Press Statement Nos. 1–17 [undated]," box 3, series 5H, USFA Collection, Hoover Institution. Before the war, bakers had routinely resold stale bread at bargain prices to pet-owners, but the Food Administration decreed that bakeries could no longer give credit to retailers for unsold bread, an attempt to force bakers and grocers to calculate their needs more precisely, erring on the side of underproduction. "Lessons in Community and National Life," Community Leaflet no. 12, *Department of the Interior, Bureau of Education in Cooperation with the United States Food Administration* (Washington, D.C.: GPO, January 1918), 31–32.

115. "Resolutions Unanimously adopted at the first meeting of the United States Live-Stock Industry Committee appointed by the Secretary of Agriculture and the Food Administrator, Washington, D.C.," 5–7 September 1917, 9, folder "FA I-A/Organizations & Societies, Resolutions," box 2, USFA Collection, Hoover Library; "Useless Dogs Should Be Done Away With," 9 January 1918, folder "Hastings Times News (ND)," box 568, RG 4, NARA.

116. "Quit Waste, Eat Dog and Cat, Says Wiley," 27 March 1918, folder "Philadelphia Bulletin News (PA)," box 568, RG 4, NARA.

117. "Eliminate Pets to Save the Food," 6 November 1917, folder "Richmond News Edit (CA)," box 530, RG 4, NARA.

118. "A Friend of the Dog," 16 November 1917, folder, "Fresno Herald Edit (CA)," box 530, RG 4, NARA.

119. Eugene Brown, "Dog-Gone Tough," 12 November 1917, folder "Los Angeles Times Edit (CA)," box 567, RG 4, NARA.

120. Small-animal veterinarians only became regular features in American life starting in the late 1920s and 1930s, when horses disappeared from city streets and former large-animal veterinarians turned to the domestic pet market for their livelihood. Before that time, very few people knew how to spay female dogs and cats, and the casual neutering of male animals resulted often enough in infection and death that pet owners generally preferred to leave their animals intact. The result, naturally, was that female pets routinely bore litters, and responsible pet owners considered it their

duty to kill most or all of the puppies and kittens that resulted. Grier, *Pets in America*, 10–14, 78–80.

121. Ibid., 14.

122. Hoover, "Grain and Live Stock," USFA bulletin no. 10, 25 October 1917, 14, bound folder "Addresses, Letters, Magazine Articles, Press Statements, Etc. Inclusive Dates: February 1, 1917–April 6, 1918," vol. I, part 1, box 93, Hoover Collection, Hoover Institution.

123. "Elephant Steak," no. 72, 19 January 1918, States Publicity Section, USFA Public Information Division, folder "Press Releases, States Section, Educational Division #1–99," box 9, USFA Collection, Hoover Library.

124. "Poor Belgium: Dog Meat a Luxury, Cats Are Slaughtered for the Table," *Chicago Daily Tribune*, 26 May 1918, 3, PQHN.

125. "Reject Peace Terms," *Washington Post*, 11 January 1918, 1, PQHN.

126. Harvey Wiley, in Maddocks, *Pure Food Cook Book*, 185.

127. Wiley, *Not by Bread Alone*, vi; Harvey Wiley, questionnaire attached to "The Chemistry, Nutritive Value and Economy of Foods," Lecture IV, Westbrook Free Lectureship, Philadelphia, March 1918, folder "1918," box 126, Harvey Wiley Papers, LOC.

128. Letter from Harvey Wiley to Mr. C. F. Fisher, Sheridan, Wyo., 11 March 1918, folder "1918," box 126, Harvey Wiley Papers, LOC.

CHAPTER THREE

1. Hoover, "America's Obligations in Belgian Relief—Address before the Chamber of Commerce in the State of New York," 15, 1 February 1917, bound folder "Addresses, Letters, Magazine Articles, Press Statements, Etc. Inclusive Dates: February 1, 1917–April 6, 1918," vol. I, part 1, box 93, Hoover Collection, Hoover Institution.

2. Emphasis added. Hoover, "Belgian Relief—Message to American People," March 14, 1917, bound folder "Addresses, Letters, Magazine Articles, Press Statements, Etc. Inclusive Dates: February 1, 1917–April 6, 1918," vol. 1, part 1, box 93, Hoover Collection, Hoover Institution; Kennedy, *Over Here*, v, 45.

3. "What America Has Done in Feeding the Allies," bulletin no. 772, 23 February 1918, Food Administration Statistical Department Information Service, folder "FA I-A/Statistical Department Information Service, Bulletins #650–859, 1918 Incomplete," box 4, USFA Collection, Hoover Library. At the time, there were roughly 46 million people in Great Britain, 40 million in France, 35 million in Italy, and 125 million in Russia, which received a small percentage of aid early in the war.

4. The United States in the past had given food to countries experiencing severe shortages, as when the government donated food to Ireland during the potato famine and to India in 1899, but it had never before done so through a formal aid program. Ahlberg, *Transplanting the Great Society*, 15.

5. See Cullather, *Hungry World*; Ahlberg, *Transplanting the Great Society*; Patenaude, *Big Show in Bololand*; and Wallerstein, *Food for War*.

6. Clements, *Hoover, Conservation, and Consumerism*, 32–33.

7. Hoover, introduction to Mullendore, *History of the United States Food Administration*, 9.

8. Nash, *Life of Herbert Hoover: Master of Emergencies*, 6.

9. Rothbard, "Hoover's 1919 Food Diplomacy."

10. W. A. M. Goode, "Relief Work in Belgium," *Royal Society of Arts Journal* 65, no. 3349 (26 January 1917): 178–89, 186, folder "Jan 26, 1917. Relief work in Belgium," box 11, Hoover Library.

11. "Billy Sunday's Sermon Yesterday: 'Present Your Bodies,'" 28 March 1918, folder, "Chicago Herald News," box 554, RG 4, NARA.

12. See Belasco, *Meals to Come*, 26–8.

13. The United States was more than ten times as large as France and more than twenty times as large as Britain. Pearl and Matchett, *Reference Handbook of Food Statistics in Relation to the War*, 9, folder "Statistics: Prices, Fish, General," box 5, USFA Collection, Hoover Library.

14. "Interesting Westerners: The Americans of the Hour in Europe," no author, *Sunset Magazine* 34 (June 1915): 1175–79, box 219, Hoover Collection, Hoover Institution.

15. The Food Administration delivered the bulk of its food aid calories to Britain, France, and Italy, in that order, but France actually received the most total aid. The reason was that Great Britain had made an agreement with France in 1916 to ship it food, so the British actually shipped some of the American food they received to France. Britain was the recipient of just over half of the calories that the Food Administration shipped. France got 28 percent; Italy, 19.4 percent; and Russia, less than 1 percent. "What America Has Done in Feeding the Allies," bulletin no. 772, 23 February 1918, 1–5, Food Administration Statistical Department Information Service, folder "FA I-A/Statistical Department Information Service, Bulletins #650–859, 1918 Incomplete," box 4, USFA Collection, Hoover Library. See also Surface, *American Food*. France relied on the United States for more than half of its wheat supply. Food Conservation Notes, no. 21, 17 August 1918, folder "FA-II/Food Conservation Notes," box 8, USFA Collection, Hoover Library.

16. Sir William Goode, "Food from America: What It Means to Us and How We Get It," April 1918, *World's Work*, folder "April 1918. Food from America," box 14, Hoover Library.

17. Offer, *First World War*, 81.

18. Before the war, imported food accounted for somewhere between 6 and 12 percent of French national consumption. Gervais, Jollivet, and Tavernier, *La fin de la France paysanne depuis 1914*, 23–24, 29.

19. Ironically, this quest was hindered by the fact that France had been largely self-sufficient before the war; it meant it did not have the ships, warehouses, refrigerators, and other infrastructure in place to transport and store the food it needed. Legendre, *Alimentation et ravitaillement*, 5, 3, BNF.

20. In contrast, bread made up about 30 percent of average American diets. "Consumption of Grains as Bread in the United States and France," bulletin no. 828, 9 March 1918, Food Administration Statistical Department Information Service, folder "FA I-A/Statistical Department Information Service, Bulletins #650–859, 1918 Incomplete," box 4, USFA Collection, Hoover Library.

21. Bonzon and Davis, "Feeding the Cities," 327; *L'effort du ravitaillement français*, 59–60, BNF.

22. Augé-Laribé, *Agriculture and Food Supply*, 70–71.

23. John Simpson, "Food Problems in France," draft, 31 August 1918, 1, folder "France. Food Administration (U.S.) Correspondence. Simpson, John L," box 114, USFA Collection, Hoover Institution. Another factor that hobbled French peoples' ability to feed themselves during the war was that a growing number of French acres had been turned over from wheat farming to cattle ranching earlier in the twentieth century. While ranching could be profitable for those directly involved, the turn to cattle had decreased French agricultural productivity overall, since it takes many more resources to produce calories from meat than it does from grains or vegetables. Gervais, Jollivet, and Tavernier, *La fin de la France paysanne depuis 1914*, 22–23; "Resume of Important Rulings and Letters Sent to Federal Food Administrators May 15th to June 1st," folder "FA I-A/Resume of Important Rulings, for district & county Administrators, April–Aug. 1918," box 3, USFA Collection, Hoover Library.

24. A. M. Thackara, "Measures to Restrict Food Consumption in France," from typed report marked "Confidential: The Food Situation in France," 1 July 1917, Paris, folder "Food Reports from A. M. Thackara, American Consul General, Paris," box 116, USFA Collection, Hoover Institution.

25. "Pain Rassis" (or "Stale Bread"), *Le Progrès de la Somme*, 26 February 1917, Amiens, France, 259 PER 106 (1 Jan 1917–30 April 1917), ADS.

26. *L'effort du ravitaillement français*, 61.

27. Bonzon and Davis, "Feeding the Cities," 327.

28. Starting in 1918, restaurants in France could serve no butter or milk after 9 A.M., and the state raised the mandatory number of meatless days to three a week. The government enforced the meatless days by allowing individuals to purchase a maximum of 200 grams of meat every four days. Moreover, these restrictions lasted through mid-1919. Bonzon and Davis, "Feeding the Cities," 318. The meat ration for France was about a pound a week, including horsemeat, the consumption of which increased significantly during the war. "Resume of Important Rulings and Letters Sent to Federal Food Administrators May 15th to June 1st," folder "FA I-A/Resume of Important Rulings, for district & county Administrators, April–Aug. 1918," box 3, USFA Collection, Hoover Library.

29. John Simpson, "Report on Department 'Puy-de-Dome,'" typed report, 20 August 1918, 8, folder "R 37–44 Food Conditions in Various Sections of France," box 115, USFA Collection, Hoover Institution.

30. Legendre, *Alimentation et ravitaillement*, 141.

31. John Simpson, "Report on Department 'Puy-de-Dome,'" typed report, 20 August 1918, 8, folder "R 37–44 Food Conditions in Various Sections of France," box 115, USFA Collection, Hoover Institution; letter from the Mayor of Laon to Monsieur le Président and to the Members of the Comité d'Alimentation du Nord de la France in Brussels, 1 July 1918, folder "4 H 177, Archives Communales, Laon—CRB—Rapports sur la situation du ravitaillement dans la region de Laon, Juin 1915–Sept 1916," ADA.

32. Alonzo Taylor, reprinted speech, Hotel Astor, New York, 8 February 1918, printed pamphlet (Roanoke, Va.: Union Printing & Manufacturing Co., 1918), 8–9, folder "FA-II/Addresses by Grew, Merrill, Pearl, Smith, Taylor, Wilbur," box 7, USFA Collection, Hoover Library; Hoover, introduction to Mullendore, *History of the United States Food Administration*, 38.

33. Winter, *Great War and the British People*; Bonzon and Davis, "Feeding the Cities," 315; Offer, *First World War*, 54.

34. Telegram from King Albert of Belgium to Hoover, 22 October 1918, reprinted in Official Statement of the United States Food Administration, no. 6, 1 November 1918, Washington, D.C., folder "FA I-A/Official Statements #1-18, 1918-1919," box 2, USFA Collection, Hoover Library.

35. Remarks by the Belgian Ministers [?] to the Daughters of the American Revolution at Memorial Continental Hall, Washington, D.C., 15 April 1918, folder "Belgium," box 89, USFA Collection, Hoover Institution.

36. Letter from Maurice Viollette to M. le Président, 3 May 1917, "Céréales, farines, pain, loi, circulaires et instructions. 1915-1918," 132 M 20, Archives Départementales de la Marne. Likewise, Victor Boret, the French Food Controller, said in May 1918 that the Allies would be grateful for their eventual victory to two people, the French general and Hoover. Guerrier, *We Pledged Allegiance*, 119.

37. Legendre, *Alimentation et ravitaillement*, 4.

38. Untitled press release no. 304, 1 July 1918, States Publicity Section, USFA Public Information Division, folder "Press Releases, States Section, Educational Division #300-399," box 10, USFA Collection, Hoover Library.

39. "Herbert C. Hoover—How He Made His Millions," 3 June 1917, folder "San Francisco Examiner Edit (CA)," box 530, RG 4, NARA.

40. Alonzo Taylor, reprinted speech, Hotel Astor, New York, 8 February 1918, printed pamphlet (Roanoke, Va.: Union Printing & Manufacturing Co., 1918), 8-9, folder "FA-II/Addresses by Grew, Merrill, Pearl, Smith, Taylor, Wilbur," box 7, USFA Collection, Hoover Library.

41. "Love for America Growing in France," 26 June 1918, folder "Boston Herald News (MA)," box 557, RG 4, NARA.

42. "Note to the Educational Director," no. 451, 2 November 1918, States Publicity Section, USFA Public Information Division, folder "Press Releases, States Section, Educational Division #400-470," box 10, USFA Collection, Hoover Library.

43. John Simpson, letters on trip of investigation in the departments of the Isere, Rhone, and Loire, 3 July 1918, typed report, Paris, 26 September 1918, folder "R 37-44 Food Conditions in Various Sections of France," box 115, USFA Collection, Hoover Institution.

44. Untitled press release no. 240, 22 May 1918, States Publicity Section, USFA Public Information Division, folder "Press Releases, States Section, Educational Division #200-249," box 9, USFA Collection, Hoover Library.

45. "European Food Condition," 18[?] May 1918, folder "Grand Forks Herald Edit (ND)," box 568, RG 4, NARA; Food Administration Bulletin for Massachusetts, no. 28, 1 August 1918, Boston, folder "Massachusetts," box 14, series 6H, USFA Collection, Hoover Institution; untitled press release no. 467, 6 December 1918, States Publicity Section, USFA Public Information Division, folder "Press Releases, States Section, Educational Division #400-470," box 10, USFA Collection, Hoover Library.

46. "Belgian Relief Commission Food and Clothing Program Announced for Coming Year," Official Statement of the United States Food Administration, no. 5, 1 October

1918, Washington, D.C., folder "FA I-A/Official Statements #1–18, 1918–1919," box 2, USFA Collection, Hoover Library.

47. Ballesteros, *La Guerra Europea y la Neutralidad Española*, 70–71, BNE.

48. Alcalá Galiano y Osma, *El Fin de la Tragedia*, 151–52, 149–50, BNE.

49. Emphasis added. "The Allied Restaurant," cartoon, Official Bulletin for Colorado, USFA for Colorado, no. 1, September 1918, folder "Colorado," box 12, series 6H, USFA Collection, Hoover Institution.

50. "Rice the Food of Millions," press release for farm journals, n.d., folder "Farm Journals Section. Press Releases. Undated," box 41, series 12H, USFA Collection, Hoover Institution; *Food Saving and Sharing*, 4–5; "Food Conservation Week," *National School Service* 1, no. 7, Special Food Conservation Number, 1 December 1918, Washington, D.C.: The Committee on Public Information, folder "FA I-A/Annual Report, 1918; Report to Feb. 1918; Food Program for 1919," box 1, USFA Collection, Hoover Library; Lansing and Gulick, *Food and Life*, 154; "American Food to Save World," 6 November 1918, folder "Erie Times News (PA)," box 568, RG 4, NARA.

51. "A Universal Bread," *Food and the War: Federal Food Administration for South Dakota* 1, no. 13 (October 1918), folder "South Dakota," box 30, USFA Collection, Hoover Institution.

52. "World's Food Now Chief Peace Issue, Says Jane Addams," December 1918, folder "New York Tribune News No. 2 (NY)," box 566, RG 4, NARA; David Franklin Houston, "Program for Food Production and Conservation," *The American-Food Journal*, vol. 12, no. 5, New York: American Food Journal, Inc., May 1917, "HEARTH," Cornell University Library, online resource; Goudiss and Goudiss, *Foods That Will Win the War*, 16; Hoover, "Food Conference of Pennsylvania Public Safety Committee, Philadelphia—Address," bound folder "Addresses, Letters, Magazine Articles, Press Statements, Etc. Inclusive Dates: February 1, 1917–April 6, 1918," vol. 1, part 1, box 93, Hoover Collection, Hoover Institution.

53. Sarah Louise Arnold, "Learning the Lesson of Food Conservation," *The Journal of Home Economics* 10, no. 6 (June 1918), folder "Number of the Journal of Home Economics, June 1918," box 5, series 5H, USFA Collection, Hoover Institution.

54. "Rice," USDA press release no. 90, 21 January 1918, States Publicity Section, USFA Public Information Division, folder "Press Releases, States Section, Educational Division #1–99," box 9, USFA Collection, Hoover Library.

55. Goudiss and Goudiss, *Foods That Will Win the War*, 12; "Heavy Eater Is a Traitor," 29 October 1917, folder "Detroit Free Press News (MI)," box 537, RG 4, NARA.

56. Spelling and grammar original. "N'oubliez pas que la France a Besoin de Sucre," reprinted poster by Michigan high school student, March 1918, in *Food: News Notes for Public Libraries* 1, no. 1 (Oct. 1917–Oct. 1918), 3.

57. Emphasis original. "Are You a Slacker in Your Kitchen," 2, typed article, folder "L-M 87 Nov. 1," box 301, RG 4, NARA; Ray Wilbur, "Five Minute Speech for Movies, Etc.," n.d., folder "Dr. Wilbur. Speeches. Articles. Statements. Notes. I-1917," box 2, series 5H, USFA Collection, Hoover Institution.

58. "Milk," unlabeled script for demonstration, n.d., folder 9, box 1, series 5H, USFA Collection, Hoover Institution.

59. "Graphic Exhibits on Food Conservation at Fairs and Exhibition," USFA bulletin, September 1917, 12, folder "Exhibit and Campaign Methods. John H. Cover," box 4, series 5H, USFA Collection, Hoover Institution.

60. Hoover, "The World's Food Shortage—Address Delivered at the Smithsonian Institution, Washington, D.C. (U.S. Food Administration. Bull. 7.)," folder "Addresses, Letters, Magazine Articles, Press Statements, Etc. Inclusive Dates: February 1, 1917–April 6, 1918," vol. I, part 1, box 93, Hoover Collection, Hoover Institution; photographs of food conservation exhibits, folder "Exhibit and Campaign Methods. John H. Cover," box 4, series 5H, USFA Collection, Hoover Institution; "Food and the Undergraduate," *The Stanford Illustrated Review*, ed. Goodwin Knight and Anita Allen, November 1917, box 219, Hoover Collection, Hoover Institution; Hoover, "Food and the War," *The Day's Food in War and Peace*, 11, bound folder "Addresses, Letters, Magazine Articles, Press Statements, Etc. Inclusive Dates: February 1, 1917–April 6, 1918," vol. 1, part 1, box 93, Hoover Collection, Hoover Institution; Goudiss and Goudiss, *Foods That Will Win the War*, 5; "Objectives in the Division of Food Conservation/USFA, 1918," typed document, folder 60, box 17, NYSCHER, #23-2-749, DRMC; "The Blade," 13 December 1918, spoof paper from Educational Division of USFA, folder "Ben S. Allen. Memoranda for Mr. Rickard 'Week ending' 6 April–25 May 1918," box 39, series 12H, Education Division, USFA Collection, Hoover Institution.

61. Indeed, the new language about the collective impact of the American millions was so pervasive in the war era that some credited it with creating a new form of national consciousness, a break from inward-looking individualism. Don Herold, "Little Drops of Water Make the Mighty Ocean," 22 July 1918, One-Minute Food Talks, folder "Indiana," box 13, series 6H, States Administration, USFA Collection, Hoover Institution.

62. "Are You a Slacker in Your Kitchen," typed article, 1, folder "L-M 87 Nov. 1," box 301, RG 4, NARA.

63. Farmer, *Catering for Special Occasions*, vii. See also Hoganson, *Consumers' Imperium*, 110–20.

64. Elizabeth Watson, "Why Food Conservation Is Necessary," USFA exhibit, December 1917, folder "Exhibit and Campaign Methods. John H. Cover," box 4, series 5H, USFA Collection, Hoover Institution.

65. Grammar original. Helen Dare, "Here's the Greatest Opportunity for Women in the History of the World," press release no. 438, 26 October 1918, 1–2, States Publicity Section, USFA Public Information Division, folder "Press Releases, States Section, Educational Division #400–470," box 10, USFA Collection, Hoover Library.

66. Lou Henry Hoover, "Mrs. Hoover Writes of Relief Work," *The Examiner*, 1 January 1915, typed document, folder "January 1, 1915, Mrs. Hoover Writes of relief work," box 10, Hoover Library.

67. Emphasis added. Ray Wilbur, "Five Minute Speech for Movies, Etc.," n.d., folder "Dr. Wilbur. Speeches. Articles. Statements. Notes. I-1917," box 2, series 5H, USFA Collection, Hoover Institution.

68. "Most Extravagant" was originally capitalized. "Most Extravagant People on Earth," 22 January 1918, folder, "Hagerstown Globe News (MD)," box 557, RG 4, NARA; "Terms Food Rulers Lenient," 24 March 1918, folder "Cleveland Plaindealer News

(OH)," box 567, RG 4, NARA; Prof. Stoughton Holburn, "The Kitchen in England," 28 February 1918, folder "East Stroudsburg Press News (PA)," box 568, RG 4, NARA; "Tourists Criticize U.S. Food Waste," 17 June 1918, folder "Philadelphia Enquirer [*sic*] News No. 2 (PA)," box 568, RG 4, NARA; letter from Alonzo Taylor to Miss Stephenson, no place or first name given, duplicate, 25 May 1918, folder "Medical Questions," box 150, USFA Collection, Hoover Institution.

69. Frederic J. Haskin, "Lean Europe and Fat America," 1 June 1917, folder "Lexington Herald Editorials (KY)," box 535, RG 4, NARA; William Frederick Bigelow, "What the Editor Has to Say," *Good Housekeeping*, October 1917, folder "October 1917. What the editor has to say," box 13, Hoover Library; A. M. Thackara, "Agricultural Inducements in the Department Seine-et-Marne," from typed report marked "Confidential: The Food Situation in France," Paris, 1 July 1917, folder "Food Reports from A. M. Thackara, American Consul General, Paris," box 116, USFA Collection, Hoover Institution; "Doubling the Cheese Ration," press release no. 296, 27 May 1918, States Publicity Section, USFA Public Information Division, folder "Press Releases, States Section, Educational Division #250–299," box 9, USFA Collection, Hoover Library.

70. Defenses of rustic French cuisine had circulated in the United States since the 1870s, as Levenstein points out, but the wartime focus on aggressively unsophisticated French foods was unprecedented. Levenstein, *Revolution at the Table*, 11.

71. Americans have a long history of resisting French haute cuisine. Haley, *Turning the Tables*.

72. *Malone Cook Book*; "Win the War with Snails," 3 February 1918, folder "Dayton News Editorial (Ohio)," box 567, RG 4, NARA; "Eat the Cheap Rooster," press release for the women's pages of farm journals for week ending 2 February 1918, folder "Farm Journals Sections. Press Releases. 1918," box 41, series 12H, USFA Collection, Hoover Institution; letter from C. V. Ashburn, Southern Pacific Co., to USFA, 25 May 1918, folder "C 22 March 1," box 298, RG 4, NARA; letter from Edward Y. Breck, Pittsburgh, to USFA, 12 October 1917, folder "53 Breck, Edward Y.," box 299, RG 4, NARA.

73. Wilson, *Mrs. Wilson's Cook Book*.

74. Cora Moore, "Little French Dinners for a Week," 10 March 1918, folder "New York Tribune News No. 2 (NY)," box 566, RG 4, NARA; *Malone Cook Book*, 286.

75. Edward Penfield, "Will you help the women of France?," 1918, Prints and Photographs Division, LOC.

76. Harris Dickson, "Save and Serve with Hoover: What Will Feed Three Will Feed Four," *Collier's: The National Weekly*, ed. Mark Sullivan, 11 August 1917, 5, folder "Writings about Hoover," box 219, Hoover Collection, Hoover Institution.

77. Marian Bonsall Davis, "War-Time Pointers from French Wives," 21 June 1917, folder "New York Leslies' Weekly Edit (NY)," box 541, RG 4, NARA.

78. Letter from Mrs. Adell Foy, Berkeley, Calif., to Hoover, 29 May 1917, folder illegible, box 290, RG 4, NARA.

79. "Be a Little Hungry!," 2 January 1918, folder "Erie Herald News (PA)," box 568, RG 4, NARA.

80. "Vegetables a la Food Administration," 12 September 1918, folder "Portland Argus Editorial (ME)," box 556, RG 4, NARA; Cuniberti, *Practical Italian Recipes*, 3.

81. Jean Prescott Adams, "The Business of Being a Housewife," 6 September 1918, printed leaflet produced by Armour & Co., folder "22 Armour & Co. Feb. 1," box 298, RG 4, NARA; "How We Americans Eat," 4 February 1918, folder "Montgomery Advertiser Editorial (AL)," box 549, RG 4, NARA.

82. Bennett, *World's Food*, 242–43.

83. Soldiers' rations in World War I also echoed these national consumption figures. In 1918, rations for American soldiers provided almost 3,800 calories, French soldiers received almost 3,500, British soldiers received about 3,000, Italian soldiers got 2,700, and German soldiers received a relatively measly 2,300. Legendre, *Alimentation et ravitaillement*, 95–96; Flour et al., *Changing Body*, 314.

84. Vernon Kellogg, "Herbert Hoover, as Individual and Type," *The Atlantic*, March 1918, box 219, Hoover Collection, Hoover Archives.

85. Ray Wilbur, speech at University Club of Los Angeles, 18 January 1918, folder "Dr. Wilbur. Speeches. Articles. Statements. Notes. II-1918," box 2, series 5H, USFA Collection, Hoover Institution; Harris Dickson, "Save and Serve with Hoover: What Will Feed Three Will Feed Four," *Collier's: The National Weekly*, ed. Mark Sullivan, 11 August 1917, 5, folder "Writings about Hoover," box 219, Hoover Collection, Hoover Institution.

86. "A Woman's War Pictures," no. 6, 28 November 1917, States Publicity Section, USFA Public Information Division, folder "Press Releases, States Section, Educational Division #1–99," box 9, USFA Collection, Hoover Library.

87. "The Week's Food Fact," 28 December 1917, folder "St. Cloud Journal Press Edit (MN)," box 538, RG 4, NARA.

88. "Help the Little People of France," *The Union Signal* 43, no. 37 (27 September 1917): 16; "Help for 1,000,000 Underfed Belgian Children," April 1917[?], typed document, folder "Belgium," box 89, USFA Collection, Hoover Archives.

89. Letter from the Morain, Ministre de l'Interieur, Bordeaux, to the Prefects of France, 24 November 1914, folder "Cadeaux offerts par le gouvernement Américain à l'occasion de Noël," 203 M 212, ADM.

90. "A Queer Welcome Home," *National School Service* 1, no. 7, Special Food Conservation Number, 1 December 1918, folder "FA I-A/Annual Report, 1918. Report to Feb. 1918; Food Program for 1919," box 1, USFA Collection, Hoover Library.

91. Costigliola, *Awkward Dominion*, 42; Hoover, *Memoirs of Herbert Hoover*, 321.

92. Hoover, "Bind the Wounds of France," typed text of article for *National Geographic*, May 1917, folder "Addresses, Letters, Magazine Articles, Press Statements, Etc. Inclusive Dates: February 1, 1917–April 6, 1918," box 93, Hoover Collection, Hoover Institution.

93. Emphasis original. Hoover, "The Weapon of Food," *National Geographic*, September 1917, 197, folder "September 1917. The weapon of food," box 13, USFA Collection, Hoover Library.

94. "The American Weapon," 17 July 1917, folder, "Boston Post Edit (MA)," box 537, RG 4, NARA; "Starvation Is Weapon to Win War, Declares U.S. Food Controller," 20 September 1917, folder "Sacramento Bee News (CA)," box 531, RG 4, NARA; "Famine Will Win War, Says Hoover," 20 September 1917, folder "San Francisco Examiner News (CA)," box 531, RG 4, NARA.

95. Offer, *First World War*, 54; Bonzon and Davis, "Feeding the Cities," 324; "Germany Becomes Hungrier Each Day," 17 June 1918, folder "Philadelphia Public Ledger News No. 3 (PA)," box 569, RG 4, NARA; "German Food Substitutes," 7 February 1918, folder "Rockland Courier Gazette News (ME)," box 556, RG 4, NARA; "German Government to Seize All Food," *Boston Daily Globe*, 16 August 1917, 9, PQHN.

96. Offer, *First World War*, 59–60.

97. Inflation was another scourge, and by the fall of 1917 food prices in Germany were four to five times higher than those in the United States. "Food Prices in Germany— September 1917," bulletin no. 555, 3 January 1918, folder "FA I-A/Statistical Department Information Service, Bulletins #400–569, 1917–1918 Incomplete," box 3, USFA Collection, Hoover Library.

98. Offer, *First World War*, 63.

99. Bonzon and Davis, "Feeding the Cities," 316.

100. Offer, *First World War*, 66.

101. Ibid., 54–55; Allen, "Sharing Scarcity," 373; Erich Dombrowski, "The Starveling's Belt—The Pause Before the Harvest," 22, from the *Berlin Tagelblatt*, Official Statement of the USFA, no. 5, 1 October 1918, folder "FA I-A/Official Statements #1–18, 1918–1919," box 2, USFA Collection, Hoover Library.

102. Contemporaries estimated that the German population lost a collective half million tons of body weight. Offer, *First World War*, 31–33; Allen, "Sharing Scarcity," 380–81.

103. American newspapers publicized the fact that Germans supplemented their official rations with black market purchases, and some disapprovingly referred to it as "crooked" or "illegal trading." "Germany Gets Food by Crooked Means," 18 September 1918, folder "Philadelphia Public Ledger News No. 3 (PA)," box 569, RG 4, NARA.

104. "Cutting Germany in Two," 15 September 1918, folder "New York Tribune News No. 2 (NY)," box 566, RG 4, NARA.

105. "Indian Warfare Revived," 13 August 1917, folder "Des Moines Register News (IA)," box 535, RG 4, NARA.

106. Ruth Dennen, "Germans' Hooverizing Instinct Aid in War," December 1917, folder "Los Angeles Express News (CA)," box 530, RG 4, NARA.

107. "Russians Starving, Reason," 13 March 1918, from *The Huntington Journal*, folder "Pennsylvania Miscellaneous," box 570, RG 4, NARA. The Allies actually sent thousands of propaganda leaflets titled "Slow Starvation" over the lines to inform German soldiers that civilians back home were gradually starving. Bruntz, *Allied Propaganda*, 161–62.

108. Offer, *First World War*, 59–60; "Children Starved to Feed Soldiers," 27 August 1917, folder "New York World News (NY)," box 543, RG 4, NARA.

109. Will Irwin, "The Babes of Belgium," in *The Need of Belgium*, 3d ed. (New York: The Commission for Relief in Belgium, n.d.), Beinecke Library, Yale University, New Haven, Conn.

110. Hoover, "To All Who Have Co-operated in the Work of the United States Food Administration," in "Information for Speakers: Conservation Week for World Relief," 1 December 1918, USFA for California, folder "California," box 12, series 6H, USFA Collection, Hoover Institution.

111. Letter from Martha Van Renssalaer, D.C., to Home Conservation Workers, 11 November 1918, folder "54," box 17, NYSCHER.

112. "A Nation Prepared," 15 November 1918, folder "Toledo Blade Editorial (OH)," box 567, RG 4, NARA.

113. "After Hoover What?," 20 November 1918, folder, "Greensburg Tribune Editorial (PA)," box 568, RG 4, NARA; "The Hungry World," 29 November 1918, folder "Waterbury American Editorial (CT)," box 550, RG 4, NARA.

114. Hoover, introduction to Mullendore, *History of the United States Food Administration*, 35–36.

115. "Food Questions and Answers," bulletin, "Information for Speakers: Conservation Week for World Relief," 1 December 1918, USFA for California, folder "California," box 12, series 6H, USFA Collection, Hoover Institution.

116. Hoover quoted in press release no. 463, 20 November 1918, States Publicity Section, USFA Public Information Division, folder "Press Releases, States Section, Educational Division #400–470," box 10, USFA Collection, Hoover Library.

117. Offer, *First World War*, 393–94; Surface, *American Food*, 9. See also Vincent, *Politics of Hunger*.

118. Hoover, *Memoirs of Herbert Hoover: Years of Adventure*, 321.

119. Hoover, "Why We Are Feeding Germany—Press Statement," 21 March 1919, folder "Addresses, Letters, Magazine Articles, Press Statements, Etc. Inclusive Dates: April 30, 1918–September 16, 1919," box 93, Hoover Collection, Hoover Institution.

120. More then twenty years later, Hoover disavowed his position and claimed to have wanted almost immediate dissolution of the Food Administration in the name of limited government: "The return of business to normal was imperative and the reduction of national expenditure essential. Of even more importance was the fact that all these measures, while necessary to enable the prosecution of the war, became in peace a strangulation of initiative and would burden the country with bureaucracy." Hoover, introduction to Mullendore, *History of the United States Food Administration*, 34–35. For more on the American Relief Administration, see Patenaude, *Big Show in Bololand*.

121. Offer, *First World War*, 390.

122. Offer argues that Germans saw the postarmistice blockade as profoundly unjust, and it allowed them to "nurture a self-righteous dream of revenge. That is how the agrarian outcomes of one great war became the origins of the next" (ibid., 395).

123. Hoover, introduction to Mullendore, *History of the United States Food Administration*, 12.

124. "It Does Us Good," 31 October 1917, folder "Wichita Eagle Edit (KS)," box 535, RG 4, NARA.

125. Herman Bernstein, "Herbert Hoover: The Man Who Brought America to the World," *McClure's Magazine*, September 1919, box 219, Hoover Collection, Hoover Institution.

126. Victoria De Grazia argues that U.S. hegemony was forged in Europe, not in America, and that it was forged by diffuse habits of mass consumption, not by military might. De Grazia, *Irresistible Empire*, 4–6. See also Fein, "Culture across Borders." During Hoover's presidential campaign a decade later, one supporter claimed that Hoover

introduced the very idea of social welfare to Europe. Kathleen Norris, "A Woman Looks at Hoover," *Collier's*, 5 May 1928, 8, box 221, Hoover Collection, Hoover Institution.

127. "The Hungry Must Be Fed," 13 November 1918, folder "Philadelphia Public Ledger Editorial (PA)," box 569, RG 4, NARA.

128. "India's Famine Worst for Century," 17 January 1919, folder "Philadelphia Public Ledger Editorial (PA)," box 569, RG 4, NARA.

129. Persia was officially neutral in the war, and representatives of the U.S. government expressed the country's goodwill to Persia, but in practice the United States "did almost nothing to provide relief for the famine or to help maintain the integrity of the nation. When the Persian government in 1918 asked the U.S. for a loan of $2,000,000 to be used solely for famine relief, Washington refused on the grounds that loans were only to be given to governments engaged in war with Germany." Some Americans did help to organize private relief organizations to Persia. Ghaneabassiri, "U.S. Foreign Policy in Persia," 162–63. See also Majd, *Great Famine and Genocide in Persia*.

130. Ahlberg, *Transplanting the Great Society*; Cullather, *Hungry World*.

CHAPTER FOUR

1. Spelling original. Letter from F. W. Burnener, Wheeling, W.V., to J. C. [*sic*] Schurman, Ithaca, N.Y., 12 February 1912, folder 26, box 33, NYSCHER. Cornell's president's name was actually J. G. Schurman.

2. Letter from Percival Bailey, Richland, N.Y., to Cornell Domestic Science Department, 5 September 1918, folder "N-S 38 Nov. 1," box 298, RG 4, NARA.

3. Emphasis added. Letter from Martha Van Renssalaer to Percival Bailey, 18 September 1918, folder "N-S 38 Nov. 1," box 298, RG 4, NARA.

4. Before the twentieth century, the single most common paid job for women was domestic service. Kessler-Harris, *Out to Work*, 71, 258; Norton and Alexander, "Women Work and Work Culture," 260; Fritschner, *Rise and Fall of Home Economics*, 224–25. See also Kessler-Harris, *Gendering Labor History*; Cowan, *More Work for Mother*; Boris and Daniels, *Homework*; and Goldin, *Understanding the Gender Gap*.

5. Glenna Matthews discusses the importance of the managerial housewife in the mid-nineteenth century, revitalized in that era by the idea of separate spheres. Matthews, *"Just a Housewife"*; Beecher, *Treatise on Domestic Economy*; White, *Beecher Sisters*, 43–44; Holland, "Lydia Maria Child," 159. Other works, like William A. Alcott's 1837 *Young Housekeeper* and Joseph and Laura Lyman's 1867 *The Philosophy of House-Keeping* rehearsed what would become the central themes of the home economics movement.

6. Katzman, *Seven Days a Week*, 223. See also Ryan, *Love, Wages, Slavery*; Palmer, *Domesticity and Dirt*; Dudden, *Serving Women*; and Sutherland, *Americans and their Servants*.

7. See Ryan, *Love, Wages, Slavery*.

8. Purdy, *Food and Freedom*, ii.

9. Pattison, "Scientific Management in Home-Making," 96; Cocroft, *What to Eat and When*, 185; Sutherland, *Americans and Their Servants*.

10. "Where Cooks Go," 430.

11. Deutsch, *Women and the City*, 66.

12. Similarly, writing about the Civil War era, the historian Drew Gilpin Faust clarifies that claims about the helplessness of southern belles went beyond performative femininity, because elite southern women who had grown up surrounded by slaves genuinely lacked knowledge about how to carry out even the simplest domestic tasks. Faust, *Mothers of Invention*, 78.

13. Unlike many women whose servants left them, Griffin fired her servants herself because they refused to follow food conservation guidelines, and she planned to hire new servants the next day. "Ousts Servants Who Spurn Food Cards," 30 October 1917, folder "New York Times News (NY)," box 541, RG 4, NARA.

14. Harvey Levenstein argues that home economics flourished in large part because it seemed to offer a solution to the servant problem. Levenstein, *Revolution at the Table*, 60–71.

15. Buell, "Household Adjustment," 94.

16. Cocroft, *What to Eat and When*, 185.

17. Stigler, *Domestic Servants in the United States*, 28–29.

18. Nye, *Electrifying America*, 16. See also Strasser, *Never Done*, and Fox, "Selling the Mechanized Household."

19. "Don't Be a Machine," 10 February 1918, folder "Augusta Herald News (GA)," box 553, RG 4, NARA; De Grazia, *Irresistible Empire*, 437; Du Vall, *Domestic Technology*, 443, 449.

20. "How to Choose a Vacuum Cleaner," The Hoover Suction Sweeping Company (New Berlin, Ohio: ca. 1917–18), folder "Mag-May Correspondence," box 147, USFA Collection, Hoover Institution; Harvey Wiley, "What Does the Housewife Get out of the Eight Hour Law?," January 1917, folder "Jan. 1917," box 163, Harvey Wiley Papers, LOC.

21. On the bottom of a letter endorsing the Hoover vacuum on behalf of the Massachusetts State Federation of Women's Clubs, an anonymous handwritten comment read: "Pretty cheap business for Mr. Hoover to let his name be attached to these kinds of business propositions." Reproduction of letter from Florence Perkins to the Hoover Suction Sweeper Co., n.d., folder "Mag-May Correspondence," box 147, USFA Collection, Hoover Institution.

22. See Bederman, *Manliness & Civilization*.

23. Emphasis added. Wilbur, typed text of article for *Ladies' Home Journal*, 4[?] June 1917, folder "Dr. Wilbur. Speeches. Articles. Statements. Notes. I-1917," box 2, series 5H, USFA Collection, Hoover Institution; Pattison, "Scientific Management in Home-Making," 97.

24. Report on a trip to Philadelphia to visit Pennsylvania Food Administration, n.a., folder 42, box 17, NYSCHER; Louise Arnold, "Learning the Lesson of Food Conservation," *The Journal of Home Economics* 10, no. 6 (June 1918), American Home Economics Association, folder "Number of the *Journal of Home Economics*, June 1918," box 5, series 5H, USFA Collection, Hoover Institution.

25. Buell, "Household Adjustment," 94. In one story about a disorganized middle-class household, the ignorant but intelligent Mrs. Barry turns out to be an "apt pupil" while her servant is hopelessly dim. "The Visiting Housekeeper," *Good Housekeeping*, September 1911, 391–93.

26. Mennell, *All Manners of Food*, 230–31.

27. Berlage, "Establishment of an Applied Social Science," 333.

28. Levenstein, *Revolution at the Table*, 96.

29. "American Womanhood Is Preparing for Big Task," 11 February 1918, folder "Birmingham Ledger News (AL)," box 549, RG 4, NARA.

30. For more on the home economics movement, see Goldstein, *Creating Consumers*; Elias, *Stir It Up*; Rutherford, *Selling Mrs. Consumer*; Berlage, "Establishment of an Applied Social Science"; Hoganson, *Consumers' Imperium*; Biltekoff, *Hidden Hunger*; Stage and Vincenti, *Rethinking Home Economics*; Leavitt, *From Catharine Beecher to Martha Stewart*; Goldstein, "From Service to Sales"; Mennell, *All Manners of Food*; and Weigley, "It Might Have Been Euthenics."

31. Text of card from Mary Lowell Stone Exhibit, traveling home economics exhibit, ca. 1902, quoted in Weigley, "It Might Have Been Euthenics," 94.

32. Pattison, "Scientific Management in Home-Making," 97; Curtis, *Mrs. Curtis's Cook Book*, 1.

33. Rose quoted in Flora Rose, Esther Stocks, and Michael Whittier, *A Growing College: Home Economics at Cornell* (Ithaca, N.Y.: Cornell University Press, 1969), 73–74, in Berlage, "Establishment of an Applied Social Science," 194.

34. Belasco, "Food Matters," 7.

35. Jean Prescott Adams, "The Business of Being a Housewife," 6 September 1918, printed leaflet produced by Armour & Co., folder "22 Armour & Co. Feb. 1," box 298, RG 4, NARA; "Care of Children," Home Demonstration in Care and Feeding of a Normally Well Child, no. 276, 2–3, Department of Home Economics, Cornell University, 1919[?], folder 2, box 18, NYSCHER.

36. "Common-Sense and Our Daily Bread," 9 February 1918, *The Bellman*, folder "Common-Sense and Our Daily Bread," box 14, Hoover Library.

37. Preston, *Fatal Years*.

38. Berlage, "Establishment of an Applied Social Science."

39. "The Visiting Housekeeper," *Good Housekeeping*, September 1911, 393; "War Inventions," 19 August 1917, folder "NY Tribune Editorial (NY)," box 541, RG 4, NARA.

40. Cullather, "Foreign Policy of the Calorie."

41. "Woman Puts Housekeeping on List of Professions," *Christian Science Monitor*, 30 January 1915, 8, PQHN.

42. Heath, "Work of the Housewives League," 123–26; Food Conservation Notes, no. 9, 25 May 1918, folder "FA-II/Food Conservation Notes," box 8, USFA Collection, Hoover Library.

43. Other professional-style manuals included ones like *Library of Home Economics*; Pattison, *Principles of Domestic Engineering*; MacLeod, *Housekeeper's Handbook of Cleaning*; Fisher, *Twenty Lessons in Domestic Science*; Holt, *Complete Housekeeper*; Donham, *Marketing and Housework Manual*; and Balderston, *Housewifery*.

44. Green, *Effective Small Home*, 114–15.

45. "Managing a Household Efficiently," *New York Times*, 13 January 1915, SM6, PQHN.

46. Pattison, "Scientific Management in Home-Making"; Lancaster, *Making Time*.

47. See Wiebe, *Search for Order*.

48. Kessler-Harris, *Out to Work*, 116.

49. Eliza W. M. Bridges, "A Plea for Disorder," letter to the editor, "The Family Conference," *Good Housekeeping*, March 1911, 373–76, 374.

50. "Graphic Exhibits on Food Conservation at Fairs & Exhibition," USFA bulletin, September 1917, 47, folder "Exhibit and Campaign Methods. John H. Cover," box 4, series 5H, USFA Collection, Hoover Institution; abstract of unsigned memo to Ray Wilbur, 20 July 1917, folder "How the People of the Country Criticize the Policies of the Food Administration," box 3, series 5H, USFA Collection, Hoover Institution.

51. Photographs, folder "Miscellaneous Illustrations," box 5, series 5H, Home Conservation Division, USFA Collection, Hoover Institution.

52. "Uniforms for Housewives," 26 June 1917, folder "Savannah News Editorials (GA)," box 533, RG 4, NARA.

53. For instance, in a typical short story from 1915, a young married woman named Mollie thinks of cooking as "fun" and longs to do it, but her millionaire husband forbids her to do such "servant's work." Things change when her husband's aristocratic English relatives visit and the servant-cooked meals are disastrously bad. Secretly and "blissfully," Mollie begins to cook herself, producing delectable meals that amaze her husband's aunt, a haughty duchess. The story ends with the revelation that it is Mollie who has been doing the cooking, and with the approving duchess praising the "intellect" needed to cook well. Mabel S. Merrill, "The Pie of Her Dreams," *American Cookery*, March 1915, 592–95; "Sacrifices Today and in the '60s," 26 October 1917, folder "Columbia State News (SC)," box 547, RG 4, NARA.

54. "Cooking for the Fun of It," 3 February 1918, folder "Youngstown Vindicator Edit (OH)," box 567, RG 4, NARA; "Fun in the Kitchen," February 1918, folder "Cleveland Plaindealer Edit (OH)," box 567, RG 4, NARA.

55. In the late 1920s, Martha Van Renssalaer wrote to Carrie Chapman Catt, who had asked about the possibility of devising a system to compensate housewives for their work. Van Renssalaer acknowledged that compensation was important, but she said that most people with salaries had very little money left after paying for their clothing, food, and housing—and didn't the housewife get these things anyway? She also said that housewives received a "psychic income" in the form of satisfaction and family love that sufficed for compensation. Letter from Van Renssalaer, Ithaca, N.Y., to Carrie Chapman Catt, New Rochelle, N.Y., 23 June 1928, folder 25, box 33, NYSCHER.

56. Letter from Van Renssalaer, D.C., to Mrs. Iris Bassett Coville, Doylestown, Pa., 10 September 1918, folder "H-I 85 Mar. 1," box 301, Home Conservation Division, General Office, General Correspondence, April–August 1917, RG 4, NARA.

57. Gilman, "Housekeeper and the Food Problem." In her 1903 book *The Home: Its Work and Influence*, Gilman had urged Americans to banish "primitive industries" like cooking from their homes. See "The Ideal Home," reprinted from *New York Times*, 26 December 1903, K3, in Karpinski, *Critical Essays*; and Allen, *Building Domestic Liberty*. For more on Gilman, see also Rudd and Gough, *Charlotte Perkins Gilman*; Davis, *Charlotte Perkins Gilman*; and Allen, *Feminism of Charlotte Perkins Gilman*.

58. Gilman, "Housekeeper and the Food Problem," 125–28; "Feminist Dooms 'Home Cooking': Mrs. Gilman Says 'Liberate Wives and Professionalize Housework,'" *New-York Tribune*, 12 March 1914, 9, PQHN; Allen, *Building Domestic Liberty*, 69.

59. Matthews, *"Just a Housewife,"* 97–98. See also Levenstein, *Revolution at the Table*, and Hayden, *Grand Domestic Revolution*.

60. Bellamy, *Looking Backward*.

61. "Now It's a Hot Meal by Auto," 27 December 1917, folder "NY Evening Sun News (NY)," box 541, RG 4, NARA.

62. Levenstein, *Revolution at the Table*, 50–55.

63. "Says Home Baking Causes Serious Waste," 19 November 1917, folder "Scranton Scrantonian Edit (RI)," box 547, RG 4, NARA.

64. "Resume of Important Rulings and Letters Sent to Federal Food Administrators, July 1–15," folder "FA I-A/Resume of Important Rulings, for district & county Administrators, April-Aug. 1918," box 3, USFA Collection, Hoover Library; "Britain's National Kitchens," 7 June 1918, folder "Philadelphia Bulletin News (PA)," box 568, RG 4, NARA.

65. Letter from Helen Atwater to Vernon Kellogg, 25 June 1918, folder "Dr. Vernon Kellogg #4 (2)," box 58, series 27H, USFA Collection, Hoover Institution; memo from Van Renssalaer to conservation workers, 30 November 1918, folder 54, box 17, NYSCHER.

66. Typed report, 2 December 1918, folder 54, box 17, NYSCHER.

67. Food Conservation Notes, folder "FA-II/Food Conservation Notes," box 8, USFA Collection, Hoover Library.

68. "Now It's a Hot Meal by Auto," 27 December 1917, folder "NY Evening Sun News (NY)," box 541, RG 4, NARA. Designed with the servant problem in mind, the American Cooked Food Service Company had planned to provide food for a few hundred families, but within months of opening, company officials were overwhelmed with 2,000 subscription requests. The service also claimed to adhere to all Food Administration guidelines. "Complete Cooked Meals Brought to Your Door," *New York Times*, 28 July 1918, 54, PQHN.

69. Wilma Wilcox, "Futurist Domestic Science Will Improve Home Control," 7 November 1917, folder "Lansing State Journal Editorial (MI)," box 538, RG 4, NARA.

70. E. K. Wolley, "Housewifery vs. Stenography," *Boston Daily Globe*, 7 April 1915, 12, PQHN.

71. Wilma Wilcox, "Futurist Domestic Science Will Improve Home Control," 7 November 1917, folder "Lansing State Journal Editorial (MI)," box 538, RG 4, NARA.

72. Ryan, *Love, Wages, Slavery*, 1. The familial rhetoric was part of the impetus behind familial honorifics for slaves and free African Americans like "Aunt" and "Uncle."

73. Ryan, *Love, Wages, Slavery*.

74. Grammar original. Letter from Mrs. Ada M. Buxton, D.C., to Hoover, 12 July 1917, folder illegible, box 288, RG 4, NARA.

75. Rossiter, *Women Scientists in America*, 120.

76. Program for "Agricultural War Dinner," 12 January 1918, folder 62, box 17, NYSCHER.

77. Shapiro, *Perfection Salad*, 206.

78. Experiment sheets for "Cereal Flour Muffins," folder 46, box 17, NYSCHER; report, unsigned and undated but on official USFA stationery, folder 43, box 17, NYSCHER.

79. Members of Committee on Home Economics, folder "Advisory Committee on Home Economics," box 3, series 5H, USFA Collection, Hoover Institution; "Resume

of Important Rulings and Letters Sent to Federal Food Administrators August 15th to September 1st," folder "FA I-A/Resume of Important Rulings, for district & county Administrators, April–Aug. 1918," box 3, USFA Collection, Hoover Library.

80. Spelling original. Copy of letter from Hoover to Departments of Home Economics in the Colleges and Universities, n.d., folder "Collegiate Section (after Oct 1, 1918 the School and College Section)," box 40, series 12H, USFA Collection, Hoover Institution.

81. Linn Ball, painting, from Exhibit Sent to State and County Fairs by USFA, Summer 1918, folder "Press Releases 1–1400," box 42, series 12H, USFA Collection, Hoover Institution.

82. Emphasis added. Untitled article, 19 January 1918, folder "Baltimore Star News (MD)," box 556, RG 4, NARA.

83. Alice Chittenden, quoted in George MacAdam, "Getting Behind Hoover in the Kitchen," *New York Times Magazine*, 17 June 1917, folder illegible, box 296, RG 4, NARA.

84. Letter from Charles H. Armstrong, Shelbyville, Tenn., to Hoover, 25 June 1917, folder illegible, box 288, RG 4, NARA; "Some Suggestions in Regard to Food Conservation," typed memo from R. F. Campbell, Asheville, N.C., 6 August 1917, folder illegible, box 289, RG 4, NARA.

85. Abstract of letter from Cally Ryland, Richmond, Va., to USFA, folder "R 30, 31," box 328, RG 4, NARA.

86. "Feeding the Fighting Men," 1 November 1917, folder "Birmingham News Edit (AL)," box 529, RG 4, NARA.

87. While administrators invoked images of women as competent state actors, they also created ominous images of the New Woman as a "pleasure-seeking sugar consumer" (Merleaux, "Sweet Innocence").

88. Letter from South Dakota farm woman to Hoover, folder 37, box 288, RG 4, NARA.

89. Letter from El Paso farm woman to Hoover, folder 11, box 288, RG 4, NARA.

90. Letter from Helen Moore, Milwaukee, Wisc., to USFA, 25 January 1918, folder 41, box 17, NYSCHER.

91. See Bentley, *Eating for Victory*, 5.

92. Letter from Mrs. Helen Dortch Longstreet, D.C., to Hoover, 30 July 1917, folder "HI—225," box 292, RG 4, NARA.

93. Cynthia Enloe argues that nationalism has often been empowering for women, despite the limited roles to which it tended to consign them. Enloe, *Bananas, Beaches & Bases*, 61.

94. Rose, *Everyday Foods in War Time*, 12.

95. Goudiss and Goudiss, *Foods That Will Win the War*, 33.

96. "Food Fillers," press release for farm journals for week ending 5 August 1918, folder "Farm Journals Sections. Press Releases. 1918," box 41, series 12H, USFA Collection, Hoover Institution; Pennybacker, "What Our Country Asks of Its Young Women." Amy Bentley writes that even as the food campaigns of World War II likewise made "the family dinner . . . a weapon of war, and the kitchen a woman's battlefront," the campaigns also "perpetuated stereotypical notions of gender by maintaining segregated

'gendered spaces' and portraying women as subordinates whose primary duty was to cook and serve food" (*Eating for Victory*, 5).

97. Its editor, Sarah Splint, was a home economist who later served as co-chief of the Home Conservation Division in the Food Administration. The magazine kept the title until May 1927. "Today's Housewife," LOC.

98. "Home woman" was from Bertha Baur, "Why American Women of German Descent Should Vote for Hoover," *The Progressive Magazine*, 1928, box 221, folder "Writings about Hoover," Hoover Collection, Hoover Institution; J. W. Sullivan, "The Bread Problem in the Food Administration," report to Samuel Gompers, March 1918, folder "The Bread Problem in the Food Administration," box 64, series 33H, USFA Collection, Hoover Institution. "House-mother" was from Hitchcock, "Relation of the Housewife to the Food Problem." "Householder," more or less a literal translation of "husband," an Old English word meaning the master or holder of a house, appeared especially frequently in Food Administration documents. USFA press release no. 610, 29 January 1918, folder "New York—Rationing," box 18, series 6H, States Division, USFA Collection, Hoover Institution; "Rules for Householders," USFA, 11 June 1918, folder 9, box 1, series 5H, USFA Collection, Hoover Institution; "Present Food Regulations for Householders Briefly Stated," Federal Food Administrator for New York State, bulletin no. 25, 8 April 1918, folder "New York, Bulletins 4–100," box 15, series 6H, USFA Collection, Hoover Institution. Among other places, "house manager" appeared in one propaganda poster by Charles Dana Gibson, creator of the turn-of-the-century Gibson Girls. See Charles Dana Gibson, illustrated postcard, created by Kream Krisp shortening, 23 February 1918, folder 9, box 1, series 5H, USFA Collection, Hoover Institution. "Home manager" was a variation on this term, appearing, for example, in Mrs. Alice Gitchell Kirk, "Buying Food Is Home Manager's Problem," February [?] 1918, folder "Cleveland Plaindealer News (OH)," box 567, RG 4, NARA.

99. Letter from J. A. Derome, Sioux Falls, S.D., to Hoover, 7 August 1917, folder illegible, box 289, RG 4, NARA.

100. "Rice," USFA press release no. 90, 21 January 1918, States Publicity Section, USFA Public Information Division, folder "Press Releases, States Section, Educational Division #1–99," box 9, USFA Collection, Hoover Library; "Plenty of Corn—Save It by Eating It," no author, Official Food Bulletin, USFA for California, no. 13, San Francisco, 25 June 1918, folder "Dr. Wilbur. Speeches. Articles. Statements. Notes. II-1918," box 2, series 5H, USFA Collection, Hoover Institution; *The Blade*, spoof paper from Educational Division of USFA, 13 December 1918, folder "Ben S. Allen. Memoranda for Mr. Rickard 'Week ending' 6 April–25 May 1918," box 39, series 12H, USFA Collection, Hoover Institution.

101. Abstract of unsigned letter to Hoover, 13 August 1917, folder "U 37," box 328, Home Conservation Division, General Office, Abstracts of Letters on Food Conservation & Pledge Card Campaign, RG 4, NARA.

102. Emphasis original. "Enumeration and Classification of Occupations at the Thirteenth Census," U.S. 1910 Census of Population and Housing, accessed online. The 1930 census changed the wording only enough to stress, peevishly, that this confusion between housewives, housekeepers, and other servants had by then occurred for three consecutive decades. 1930 Census of Population and Housing, "Enumeration

and Classification of Occupations," 9, Ancestry Library Edition, accessed online. By 1940, however, the confusion seemingly became less acute. Neither the 1940 census nor any of the censuses that followed mentioned any confusion between housewives and servants.

103. "Huswife" dates back at least to the ninth century, and the modern spelling of "housewife" emerged in the eighteenth century. By contrast, "husband" kept its Old English prefix. Barnhart, *Barnhart Concise Dictionary of Etymology*, 362, 366. "Huswife" was the source of the word hussy, which originally meant just girl or woman and only became a derogatory term in the nineteenth century. *Oxford English Dictionary Online*, s.vv. "housewife, v.," "husband, v."

104. Letter from H. F. Merrill, Cambridge, Mass., to Hoover, July 1917, folder "HI-245," box 293, RG 4, NARA; unsigned letter to Ray Wilbur, n.d., "Dr. Ray Lyman Wilbur, 17 May–24 November 1917," folder 8, box 1, series 5H, USFA Collection, Hoover Institution.

105. Letter from Ray Wilbur to David Harvey, N.Y., 7 July 1917, folder illegible, box 291, RG 4, NARA.

106. H. E. Barnard, "War Restoring Kitchen to Its Pioneer Place as Center of Home," 16 January[?] 1918, folder "Chagrin Express News (OH)," box 566, RG 4, NARA.

107. Frederick Howe, paraphrased in Buell, "Household Adjustment," 98; Helen Guthrie Miller, "The Thrift Division of the Suffrage Army," National Suffrage News, New York: National American Woman Suffrage Association, 1917, folder illegible, box 296, RG 4, NARA.

108. Barker, *Wanted*, 5.

109. Kennedy, *Over Here*, 30.

110. Scott, *Natural Allies*, 124.

111. According to Wiley, the "feeding of man" would be the "great economic problem of the near future," and only the vote would enable American women to help solve it. Wiley, *Not by Bread Alone*, 15.

112. Letter from Ada L. James, Richland Center, Wisc., to Mina Van Winkle, D.C., 25 July 1917, folder illegible, box 292, RG 4, NARA.

113. Letter from Anna Brann, Chicago, to Hoover, 20 July 1917, folder illegible, box 288, RG 4, NARA.

114. Abstract of letter from Miss Mary T. Aiken, Witherby Farm, Mass., to USFA, 30 July 1917, folder "How the People of the Country Criticize the Policies of the Food Administration," box 3, series 5H, USFA Collection, Hoover Institution; letter from Mrs. Anna M. Veit, Philadelphia, to Hoover, 12 July 1917, folder illegible, box 296, RG 4, NARA.

115. Letter from Harriet Stanton Blatch, N.Y., to Ray Wilbur, 6 July 1917, folder illegible, box 288, RG 4, NARA; list of volunteers in leadership positions for the Food Conservation Department, n.d., folder illegible, box 288, RG 4, NARA; "Lecture on Food Conservation and Thrift," printed leaflet, May 1917, folder illegible, box 296, RG 4, NARA.

116. Letter from Carrie Chapman Catt to Mina Van Winkle, 3 July 1917, folder illegible, box 288, RG 4, NARA; letter from Laura Clay, Lexington, Ky., to Mina Van Winkle, 12 July 1917, folder illegible, box 296, RG 4, NARA.

117. Letter to Gertrude Lane from Rose Young, N.Y., 4 August 1917, folder illegible, box 296, RG 4, NARA.

118. The connection between women's work with food and women's political rights was not unprecedented. In 1915, for example, a suffrage organization in Pennsylvania had published *The Suffrage Cook Book*, with recipes like "pie for a suffragist's doubting husband," in part to demonstrate that woman suffrage was not as radical a prospect as it might seem. Its contributors included Jane Addams, Anna Shaw, Julia Lathrop, and Charlotte Perkins Gilman, among others. See *Suffrage Cook Book*. After the war and the passage of the Nineteenth Amendment granting woman suffrage, the Virginia League of Women Voters produced a cookbook designed to demonstrate the league's "interest in the question of Food Supply and Demand" and the fact that "the woman voter is none the less the efficient housewife" (*Virginia Cookery Book*, 11).

119. Adams and Keene, *Alice Paul*, 157–214.

120. "Suffrage Address Made by Dr. Harvey W. Wiley," clipping from the *Richmond Times-Dispatch*, 4 April 1918, folder "1918," box 179, Harvey Wiley Papers, LOC.

121. "Comments on Women' [*sic*] Prisoners' Fare at Occoquan Workhouse," attached to letter from Katharine R. Fisher, D.C., to Wiley, 25 October 1917, folder "1917," box 125, Harvey Wiley Papers, LOC; letter from Harvey Wiley to Ulric Z. Wiley, Indianapolis, 15 November 1917, folder "1917," box 125, Harvey Wiley Papers, LOC; letter from Wiley to Honorable Lewis Brownlow, D.C., 25 November 1917, folder "1917," box 125, Harvey Wiley Papers, LOC; letter from Wiley to Mrs. Amos W. Walker, Chicago, 14 November 1917, folder "1917," box 125, Harvey Wiley Papers, LOC. "A Diet of Worms won one reformation," Wiley quipped in a public statement, "and I expect it will win another" (press release or copy of speech included in letter from Wiley to George M. Kober, 27[?] October 1917, folder "1917," box 125, Harvey Wiley Papers, LOC). As reports of the mistreatment of jailed suffragists made front-page headlines through the fall, national sympathy for the women mounted, predicated in part on the assumption that, as women, they were less able to endure physical distress. But many remained unsympathetic.

122. Original spelling. Letter from Mrs. Anna M. Veit, Philadelphia, to Hoover, D.C., 12 July 1917, folder illegible, box 296, RG 4, NARA; abstract of letter from Mrs. Kate Richards O'Hare, Ruskin, Fla., to USFA, n.d., folder "How the People of the Country Criticize the Policies of the Food Administration," box 3, series 5H, USFA Collection, Hoover Institution. O'Hare was arrested in July 1917 in North Dakota for making antiwar speeches and indicted under the Espionage Act. She was sentenced to five years, which she began serving in 1919, though her sentence was commuted in 1920. She later spent most of her energies on prison reform. See Miller, *From Prairie to Prison*.

123. Letter from Alice Hill Chittenden, N.Y.C., representing the N.Y. State Association Opposed to Woman Suffrage, to Hoover, 13 July 1917, folder illegible, box 296, RG 4, NARA; letter from Mrs. Ada M. Buxton, D.C., to Hoover, 12 July 1917, folder illegible, box 288, RG 4, NARA; letter from Mrs. Francis E. Day, Milwaukee, Wisc., to Wilson, 28 July 1917, folder illegible, box 289, RG 4, NARA.

124. Letter from Mrs. Agnes Bourelle, Richmond, Minn., to USFA, 3 September 1917, folder "41 Bourelle, Mrs. Agnes/Minn," box 299, RG 4, NARA; letter of reference for

Ruth Underhill White from Benjamin B. Lawrence to Edgar Rickard, D.C., 14 July 1917, folder illegible, box 296, RG 4, NARA; telegram from Mrs. Harold T. White, White Plains, N.Y., to Hoover, 14 July 1917, folder illegible, box 296, RG 4, NARA.

125. Chittenden, quoted in George MacAdam, "Getting Behind Hoover in the Kitchen," from *New York Times Magazine*, 17 June 1917, folder illegible, box 296, RG 4, NARA. Like other leading antisuffragists, of course, Chittenden condemned women for public speechifying and political meddling while doing essentially those same things herself.

126. "Anti-Suffragists Invite Men in Service to Piefest," 20 November 1917, folder "Boston Herald News (MA)," box 536, RG 4, NARA.

127. A. D. Condo, Everett True Cartoon, from unnamed Food Administration bulletin, folder "Cartoons," box 325, RG 4, NARA.

128. "Two Housewives, Which Is Right?," 8 November 1918, folder "Baltimore Sun Edit (MD)," box 557, RG 4, NARA.

129. For more on the complex motivations behind the antisuffrage campaign, see Camhi, *Women against Women*.

130. "Internal Management of Home Conservation Division," List of Food Conservation Staff, folder 53, box 17, NYSCHER.

131. Seaton Taylor Purdon, "Hooverist: Experiences of One Who Objects to Term Cook," 25 November 1917, folder "Macon Telegraph Edit (GA)," box 533, RG 4, NARA.

CHAPTER FIVE

1. "Throngs Enjoy Many Features at Traveler-Herald Food Show," 2 April 1918, folder "Boston Post News (MA)," box 557, RG 4, NARA; "Befo' the War Corn Recipes Demonstration," 22 January 1918, folder "Taunton Gazette News (MA)," box 537, RG 4, NARA.

2. "Befo' the War Corn Recipes Demonstration," 22 January 1918, folder "Taunton Gazette News (MA)," box 537, RG 4, NARA.

3. "Food Demonstration by Aunt Portia Smiley," 28 April 1918, folder "Providence Journal News (RI)," box 570, RG 4, NARA; Williams-Forson, *Building Houses out of Chicken Legs*, 80–113. Micki McElya demonstrates that affection for "Mammy" and other caricatures of devoted slaves, along with nostalgia for antebellum paternalism in general, was a powerful and growing force among white Americans in the late nineteenth and twentieth centuries. McElya, *Clinging to Mammy*.

4. "Food Demonstration by Aunt Portia Smiley," 28 April 1918, folder "Providence Journal News (RI)," box 570, RG 4, NARA.

5. Emphasis added. "Befo' the War Corn Recipes Demonstration," 22 January 1918, folder "Taunton Gazette News (MA)," box 537, RG 4, NARA.

6. "Throngs Enjoy Many Features at Traveler-Herald Food Show," 2 April 1918, folder "Boston Post News (MA)," box 557, RG 4, NARA.

7. Most of Smiley's demonstrations were "under the auspices" of local committees connected to the Food Administration or the Women's Committee of the Council on National Defense. "Food Demonstration by Aunt Portia Smiley," 28 April 1918, folder "Providence Journal News (RI)," box 570, RG 4, NARA.

8. L. Harper Leech, "War Diet Real Health Saver," October 1917, folder, "Waterloo Times Tribune News (IA)," box 535, RG 4, NARA.

9. Ward, "Eugenics, Euthenics, and Eudemics," 739. See also Kevles, *In the Name of Eugenics*; Dorr, *Segregation's Science*; Largent, *Breeding Contempt*; Dain, *Hideous Monster of the Mind*; Paul, *Politics of Heredity*; Pernick, *Black Stork*; and Cowan, *Sir Francis Galton*.

10. Ward, "Eugenics, Euthenics, and Eudemics," 737.

11. Mrs. Melvin Dewey, quoted in "A Better Race in the Making," *Los Angeles Times*, 11 January 1914, I4, PQHN.

12. Weigley, "It Might Have Been Euthenics"; Richards and Norton, *Cost of Food*, 9; Greer, *Food*, iii–iv.

13. Eaves, *Food of Working Women in Boston*, 3–4.

14. Hunger itself had propelled many migrants from Europe to the United States. The historian Hasia Diner argues that even what looked like a meager diet in the United States was plentiful by the standards of European poverty. Diner, *Hungering for America*, 10, 12.

15. Christian, "Food and Morality," 12, 9–10; Armitage, *Diet and Race*.

16. Cocroft, *What to Eat and When*, v; "Dr. Wiley Predicts German Race of Weaklings While Americans Become Strong," n.d., folder "Washington Herald News No. 2 (DC)," box 552, RG 4, NARA. However, others were sure that modern diets made people weak; one scientist argued that civilized people were eating so much soft, processed food that their unused jaws were visibly receding. "Wisdom Teeth Exception to Rule," *Washington Post*, 29 August 1915, C4, PQHN.

17. "Dr. Wiley Predicts German Race of Weaklings While Americans Become Strong," n.d., folder "Washington Herald News No. 2 (DC)," box 552, RG 4, NARA; "Registered as Human Thoroughbred," *Boston Daily Globe*, 27 August 1916, 38, PQHN.

18. Joseph T. Mannix, "Milling in China," *Weekly Northwestern Miller* 43, no. 26 (June 25, 1897), 946; "Negro Diet of Snakes: Queer Things Eaten in Region of Great Dismal Swamp," *Washington Post*, 5 August 1900, 13, PQHN.

19. Christian, "Food and Morality"; Armitage, *Diet and Race*, 17–23.

20. Macleod notes that popular convictions that white people needed meat exacerbated concerns about rising meat prices in this era. Macleod, "Food Prices," 376.

21. Luff, *Gout*, 247–48; Ritvo, *Platypus and the Mermaid*, 200.

22. "Wisdom Teeth Exception to Rule," *Washington Post*, 29 August 1915, C4, PQHN; Lorand, *Health through Rational Diet*, 374.

23. L. Harper Leech, "War Diet Real Health Saver," October 1917, folder "Waterloo Times Tribune News (IA)," box 535, RG 4, NARA; "American People Are Born Meat Eaters; They Miss It," 25 December 1917, folder "La Fayette Journal Edit (IN)," box 535, RG 4, NARA.

24. "Vegetarian Slackers," 1 August 1917, folder "Mobile Item Edit (AL)," box 529, RG 4, NARA; "Disproving Their Own Case," Topics of the Times, *New York Times*, 6 April 1916, 12, PQHN.

25. Brewster and Brewster, *Nutrition of a Household*.

26. "War*Time*Cook*Book," press release to farm journals, 1 December 1917, folder "Press Releases, to Farm Journals," box 12, USFA Collection, Hoover Library.

27. "Mexican Diet: Not Conductive to American Energy," *Christian Observer*, 14 October 1908, 17, PQHN; "Chinese Yellow Because of Food," *Boston Daily Globe*, 26 October 1924, 53, PQHN.

28. Lorand, *Health through Rational Diet*, 375.

29. Steiner quoted in "America Called 'God's Crucible,'" *Chicago Daily Tribune*, 25 November 1912, 13, PQHN; Gillett, *Food Primer for the Home*, 2, 4.

30. Hoganson, *Consumers' Imperium*, 133; "A Better Race in the Making," *Los Angeles Times*, 11 January 1914, I4, PQHN; Fisher, "Impending Problems of Eugenics," 219.

31. "Plan a Human Pedigree Book," *Washington Post*, 19 April 1914, M1, PQHN.

32. "Registered as Human Thoroughbred," *Boston Daily Globe*, 27 August 1916, 38, PQHN; "'End the Wild Oats Days of Men': Perfect Woman Gives Views on Eugenics," *Washington Post*, 28 January 1917, ES10, PQHN.

33. "A Better Race in the Making," *Los Angeles Times*, 11 January 1914, I4, PQHN.

34. Cocroft, *What to Eat and When*, vii, viii; Gillett, *Food Primer for the Home*, 2, 4.

35. Richards and Norton, *Cost of Food*, 9.

36. Tucker, "Distribution of Men Physically Unfit," 378–79.

37. McCann, *This Famishing World*, 21.

38. The writer was Paul Popenoe, the elder brother of the cat-eating Herbert Popenoe. Popenoe, *Applied Eugenics*, xi.

39. McCann, *This Famishing World*, 21; Love and Davenport, *Defects Found in Drafted Men*, 27, 28–29.

40. Dickson, *Food Front in World War I*, 18.

41. Harvey Wiley, "The Chemistry, Nutritive Value and Economy of Foods," lecture IV, Westbrook Free Lectureship, Philadelphia, March 1918, folder "1918," box 126, Harvey Wiley Papers, LOC.

42. "Rice the Food of Millions," press release for farm journals, n.d., folder "Farm Journals Section. Press Releases. Undated," box 41, series 12H, USFA Collection, Hoover Institution; Alonzo Taylor, reprinted speech, Hotel Astor, New York, 8 February 1918, printed pamphlet (Roanoke, Va.: Union Printing & Manufacturing Co., 1918), 4–5, folder "FA-II/Addresses by Grew, Merrill, Pearl, Smith, Taylor, Wilbur," box 7, USFA Collection, Hoover Library; Katherine Blunt, Frances L. Swain, and Florence Powdermaker, *Food Guide for War Service at Home*, Collegiate Section of the USFA (New York: Charles Scribner's Sons, 1918), folder "FA-II/Food Saving & Sharing, Food Guide (booklets)," box 8, USFA Collection, Hoover Library.

43. Wiley, "The Chemistry, Nutritive Value and Economy of Foods," Lecture IV, Westbrook Free Lectureship, Philadelphia, March 1918, folder "1918," box 126, Harvey Wiley Papers, LOC.

44. Phrasing original. "White-Bread for the Trenches," 4 February 1918, folder "Birmingham News News (AL)," box 549, RG 4, NARA.

45. Sir William Crookes, "Presidential Address on the Wheat-Supply of the World, the Latest Achievements of Science, and the Position of Psychical Research," *Lancet* (10 September 1898): 669–78, 670; Mendel, *Changes in the Food Supply*, 3.

46. Mrs. Frank J. Belot, "Requires 'Know-How' to Make Bread," clipping from unnamed Fort Wayne, Ind., paper, June 1918, folder "F-G 44 May," box 299, RG 4, NARA.

47. Charles Betts, "Wheat the Grain of Civilization," reprinted from *State Service* magazine, 42, November 1918, Albany, N.Y., folder "FA-IA/Bulletins, Notices, Zones, Instructions, Misc.," box 6, USFA Collection, Hoover Library.

48. "Rice," U.S. Food Leaflet no. 18, n.d., folder "Publications," box 5, series 5H, USFA Collection, Hoover Institution. See also McWilliams, *Revolution in Eating*, and Carney, *Black Rice*.

49. The Food Administration released inconsistent figures about domestic rice consumption, ranging from eight pounds per capita to over seventeen. "People Eat Rice," 19 October 1917, folder "San Francisco Retail Grocers Adv. Edit (CA)," box 531, RG 4, NARA.

50. About 361,000 acres were devoted to rice production in 1900; by 1920, U.S. acreage had jumped to 1,299,000. It would not reach that height again until the middle of World War II. "Rice, oats, sorghum, and soybeans-acreage, production, and price: 1866–1998," table Da667-678, in Carter et al., Historical Statistics. According to contemporary estimates, U.S. farms produced over a billion pounds of cleaned rice, a jump of more than 40 percent over the average from the previous four years. "Rice the Food of Millions," press release for farm journals, n.d., folder "Farm Journals Section. Press Releases. Undated," box 41, series 12H, USFA Collection, Hoover Institution; "Carolina Rice Being Harvested," 13 September 1917, folder "Charleston Post News (SC)," box 547, RG 4, NARA; "People Eat Rice," 19 October 1917, folder "San Francisco Retail Grocers Adv. Edit (CA)," box 531, RG 4, NARA; Greer, *Food*, 158.

51. At the turn of the century, Kristin Hoganson writes, "middle-class American kitchens had become places of global encounter," and she stresses that while of course it was possible to eat or buy or cook internationally without thinking about it as an international experience, cookbook writers at this time highlighted the internationality of the experience. Hoganson, *Consumers' Imperium*, 111, 135; "The War Kitchen," ed. Timothy Hayes, n.d., folder "Columbus Dispatch News (OH)," box 567, RG 4, NARA; "Rice Can Do a Super-Bit," press release for women's pages of farm journals for week ending 12 January 1918, folder "Farm Journals Sections. Press Releases. 1918," box 41, series 12H, USFA Collection, Hoover Institution; "Rice," USDA press release no. 90, 21 January 1918, States Publicity Section, USFA Public Information Division, folder "Press Releases, States Section, Educational Division #1–99," box 9, USFA Collection, Hoover Library.

52. Nixola Greeley-Smith, "Vegetarian Diet Takes Fight Out of Men; Romantic Feeling an Evidence of Spring Fever," *Washington Post*, 2 April 1916, ES15, PQHN; "Rice the Food of Millions," press release for farm journals, n.d., folder "Farm Journals Section. Press Releases. Undated," box 41, series 12H, USFA Collection, Hoover Institution; "Marrowfat Bean Stew," *Chicago Daily Tribune*, 14 October 1917, E8, PQHN; "Rice," USDA press release no. 90, 21 January 1918, 5, States Publicity Section, USFA Public Information Division, folder "Press Releases, States Section, Educational Division #1–99," box 9, USFA Collection, Hoover Library.

53. Press release no. 1317, 23 November 1918, Public Information Division, folder "Press Releases, #130–1400," box 12, USFA Collection, Hoover Library; "Rice," U.S. Food Leaflet no. 18, n.d., folder "Publications," box 5, series 5H, USFA Collection, Hoover Institution; Wallace, *Rumford Complete Cook Book*, 88; "Rice the Food of

Millions," press release for farm journals, n.d., folder "Farm Journals Section. Press Releases. Undated," box 41, series 12H, USFA Collection, Hoover Institution.

54. Wood and Hopkins, *Food Economy in War Time*, 25.

55. "Worlds [*sic*] Food Shortage," 9 January 1918, folder "Greenville Advocate Edit (OH)," box 567, RG 4, NARA; letter from Oliver Smith, Salem, Ohio, to Hoover, 20 January 1918, box 320, RG 4, NARA; Katherine Blunt, Frances L. Swain, and Florence Powdermaker, *Food Guide for War Service at Home*, Collegiate Section of the USFA (New York: Charles Scribner's Sons, 1918), 13, folder "FA-II/Food Saving & Sharing, Food Guide (booklets)," box 8, USFA Collection, Hoover Library.

56. "Worlds [*sic*] Food Shortage," 9 January 1918, folder "Greenville Advocate Edit (OH)," box 567, RG 4, NARA; "More Nutriment in Rice than in Wheat," 23 February 1918, folder "New Orleans Item News (LA)," box 556, RG 4, NARA. However, others suggested that Japan's growing world power was occurring precisely because Japanese people were eating more meat. Luff, *Gout*, 247–48.

57. Levenstein, *Revolution at the Table*, 24.

58. Jacobs, *Pocketbook Politics*, 40. See also Belasco, *Meals to Come*, 8–11.

59. This joke was retold in the United States in the 1930s. "Family Reunion in Lay-By Time," typed manuscript, 1, folder "'America Eats' Notes, Reports, and Essays (Louisiana)," box A831, America Eats Papers, Records of the U.S. Work Projects Administration, LOC.

60. "Rice," USFA press release no. 90, 21 January 1918, States Publicity Section, USFA Public Information Division, folder "Press Releases, States Section, Educational Division #1–99," box 9, USFA Collection, Hoover Library; Horace Fletcher, "Fat Minimum," typed document, n.d., folder, "Fletcher, Horace," box 127, USFA Collection, Hoover Institution.

61. "How We Americans Eat," 4 February 1918, folder "Montgomery Advertiser Edit (AL)," box 549, RG 4, NARA; Riley, *Rising Life Expectancy*, 23.

62. "Corn Vital Crop in this War Stress Period," 8 December 1917, folder "Grass Valley Mirror Edit (CA)," box 530, RG 4, NARA.

63. Roorbach, "World's Food Supply," 11; "The World's Normal Consumption of Cereals," Statistical Division Information Service, USFA, bulletin no. 970, 13 April 1918, folder "FA I-A/Statistical Department Information Service, Bulletins #860–999, 1918 Incomplete," box 4, USFA Collection, Hoover Library; "Corn Is King," *Bulletin for the Clergy* 1, no. 2 (January 1918), folder "Cooperating Organizations. Religious, Fraternal, Patriotic, Labor, Agricultural, Commercial, etc.," box 3, series 5H, USFA Collection, Hoover Institution.

64. Spelling original. Abstract of letter sent from Mrs. W. R. Chandler, Boyds' Creek, Tenn., to USFA, 10 November 1917, folder "C 6,7, 8," box 327, RG 4, NARA. Similarly, one Georgia woman proudly called cornbread "the best, most nourishing bread in the world except for Yankee [*sic*] and foreigners who do not know how to prepare it." Corra Harris, "All Days Wheatless There," excerpted from *New York Independent*, 19 January 1918, folder "Mobile Item News (AL)," box 549, RG 4, NARA.

65. "The World's Normal Consumption of Cereals," Statistical Division Information Service, USFA, bulletin no. 970, 13 April 1918, folder "FA I-A/Statistical Department Information Service, Bulletins #860–999, 1918 Incomplete," box 4, USFA Collection,

Hoover Library; "Corn Is King," *Bulletin for the Clergy* 1, no. 2 (January 1918), folder "Cooperating Organizations. Religious, Fraternal, Patriotic, Labor, Agricultural, Commercial, etc.," box 3, series 5H, USFA Collection, Hoover Institution.

66. "The Cornbread Breakfast," June 1917, folder "Montgomery Advertiser Edit (AL)," box 529, RG 4, NARA. Or as another journalist wrote, when southerners "got up in the world they felt they must have white bread." "The White Flour Habit," 28 August 1917, folder "Lodi Sentinel Edit (CA)," box 530, RG 4, NARA.

67. Letter from A. W. Douglas, St. Louis, to Hoover, 27 June 1917, folder illegible, box 289, RG 4, NARA; letter from Mrs. Frank Ashcraft, Monroe, N.C., to Hoover, 15 October 1917, folder "F-G 24 Oct. 1," box 298, RG 4, NARA.

68. "The Poor Man's Corn," 18 October 1917, folder "Memphis Commercial Appeal Edit (TN)," box 547, RG 4, NARA. Joel Chandler Harris, author of the B'rer Rabbit stories, championed corn and said such anti-corn snobbery was misplaced. Harris, "Cornmeal and What It Means, as Told by Joel Chandler Harris," 18 November 1917, folder "Springfield Morning Union Edit (MA)," box 537, RG 4, NARA.

69. After the completion of the experiment, the governor of Mississippi pardoned the prisoners who had participated. Gratzer, *Terrors of the Table*, 144–48; Cummings, *American and His Food*, 174. See also McCollum, "Some Essentials to a Safe Diet."

70. Bradley, *Cook Book*, 11; recipes, 4 January 1918, folder "Columbus Dispatch News (OH)," box 567, RG 4, NARA; Nettleton, *One Hundred-Portion War Time Recipes*, 9.

71. "Just Plain Cornbread," press release for women's pages of farm journals for week ending 26 January 1918, folder "Farm Journals Sections. Press Releases. 1918," box 41, series 5H, USFA Collection, Hoover Institution.

72. "Women of the North Urged to Use Meal Like Those in the South," 21 January 1918, folder "Columbus State Journal News (OH)," box 567, RG 4, NARA.

73. "Conquer with Corn," June 1917, folder "Boston Record Edit (MA)," box 537, RG 4, NARA.

74. Letter from Mrs. M. S. Crary, Boone, Iowa, to Hoover, 2 November 1917, folder "L-M 87 Nov. 1," box 301, Home Conservation Division, General Office, General Correspondence, April–August 1917, RG 4, NARA; letter from Lenna Frances Cooper to A. L. Marlatt, 7 July 1917, folder illegible, box 288, RG 4, NARA; "Corn Bread Contest Next Wednesday," 4 February 1918, folder "Allentown Chronicle and News (PA)," box 568, RG 4, NARA; letter from Richard H. Edmonds, Baltimore, to Hoover, 31 July 1917, folder "N.S. 238," box 293, RG 4, NARA; letter from T. M. Alexander of New York City to Hoover, 22 June 1917, folder illegible, box 288, RG 4, NARA.

75. Pilcher, *Que Vivan los Tamales!*

76. Paul Laurence Dunbar, "When De Co'n Pone's Hot," *Li'l' Gal* (1896; New York: Dodd Mead, 1904), 47–50.

77. Thomas J. McKie, M.D., "A Brief History of Insanity and Tuberculosis in the Southern Negro," *Journal of the American Medical Association* (March 1897): 538; "Don't Cut the Rope," USFA bulletin, October 1918, 4, folder "Negro Press. A. U. Craig," box 42, series 12H, USFA Collection, Hoover Institution.

78. Letter from I. E. Barwick, Gillette, Fla., to Martha Van Renssalaer, 11 March 1918, folder "35 Barwick, I.E.," box 298, RG 4, NARA; interoffice memo paraphrasing

Hoover from L. L. Strauss[?] to Paul Boden, 12 April 1918, folder "P. B. Boden," Hotels and Restaurants Division, box 74, series 43H, USFA Collection, Hoover Institution.

79. "'Fifty Ways of Using Corn Meal' by Cousin Angelina," leaflet (Newark, N.J.: L. Bamberger & Co., 1918), folder "L-M 37 April 1," box 298, RG 4, NARA; "'Cohn Pone': 'Marse Henry' Tells How to Make Real Corn Bread," excerpted from *Topeka State Journal*, 24 January 1918, folder "Garnette Review News (KS)," box 555, RG 4, NARA.

80. "Hoover Urges People to Eat 'Cohn Pon,'" 11 September 1917, folder "Minot Optic Republic News (ND)," box 544, RG 4, NARA.

81. Eleanor Franklin Egan, "The Modern Samaritan: How Charity Pays Its Way in Belgium," *Saturday Evening Post*, 21 October 1916, folder "Writings about Hoover," box 219, Hoover Collection, Hoover Institution.

82. Alexandre Dumas wrote that corn was a grain "qui se digère difficilement, qui pèse sur l'estomac, et qui ne convient qu'aux personnes d'un tempérament fort et robuste" (Dumas, *Grand dictionnaire de cuisine*, 383). See also Harvey Wiley, "Corn to the Rescue," *Good Housekeeping*, January 1918, 55–56, 93.

83. "Consumption of Grains as Bread in the United States and France," bulletin no. 828, 9 March 1918, Food Administration Statistical Department Information Service, folder "FA I-A/Statistical Department Information Service, Bulletins #650–859, 1918 Incomplete," box 4, USFA Collection, Hoover Library.

84. Surface, *American Food*, 9.

85. "Why Not Send the Corn Abroad," cartoon, "Graphic Exhibits on Food Conservation at Fairs and Exhibition," USFA bulletin, September 1917, folder "Exhibit and Campaign Methods. John H. Cover," box 4, series 5H, USFA Collection, Hoover Institution.

86. "Corn Vital Crop in this War Stress Period," 8 December 1917, folder "Grass Valley Mirror Edit (CA)," box 530, RG 4, NARA; "Pork in Polite Company," 14 August 1917, folder "Newark Call Edit (NJ)," box 540, RG 4, NARA; "Food Demonstration by Aunt Portia Smiley," 28 April 1918, folder "Providence Journal News (RI)," box 570, RG 4, NARA.

87. Letter from R. A. Torry, Dean of Bible Institute of Los Angeles, to USFA, 27 May 1918, folder "Prohibition Letters," box 405, RG 4, NARA; letter from Mrs. Angeline Beeson, Niagara Falls, N.Y., to Hoover, 7 June 1917, folder illegible, box 288, RG 4, NARA; letter from Miss Clare Bunce, Manhattan Beach, N.Y., to Gertrude Lane, 18 October 1917, folder "C 42," box 299, RG 4, NARA; "Indian Meal for Europe?," 20 January 1918, folder "Pittsburg Dispatch Edit (PA)," box 569, RG 4, NARA.

88. "Consumption of Grains as Bread in the United States and France," bulletin no. 828, 9 March 1918, Food Administration Statistical Department Information Service, folder "FA I-A/Statistical Department Information Service, Bulletins #650–859, 1918 Incomplete," box 4, USFA Collection, Hoover Library.

89. Bennett, *World's Food*, 165; Harriet Anderson, "Oats, Peas, Beans, and Barley Grows," draft with handwritten editing corrections, May 1918, folder "25 Anderson, Harriet, Publicity Material," box 298, RG 4, NARA; "Easy, When You Think," 7 February 1918, folder "Portland News Edit (OR)," box 570, RG 4, NARA.

90. "Corn," USFA leaflet, December 1917, folder "FA-II/Home Cards," box 8, USFA Collection, Hoover Library.

91. "Hominy," bulletin copublished by USFA and USDA, U.S. Food Leaflet no. 19, n.d., folder "Publications," box 5, series 5H, USFA Collection, Hoover Institution; "Corn," USFA leaflet, December 1917, folder "FA-II/Home Cards," box 8, USFA Collection, Hoover Library; "Fillers for the Makeup," press release for farm journals, n.d., folder "Farm Journals Section. Press Releases. Undated," box 41, series 12H, USFA Collection, Hoover Institution; "Eat Corn and Praise God," 30 March 1918, folder "Birmingham News Edit (AL)," box 549, RG 4, NARA; Dr. H.E. Horton, "Back to Indian Days—How to Use our Coming Great Corn Crop for Human Food," n.d., folder "Montgomery Advertiser News (AL)," box 529, RG 4, NARA.

92. Photograph of Library Exhibit, n.d., no location, folder "Library and Exhibits Section. Edith Guerrier," box 42, series 12H, USFA Collection, Hoover Institution; Bradley, *Cook Book*, 7.

93. "Corn," USFA leaflet, December 1917, folder "FA-II/Home Cards," box 8, USFA Collection, Hoover Library.

94. McWilliams, *Revolution in Eating*, 82; "A Corn-Fed Nation," 5 March 1918, folder "Dayton Journal News (OH)," box 567, RG 4, NARA; "King Corn for Democracy," Illinois Division of USFA Bulletin, 28 December 1917, folder "Illinois," box 12, series 6H, States Administration, USFA Collection, Hoover Institution; "Easy, When You Think," 7 February 1918, folder "Portland News Edit (OR)," box 570, RG 4, NARA; "Release Corn—The Colossus," full-page advertisement from the National Association of White Corn Millers, 8 August 1917, folder "Washington Post Edit (DC)," box 532, RG 4, NARA.

95. The "our" was originally capitalized. "Economy in War Recipes: Bliss Native Herbs: Great Laxative," printed recipe booklet (Washington, D.C.: The Alonzo O. Bliss Co., June 1918), folder "41 Bliss, The Alonzo O. Company," box 299, RG 4, NARA; "Do You Know Corn Meal?," U.S. Food Leaflet no. 2, folder "U.S. Food Administration Dept.," AAFCSR, #6578, DRMC.

96. "Economy in War Recipes: Bliss Native Herbs: Great Laxative," printed recipe booklet (Washington, D.C.: The Alonzo O. Bliss Co., June 1918), folder "41 Bliss, The Alonzo O. Company," box 299, RG 4, NARA; "A Wheat Saving Way for Every Day," leaflet produced by Baltimore Pearl Hominy Co., Baltimore, June 1917, folder "L-M 37 April 1," box 298, RG 4, NARA.

97. "Conquer with Corn," June 1917, folder "Boston Record Edit (MA)," box 537, RG 4, NARA; "Corn," USFA leaflet, December 1917, folder "FA-II/Home Cards," box 8, USFA Collection, Hoover Library; "King Corn for Democracy," Illinois Division of USFA Bulletin, 28 December 1917, folder "Illinois," box 12, series 6H, USFA Collection, Hoover Institution; photograph of Library Exhibit, n.d., no location given, folder "Library and Exhibits Section. Edith Guerrier," box 42, series 12H, USFA Collection, Hoover Institution; "Corn—The Nation's Mainstay," full-page advertisement from the National Association of White Corn Millers, 18 June 1917, folder "Washington Post Edit (DC)," box 532, RG 4, NARA; "Hominy," bulletin copublished by USFA and USDA, U.S. Food Leaflet no. 19, n.d., folder "Publications," box 5, series 5H, USFA Collection, Hoover Institution; Harriet Anderson, "Oats, Peas, Beans, and Barley Grows," draft with handwritten editing corrections, May 1918, folder "25 Anderson, Harriet, Publicity Material," box 298, RG 4, NARA; "Children Should Have Candy!," full-page advertisement for

Karo corn syrup, 19 December 1917, folder "New York Herald Edit (NY)," box 541, RG 4, NARA.

98. "A Corn-Fed Nation," 5 March 1918, folder "Dayton Journal News (OH)," box 567, RG 4, NARA.

99. Laird, *Brunswick Records*, 368.

100. George G. Bradford, editorial, *Crisis*, May 1918, 7. See also Lentz-Smith, *Freedom Struggles*.

101. "How the Negro Can Help Make Food Win the War," USFA Bulletin, April 1918, folder "Negro Press. A. U. Craig," box 42, series 12H, USFA Collection, Hoover Institution.

102. Letter from USFA staff to P. M. Harding, Vicksburg, Miss., 1 April 1918, folder "C," box 405, RG 4, NARA; "Negro Food Worker on Tour of State," 23 January 1918, folder "Birmingham Ledger News (AL)," box 549, RG 4, NARA; "Conservation Campaign," USFA memorandum, October 1918, folder "FA-II/Food Conservation, General," box 8, USFA Collection, Hoover Library; "Negro Institute to Aid in Food Fight," 26 October 1917, folder "Atlanta Journal News (GA)," box 533, RG 4, NARA; "Much Food Produced at Negro Normal," October[?] 1917, folder "Nashville Tennessean News (TN)," box 548, RG 4, NARA; Cornelius C. Fitzgerald, "A Patriotic Appeal to the Colored People of the Great State of Maryland," 7 August 1918, folder "Baltimore Herald News (MD)," box 556, RG 4, NARA.

103. "Meetings," *Crisis*, May 1918, 31; "War," *Crisis*, May 1917, 37; "Negro Orphans Plant 8 Acres of Potatoes/Catholic Asylums Have Fall Gardens," 9 September 1917, folder "New Orleans States News (LA)," box 536, RG 4, NARA; "Much Food Produced at Negro Normal," October[?] 1917, folder "Nashville Tennessean News (TN)," box 548, RG 4, NARA; "Negroes to Discuss Food Conservation," 2 November 1917, folder "Pensacola News News (FL)," box 533, RG 4, NARA.

104. Craig, a former teacher at Tuskegee and a former public school teacher in Washington, D.C., asked to be able to approve all prospective division employees, so that "the work among Colored people may be most effectively done, and that the United States Food Administration may not be embarrassed" (Memorandum for Mr. Rickard, week ending 25 May 1918, folder "Ben S. Allen, Memoranda for Mr. Rickard 'Week ending' 6 April-25 May 1918," box 39, series 12H, USFA Collection, Hoover Institution). See also letter from USFA staff member to William Aery at Hampton Institute, Hampton, Va., 14 July 1917, folder illegible, box 288, Home Conservation Division, General Office, General Correspondence (5HA-A1) 1917, Am20-Br 50, RG 4, NARA; and interoffice memo from A. U. Craig to Hoover, 2 November 1917, folder "Negro Press. A. U. Craig," box 42, series 12H, USFA Collection, Hoover Institution.

105. "Food Conservation Meeting," 2 February 1918, folder "Providence Journal News (RI)," box 570, RG 4, NARA; "Ladies Will Teach Negroes How to Can," 5 August 1917, folder "Knoxville Tribune News (TN)," box 547, RG 4, NARA.

106. Spelling original. "Unconscious Insult," *Crisis*, May 1918, 9–10.

107. "Don't Cut the Rope," USFA Bulletin, October 1918, 4, folder "Negro Press. A. U. Craig," box 42, series 12H, USFA Collection, Hoover Institution; "King er de Roos,'" 24 September 1918, folder "East Stroudsburg Press News (PA)," box 568, RG 4, NARA.

108. Many of these extension agents were Jeanes teachers, trained and hired by the Negro Rural School Fund, which northern philanthropists had started funding through the Rockefeller Foundation in 1909 as the Anna T. Jeanes fund. Gilmore, *Gender and Jim Crow*, 161, 197–98.

109. Food administrators likewise believed that "colored women" should "do Home Economics work among their own people." As food administrators imagined the program, the African American women "will, of course, be under the direct supervision of the Home Economics Director of each State." "Resume of Important Rulings and Letters Sent to Federal Food Administrators August 15th to September 1st," folder "FA I-A/ Resume of Important Rulings, for district & county Administrators, April–Aug. 1918," box 3, USFA Collection, Hoover Library. See also "Attention Farmers!," 17 August 1917, folder "Florence Times News (AL)," box 529, RG 4, NARA; and "Cooking Problems as Portion of War Work Solved by N.O. Gas Company," 27 January 1918, folder "New Orleans Item News (LA)," box 556, RG 4, NARA.

110. "What the Department of Agriculture Is Doing," War Work Weekly no. 8, 15 July 1918, USDA, box 453, AAFCSR, DRMC; "Negroes Help in Food Production," 27 December 1917, folder "Raleigh News & Observer News (NC)," box 544, RG 4, NARA; Carmen Harris, "Grace Under Pressure: The Black Home Extension Service in South Carolina, 1919–1966," in Stage and Vincenti, *Rethinking Home Economics*, 203–28.

111. W. E. B. Du Bois, "Negro Education," *Crisis*, February 1918, 177.

112. John Sterling, "General Report on Hotel Restaurants/Norfolk—Charleston—Savannah—Richmond," 30 August 1918, 2, folder "General Report on Hotel Restaurants," Hotels and Restaurants Division, box 74, series 43H, USFA Collection, Hoover Institution; "Some Suggestions in Regard to Food Conservation," typed memo from R. F. Campbell, Asheville, N.C., 6 August 1917, folder illegible, box 289, RG 4, NARA; letter from Charles H. Armstrong, Shelbyville, Tenn., to Hoover, 25 June 1917, folder illegible, box 288, RG 4, NARA.

113. Harris Dickson, "Save and Serve with Hoover: What Will Feed Three Will Feed Four," *Collier's: The National Weekly*, ed. Mark Sullivan, 11 August 1917, folder "Writings about Hoover," box 219, Hoover Collection, Hoover Institution.

114. Letter from Cally Rylan, Richmond, Va., to USFA, 28 January 1918, folder 41, box 17, NYSCHER; "Husbands and Cooks," from *Food Bulletin* 1, no. 3 (August 1917), Women's City Club of New York, folder illegible, box 296, RG 4, NARA.

115. Spelling original. Untitled blurb, 6[?] June 1917, folder "Yuma Sun Edit (AZ)," box 529, RG 4, NARA.

116. Untitled article, 19 January 1918, folder "Baltimore Star News (MD)," box 556, RG 4, NARA.

117. Dudley Harmon, "Dining with the Hoovers: What a Guest Eats at the Table of the Food Administrator," March 1918, *Ladies' Home Journal*, folder "March 1918. Dining with the Hoovers," box 14, Hoover Library.

118. Author originally wrote "anti-bellmu recipes." Untitled article, 19 January 1918, folder "Baltimore Star News (MD)," box 556, RG 4, NARA. For more on white fantasies about black affection for slavery, see McElya, *Clinging to Mammy*.

119. Mitchell, introduction to Eustis, *Cooking in Old Créole Days*, xiii.

120. Letter from the Teachers and Pupils of Bremestead School, Diamond Point, Lake George, N.Y., to Hoover, 28 May 1918, folder "58 Bremestead School," folder illegible, box 300, RG 4, NARA.

121. "'Sputtered' and 'Took On,' But Hoover's Cook Now Hooverizes," 3 February 1918, folder "Philadelphia Public Ledger News. No. 1 (PA)," box 569, RG 4, NARA.

122. Sheridan, *Stag Cook Book*, 32, 105.

123. Hoover proclaimed that African Americans' single "greatest opportunity" to aid the war effort was to "save and grow food" (Hoover, "For Freedom: An Appeal to the Negroes of the United States," bound folder "Addresses, Letters, Magazine Articles, Press Statements, Etc. Inclusive Dates: April 30, 1918–September 16, 1919," box 93, Hoover Collection, Hoover Institution). See also "The Power of an Ideal," 5 January 1918, folder "Allentown Call Edit (PA)," box 568, RG 4, NARA; "How the Negro Can Help Make Food Win the War," USFA Bulletin, April 1918, folder "FA-II/Food Conservation, General," box 8, USFA Collection, Hoover Library; "Negroes Helping in Food Problems," *Philadelphia Ledger*, 9 January 1918, folder "Cooperating Organizations. Religious, Fraternal, Patriotic, Labor, Agricultural, Commercial, etc.," box 3, series 5H, USFA Collection, Hoover Institution; editorial, *Crisis*, June 1917, 59; and "Don't Cut the Rope," USFA Bulletin, October 1918, folder "Negro Press. A. U. Craig," box 42, series 12H, USFA Collection, Hoover Institution. Booker T. Washington's 1903 statement that "the race is an agricultural one" had reinforced racist beliefs that African Americans were best suited to mindless farm labor (Washington, *Character Building*, 262).

124. "308,949 Leave the South," *Washington Post*, 10 May 1917, 10, PQHN.

125. Philip Weltner, "Should Help Negro Churches to Elevate Standard of Race," *Atlanta Constitution*, 4, 30 July 1917, PQHN.

126. As one writer for the *Crisis* put it, any southern African American "who wishes to have his children educated and who wishes to be in close touch with civilization" needed to "get out of the South as soon as possible" (editorial, *Crisis*, October 1916, 270). Mobs killed almost forty African Americans in 1917, almost sixty in 1918, and over seventy in 1919. Kennedy, *Over Here*, 283. See also Gilmore, *Gender and Jim Crow*.

127. Untitled blurb, 15 August[?] 1917, folder "Knoxville Tribune Edit (NY)," box 547, RG 4, NARA; "Negro Exodus Is of Big Proportion," October[?] 1917, folder "Houston Post News (TX)," box 548, RG 4, NARA.

128. Rutkoff and Scott, *Fly Away*; Wilkerson, *Warmth of Other Suns*; Grossman, *Land of Hope*. See also Marks, *Farewell—We're Good and Gone*; Trotter, *Great Migration in Historical Perspective*; and Hahamovitch, *Fruits of Their Labor*. Using wartime food needs as their justification, whites connected to the Food Administration in Wilmington, North Carolina, a bastion of racism from which an "exodus" of African Americans had fled since the city's infamous massacre of African Americans in 1898, forced more than a thousand African American men and women to stay and work on county farms in the summer of 1917. "Negro Laborers Put on Farms in New Hanover," 24 July 1917, folder "Asheville Times Edit (NC)," box 544, RG 4, NARA; "Energetic Campaign for Increased Production/Eastern North Carolina Responding Nobly to the Needs of the Hour," *Charlotte Sunday Observer*, 24 June 1917, 23, WorldCat. The historian Cindy Hahamovitch argues that the combination of wartime labor shortages and the Great Migration put southern African Americans in a unique position of bargaining power,

and "southern planters found that they required the intervention of local, state, and federal authorities to keep black laborers at work for their accustomed wages." This marked the first time the federal government had intervened in this way since Reconstruction. Hahamovitch, *Fruits of Their Labor*, 79–80.

129. For more on the internalization of "racist evolutionary discourse," see Gaines, *Uplifting the Race*, 3, 189–90.

130. W. A. Evans, "U.S. Census Office's Life Tables," How to Keep Well, *Chicago Daily Tribune*, 6 August 1916, A4, PQHN; "The Average Man and Woman Can Now Expect to Live Fifty-Six Years," *Afro-American*, 12 October 1923, 1, PQHN.

131. "Notes," *Crisis*, May 1918, 11; "A Transformed Race," *Crisis*, July 1918, 179–80. In another *Crisis* editorial, a writer claimed that European races were "ahead" of Asian races, which were in turn "ahead" of African races ("Does Race Antagonism Serve Any Good Purpose," *Crisis*, September 1914, 233). W. E. B. Du Bois opposed the racism behind eugenic theories, but the historian Gregory Dorr argues that Du Bois's own work "reveals the subtle influence of hereditarian thought on his own social theorizing." Starting in the early 1910s, the African American eugenicist Dr. Thomas Wyatt Turner taught eugenics at Howard, Tuskegee, and Hampton University, and his favored text was Paul Popenoe's *Applied Eugenics*. Meanwhile, Marcus Garvey used eugenics "to argue for racial separatism and black racial purity" (Dorr, "Fighting Fire with Fire"). See also Dorr, *Segregation's Science*.

132. Ida Crouch-Hazlett, quoted in "Fresh Fields," *Crisis*, September 1917, 247.

133. See Stavney, "'Mothers of Tomorrow.'"

134. Dorr, "Fighting Fire with Fire." See also Dorr, *Segregation's Science*.

135. "Our Baby Pictures," *Crisis*, October 1914, 298–99; "Shadows of Light," picture caption, *Crisis*, October 1918, 286.

136. "Notes," *Crisis*, May 1918, 11.

137. "Food," *Crisis*, July 1918, 165; "The Boy Over There," *Crisis*, October 1918, 269.

138. "Faces Are Altered by Food," *Chicago Defender*, 17 June 1911, 2, PQHN.

139. "Food," *Crisis*, July 1918, 165. In contrast with African Americans' rising racial fortunes, Ida Crouch-Hazlett argued that poor southern whites *were* degenerating racially, in large part because of their wretched diets. "Fresh Fields," *Crisis*, September 1917, 247.

140. Ida Crouch-Hazlett, quoted in "Fresh Fields," *Crisis*, September 1917, 247; editorial, *Crisis*, July 1918, 111.

141. "Babies Shown at Food Show, Too," 31 January 1918, folder "Cleveland Plaindealer News (OH)," box 567, RG 4, NARA. For more on Better Baby contests, see Holt, *Linoleum, Better Babies*; Stern, "Making Better Babies"; and Curry, *Modern Mothers*.

142. Du Bois, editorial, *Crisis*, October 1919; Stavney, "'Mothers of Tomorrow,'" 540.

143. Leland S. Cozart, "Mother Williams," photo caption, *Crisis*, October 1918, 273.

144. "Our Baby Pictures," *Crisis*, October 1914, 298–99.

145. Ibid. Meanwhile, as infant mortality rates among blacks remained higher than those among whites, African American writers insisted that fresh air and pure foods

would save hundreds of thousands of African American children every year. Editorial, *Crisis*, October 1918, 267.

146. Dudley Sarent, quoted in "A Better Race in the Making," *Los Angeles Times*, 11 January 1914, I4, PQHN.

147. Cocroft, *Let's Be Healthy*, iii.

148. "Dr. Wiley Predicts German Race of Weaklings While Americans Become Strong," n.d., folder "Washington Herald News No. 2 (DC)," box 552, RG 4, NARA; "How We Americans Eat," 4 February 1918, folder "Montgomery Advertiser Edit (AL)," box 549, RG 4, NARA.

149. 1880 U.S. Census, Census Place: Augusta, Richmond, Georgia, Roll: T9_163, Family History Film: 1254163, Page: 368.2000, Enumeration District: 100, Image: 0518, Ancestry Library Edition, accessed online.

150. "Lucy Craft Laney (1854–1933)," *The Georgia Encyclopedia*, accessed online; Smiley, "Courtship Formulas of Southern Negroes," 156; Mary McLeod Bethune Papers, The Bethune Foundation Collection, part 4, Administration of Bethune-Cookman College and the Mary McLeod Bethune Foundation, 1915–55, A Guide to the Microfilm Edition of Black Studies Research Sources, xi, accessed online; Yellin and Bond, *Pen Is Ours*, 326; Harvey, *Redeeming the South*, 288.

151. Smiley, "Folk-Lore," 357.

152. 1930 U.S. Census, Brookline, Norfolk, Massachusetts, Roll: 933, Page: 9A, Enumeration District: 25, Image: 695.0, ancestry.com.

153. 1920 U.S. Census, "Smiley, Portia," Suffolk, Boston, Massachusetts, Ward 5, Roll: T625_731, Page: 1A, Enumeration District: 141, Image: 143, ancestry.com.

CHAPTER SIX

1. Holbrook, "Home Environment."

2. For more on Americanization, see Selig, *Americans All*; Dorsey, *We Are All Americans*; Pickus, *True Faith and Allegiance*; and Meyer, "Adapting the Immigrant to the Line."

3. Quote was originally in all caps. Farmer and Huntington, *Food Problems*, 39.

4. Writing about the rise of foreign food imports at the turn of the twentieth century, the historian Kristin Hoganson argues that Americans' consumption of previously exotic foods "turned the foreign into the harmless stuff of pleasure that posed no significant threats to their sense of racial, class, national, and civilizational privilege" (*Consumers' Imperium*, 135).

5. Diner, *Hungering for America*, 1.

6. About a third of the population increase from 1890 to 1920 was due to immigration. Kennedy, *Freedom from Fear*, 13–4.

7. Kennedy, *Over Here*, 24; "Country of Origin of the Foreign White Stock," 1, U.S. 1910 Census of Population and Housing, http://www2.census.gov/prod2/decennial/documents/36894832v1ch11.pdf, 8 May 2007; "Foreign Language Newspapers Help Food Administration," *Bulletin to Vernacular Press*, no. 2, USFA, form no. 150, September 1917, folder "Home Card. Vernacular," box 3, series 5H, USFA Collection, Hoover Institution.

8. See Kennedy, *Over Here*, 63.

9. Jacobson argues that when nineteenth- and early-twentieth-century Americans talked about different "races," they truly *were* talking about *races*, not just ethnicities or nationalities. See Jacobson, *Whiteness of a Different Color*.

10. Guterl, *Color of Race in America*, 5.

11. See Shapiro, *Perfection Salad*.

12. Haley, *Turning the Tables*; Gabaccia, *We Are What We Eat*, 95–96.

13. For more on the waning of French haute cuisine and the French language in American restaurant culture throughout the late nineteenth and early twentieth centuries and the roles that annoyed middle-class restaurant-goers played in their demise, see Haley, *Turning the Tables*, 194.

14. "French to Be Erased from Bills of Fare," *Atlanta Constitution*, 23 September 1910, 6, PQHN.

15. *Bean-Bag* 1, no. 2, 1918, 44.

16. "Home Card Supplement," no. 1, duplicate, October or November 1917, folder 8, "Dr. Ray Lyman Wilbur. 17 May–24 November 1917," box 1, series 5H, USFA Collection, Hoover Institution.

17. See Gabaccia, *We Are What We Eat*, 122–26.

18. Fullerton, "Long Island Home Hamper," 166.

19. Chittenden, "Foreign Lenten Dishes."

20. "No 'Red Meat' on Christmas," 19 December 1917, folder "New Haven Register News (CT)," box 532, RG 4, NARA; Fullerton, "Long Island Home Hamper."

21. "The American Cook and Pure Flavors," *Hartford Courant*, 28 January 1916, 4, PQHN; "Living to Eat and Eating to Live Discussed by an English Epicure," *Washington Post*, 20 August 1913, 12, PQHN.

22. Dr. Henrietta Grauel, "Efficient Housekeeping," *Atlanta Constitution*, 14 February 1914, 4, PQHN.

23. "Common-Sense and Our Daily Bread," 9 February 1918, *The Bellman*, folder "Common-Sense and Our Daily Bread," box 14, Hoover Library.

24. "One-Dish Dinners," reprinted from the *Portland Oregonian*, 24 February 1918, folder "Philadelphia Record Edit (PA)," box 569, RG 4, NARA.

25. Ruth Kent, "Good Seasoning Is Needed to Make War Foods Tasty," 26 June 1918, folder "Philadelphia Telegraph News (PA)," box 569, RG 4, NARA.

26. Jean Prescott Adams, "Military Life Influences Food Habits," from "The Business of Being a Housewife," 6 September 1918, printed leaflet produced by Armour & Co., folder "22 Armour & Co. Feb. 1," box 298, RG 4, NARA; "Care of Children," Home Demonstration in Care and Feeding of a Normally Well Child, no. 276, Department of Home Economics, Cornell University, 1919[?], folder 2, box 18, NYSCHER; "The American Cook and Pure Flavors," *Hartford Courant*, 28 January 1916, 4, PQHN; Luff, *Gout*, 253; Christian, "What Food Is and Its True Purpose," 1; Dr. Charles M. Sheldon, "Likes Bread and Milk," *Stag Cook Book*, 52. See also Levenstein, *Revolution at the Table*, 103.

27. See Rabinbach, *Human Motor*.

28. Rorer, "Food," 19; Cocroft, *What to Eat and When*, x–xi; "Butter Camouflage," press release for farm journals, 2 March 1918, folder "Farm Journals Sections. Press Releases. 1918," series 12H—box 41, USFA Collection, Hoover Institution.

29. Letter from Harvey Wiley to Dr. George M. Kober, D.C., 9 November 1917, folder "1917," box 125, Harvey Wiley Papers, LOC.

30. Bryce, *Modern Theories of Diet*; Levenstein, *Revolution at the Table*, 103; Griffith, *Born Again Bodies*.

31. Dr. Phillip Marvel, quoted in Stewart, "Some Dietetic Errors," 142.

32. Dr. T. J. Allen, "Diet and Health Hints," *Washington Post*, 2 February 1912, 7, PQHN.

33. "Selection of Food Important," *Chicago Defender*, 1 March 1913, 5, PQHN.

34. Emphasis added. Jean Prescott Adams, "The Business of Being a Housewife," 6 September 1918, printed leaflet produced by Armour & Co., folder "22 Armour & Co. Feb. 1," box 298, RG 4, NARA; "Care of Children," Home Demonstration in Care and Feeding of a Normally Well Child, no. 276, Home Economics Department, Cornell University, 1919[?], folder 2, box 18, NYSCHER; Norton, *Mrs. Norton's Cook-Book*, vi; Rose, *Everyday Foods in War Time*, 67; Ruth Kent, "Good Seasoning Is Needed to Make War Foods Tasty," 26 June 1918, folder "Philadelphia Telegraph News (PA)," box 569, RG 4, NARA.

35. Rose, *Everyday Foods in War Time*, 69.

36. "Rice Can Do a Super-Bit," press release for women's pages of farm journals for week ending 12 January 1918, folder "Farm Journals Sections. Press Releases. 1918," box 41, series 12H, USFA Collection, Hoover Institution.

37. Hoganson discusses Americans' growing consciousness of the foreign origins of their foods in the last decades of the nineteenth century. Hoganson, *Consumers' Imperium*, 111.

38. See ibid. and McWilliams, *Revolution in Eating*. As the historian Donna Gabaccia writes, the "American penchant to experiment with foods, to combine and mix the foods of many cultural traditions" is "a recurring theme in our history as eaters" (*We Are What We Eat*, 3).

39. Floyd and Foster, "Recipe in Its Cultural Contexts," 4–5.

40. "Living to Eat and Eating to Live Discussed by an English Epicure," *Washington Post*, 20 August 1913, 12, PQHN.

41. In many descriptions of gluttony, overeating and overseasoning were kindred sins. "Overfeeding," 13 November 1917, folder, "Quincy Patriotic Ledger Edit (MA)," box 537, RG 4, NARA.

42. Norton, *Mrs. Norton's Cook-Book*, vi.

43. "Rice," USFA press release no. 90, 21 January 1918, 2, States Publicity Section, USFA Public Information Division, folder "Press Releases, States Section, Educational Division #1–99," box 9, USFA Collection, Hoover Library.

44. Dr. T. J. Allen, "Diet and Health Hints," *Washington Post*, 2 February 1912, 7, PQHN.

45. Gabaccia, *We Are What We Eat*, 37.

46. Eyewitness, "Racial Customs Declared Cause of Sick Babies," *Chicago Daily Tribune*, 10 February 1919, 9, PQHN.

47. Ibid.; untitled blurb, 4 December 1917, folder "Westerly Sun Edit (RI)," box 547, RG 4, NARA.

48. Elene Foster, "The Americanization of Our Foreign-Born Women," *New-York Tribune*, 5 January 1919, B11, PQHN; "Diet to Guard Belgian Babies," *Daily Alaskan*,

no. 311, 4 February 1915, folder "February 4, 1915. Diet to guard Belgian babies," box 10, Hoover Library.

49. *Oxford English Dictionary*, s.v. "Americanization"; "Speak English Please," *News Letter of the Woman's Committee Council of National Defense*, no. 28, 1 September 1918, 1, folder illegible, box 320, RG 4, NARA.

50. "Foreign Groups Helped Food Conservation Work," *Atlanta Constitution*, 20 November 1918, 8, PQHN; "Americanization Work Explained," 17 July 1918, folder "Boston Advertiser News No. 2 (MA)," box 557, RG 4, NARA.

51. Letter from N. Behar, New York City, to Hoover, 23 July 1917, folder "B," box 405, RG 4, NARA.

52. "War Work for Women," 19 December 1917, folder "Benton Harbor News News (MI)," box 537, RG 4, NARA.

53. Foreign Language Home Cards, folder "Home Card. Vernacular," box 3, series 5H, USFA Collection, Hoover Institution; Food Conservation Notes, no. 21, 17 August 1918, folder "FA-II/Food Conservation Notes," box 8, USFA Collection, Hoover Library.

54. "Foreign Language Newspapers Help Food Administration," Bulletin to Vernacular Press, no. 2, USFA, form no. 150, September 1917, folder "Home Card. Vernacular," box 3, series 5H, USFA Collection, Hoover Institution.

55. Abstract of memo to Ray Wilbur, unsigned, 20 July 1917, folder "How the People of the Country Criticize the Policies of the Food Administration," box 3, series 5H, USFA Collection, Hoover Institution.

56. USDA Office of Extension Work report, August 1918, 6, box 453, AAFCSR, #6578, DRMC; "Food Demonstration for Foreign-Born Residents," 8 May 1918, folder "Harrisburgh Telegraph News (PA)," box 568, RG 4, NARA.

57. "Teaching Foreign Women Food Saving, War Economy," 1 May 1918, folder "Philadelphia Public Ledger News. No. 2 (PA)," box 569, RG 4, NARA; "Women's War Time Activities," 6 March 1918, folder "Scranton Times News (PA)," box 569, RG 4, NARA.

58. "What the Department of Agriculture Is Doing," 1 July 1918, War Work Weekly, no. 6, USDA, Office of Information, box 453, AAFCSR, #6578, DRMC.

59. "To Americanize Boston's Aliens," *Boston Daily Globe*, 21 September 1917, 3, PQHN.

60. Letter from Miss Grace Andrews, Chelsea, Mass., to USFA, 30 August 1917, folder "F-G 24," box 298, RG 4, NARA.

61. USFA interoffice memo from Willa Roberts to Martha Van Renssalaer, 4 April 1918, folder 42, box 17, NYSCHER.

62. "It Means I Mustn't Eat So Much Candy," 24 October 1917, folder "Boise Statesman News (ID)," box 533, RG 4, NARA.

63. "The Sorrows of Sylvest," 23 January 1918, folder "Somerset Democrat News (PA)," box 569, RG 4, NARA.

64. "'Katie' Finds 'Treachery' in Potato Peeling Waste," clipping from *Chicago Examiner*, folder "DE—383," box 296, RG 4, NARA.

65. Eyewitness, "Racial Customs Declared Cause of Sick Babies," *Chicago Daily Tribune*, 10 February 1919, 9, PQHN.

66. Emphasis original. Letter from Mrs. Annie Wick Stephens, Buffalo, N.Y., to Hoover, 5 November 1917, folder "A-B 351 Oct. 1," box 320, RG 4, NARA.

67. Letter from Helen Atwater, D.C., to Rev. Dr. Howard B. Grose, D.C., 27 October 1917, folder illegible, box 401, RG 4, NARA.

68. "Politics and Meatless Tuesday," 1 November 1917, folder "Los Angeles Record Edit (CA)," box 530, RG 4, NARA.

69. Wording original. "Quong Wah Gets Dope from Food Board on Making His Chop Suey," 27 October 1917, folder "Denver Post News (CO)," box 532, RG 4, NARA; press release no. 811, 5 April 1918, Public Information Division, folder "Press Releases, #800–899," box 12, USFA Collection, Hoover Library.

70. Gabaccia, *We Are What We Eat*, 36; Diner, *Hungering for America*.

71. Emphasis original. Schapiro, "Social Service Dietetics," 148.

72. Elene Foster, "The Americanization of Our Foreign-Born Women," *New-York Tribune*, 5 January 1919, B11, PQHN.

73. Eyewitness, "Racial Customs Declared Cause of Sick Babies," *Chicago Daily Tribune*, 10 February 1919, 9, PQHN; Gabaccia, *We Are What We Eat*, 54; Diner, *Hungering for America*, 78.

74. It was significant that domestic Americanization efforts were taking place against the backdrop of wartime food aid to Europe, and sometimes the very successes of European food aid contrasted with the failures of Americanization at home. "Diet to Guard Belgian Babies," 4 February 1915, *Daily Alaskan*, no. 311, folder "February 4, 1915. Diet to guard Belgian babies," box 10, Hoover Library. For the most part, however, Americans saw wartime food aid to Europe as a laboratory for trying out Americanization techniques that they could use at home to teach immigrants how to eat the right food. For instance, Americans' initial failures to get European civilians to eat cornmeal taught them to "let the ideas of foreign countries permeate us and get our sympathy, at the same time that we are trying to persuade foreigners to take our American ways" (syllabus, "135 History of Homemaking and Housekeeping or Homemaking and Housekeeping Traditions," n.d. [1920?], folder 41, box 17, NYSCHER).

75. Gabaccia, *We Are What We Eat*, 55.

76. Langworthy, *Food Customs*, 8.

77. For example, wartime volunteers encouraged native Hawaiians "to serve the old fashioned poi," made of taro, in order to reduce their wheat consumption (letter from Harriet C. Andrews, Honolulu, to Martha Van Rensselaer, folder, "25 Andrews, Harriet C.," box 298, RG 4, NARA). The historian Diana Selig argues that from the 1920s through the Second World War, Americanization efforts metamorphosed into attempts to include selected parts of immigrant cultures—cultural gifts—into mainstream American culture. Selig, *Americans All*.

78. Letter from Frances Stern, Boston, to Sarah Splint, folder "354 Stern, Miss Frances," box 321, RG 4, NARA.

79. Spelling of "gefillte" original. Isaacs, "In the Hope of the New Diaspora," 191.

80. Richards, *Cost of Food*, 91.

81. Stern and Spitz, *Food for the Worker*, 19, 17.

82. Harvey Wiley, "Dr. Wiley's Question Box," *Good Housekeeping*, August 1918, 57.

83. "Foreign Cookery at Food Exhibit," 21 May 1918, folder "Meriden Journal News (CT)," box 550, RG 4, NARA.

84. "Bright Day Adds Visitors to Show," 8 February 1918, folder "Cleveland Plain-dealer [*sic*] News (OH)," box 567, RG 4, NARA.

85. Elizabeth H. Bohn, Report on the Conservation Food Show held at the Grand Central Palace, N.Y.C., 14–22 June 1918, 6, folder "43 Bohn, Miss Elizabeth H," box 299, RG 4, NARA.

86. Mrs. Edward W. Bemis, "News of the Chicago Women's Clubs," *Chicago Daily Tribune*, 14 July 1918, C5, PQHN.

87. "War*Time*Cook*Book," press release to farm journals, 1 December 1917, folder "Press Releases, to Farm Journals," box 12, USFA Collection, Hoover Library.

88. Jean Prescott Adams, "The Business of Being a Housewife," 6 September 1918, printed leaflet produced by Armour & Co., folder "22 Armour & Co. Feb. 1," box 298, RG 4, NARA.

89. Harrison and Clergue, *Allied Cookery*; Harrison and Clergue, *Cuisine des Alliés*; letter from Dr. P. J. Byrne, Cleveland, to Newton D. Baker (Secretary of War), 8 November 1917, box 300, RG 4, NARA; letter from Anne Bogenholm Sloane, D.C., to E. D. Van Sicklen at USFA, 24 October 1917, folder "American Pen Women, League of/Washington D.C.," box 298, RG 4, NARA; "N.O. Women Learn How to Make Sauehr-Kraut [*sic*]," 13 September 1917, folder "New Orleans Item News (LA)," box 536, RG 4, NARA.

90. Mencken, *American Language*, 199–200.

91. "Bananas as Body Fuel," 22 December 1918, folder "Chicago Herald Edit (IL)," box 534, RG 4, NARA; "Fillers for the Makeup," press release for farm journals, n.d., folder "Farm Journals Section. Press Releases. Undated," box 41, series 12H, USFA Collection, Hoover Institution.

92. USFA press release no. 559, 30 December 1917, Public Information Division, folder "Press Releases, #500–599," box 11, USFA Collection, Hoover Library; USFA Potato Slip, Index E-27-5, April 1918, folder "Publications," box 5, series 5H, USFA Collection, Hoover Institution; "Worlds [*sic*] Food Shortage," 9 January 1918, folder "Greenville Advocate Edit (OH)," box 567, RG 4, NARA.

93. Spelling original. Letter from C. V. Ashburn, Southern Pacific Co., to USFA, 25 May 1918, folder "C 22 March 1," box 298, RG 4, NARA.

94. Letter from Frank Koch, Paterson, N.J., to Hoover, 13 July 1917, folder "F.G.—204," box 292, RG 4, NARA.

95. "Single Dish Dinners," 1 March 1918, folder "Georgetown News (IL)," box 554, RG 4, NARA.

96. McCann, *Thirty Cent Bread*, 64.

97. Elizabeth L. Cowan, "One-Dish Meal System Offers Way for Housekeepers to Insure Nutritious Food," 10 February 1918, folder "Terre Haute Star News (IN)," box 555, RG 4, NARA.

98. Neil, *How to Cook in Casserole Dishes*, vii.

99. Elizabeth L. Cowan, "One-Dish Meal System Offers Way for Housekeepers to Insure Nutritious Food," 10 February 1918, folder "Terre Haute Star News (IN)," box 555, RG 4, NARA; "Meat Recipes," USFA bulletin, n.d., folder 47, box 17, NYSCHER; "One Dish Dinner Is Urged for Economy," 17 January 1919, Whittier, Calif., News, unlabeled folder, box 531, RG 4, NARA; "Make a Little Meat Go a Long Way," USDA and USFA, U.S. Food Leaflet no. 5 (Washington, D.C.: GPO, 1917), folder "Meat," box 8, USFA

Collection, Hoover Library; "A Whole Dinner in One Dish," USFA and USDA, U.S. Food Leaflet no. 3, 1917, folder "Publications," box 5, series 5H, USFA Collection, Hoover Institution; "One Dish Meal Recipe," 25 January 1918, folder "Cleveland Plaindealer News (OH)," box 567, RG 4, NARA; "The Savory Stew," 6 March 1918, from *Ada [Okla.] News*, loose papers not in folder, box 568, RG 4, NARA; "Herbert Hoover Says Soup Is War Time's Greatest Economy," 4 January 1918, folder "Carrington Independent News (ND)," box 568, RG 4, NARA.

100. "One Piece Victory Meals," 14 March 1918, folder "Cambridge Jeffersonian News (OH)," box 566, RG 4, NARA.

101. Letter from N. S. Amstutz, Valparaiso, Ind., to Hoover, 19 January 1918, folder "28 Amstutz, N.S.," box 298, RG 4, NARA; Dietetic Contest blank from Porter County, Ind., January 1918, folder "28 Amstutz, N.S.," box 298, RG 4, NARA; "One-Dish Dinners," reprinted from *Portland Oregonian*, 24 February 1918, folder "Philadelphia Record Editorial," box 569, RG 4, NARA.

102. "One Dish Dinner Is Urged for Economy," 17 January 1919, Whittier, Calif., News, unlabeled folder, box 531, RG 4, NARA.

103. Letter from N. S. Amstutz, Valparaiso, Ind., to Hoover, 19 January 1918, folder "28 Amstutz, N.S.," box 298, RG 4, NARA; "One-Dish Dinners," reprinted from *Portland Oregonian*, 24 February 1918, folder "Philadelphia Record Editorial," box 569, RG 4, NARA.

104. "War Time Recipes," 29 February 1918, folder "Rockland Courier Gazette News (ME)," box 556, RG 4, NARA; "Meat Recipes," n.d., folder 47, from Home Economics division of USFA, box 17, NYSCHER; "One Dish Dinner Is Urged for Economy," 17 January 1919, Whittier, Cal., News, unlabeled folder, box 531, RG 4, NARA; letter from unnamed USFA representative to Mrs. C. E. Campbell, Madison Hall, Tenn., 10 May 1918, folder illegible, box 289, RG 4, NARA.

105. Ruth Kent, "Making a Little Meat Go as Far as Possible," 13 February 1918, folder "Philadelphia Telegraph News (PA)," box 569, RG 4, NARA; "Household Hints," 21 January 1918, folder "Phoenix Gazette News (AZ)," box 550, RG 4, NARA; "Rissoto [*sic*]," Eva Robertson and Ruetta [*sic*] Townsley Day, *The Timely Cook Book*, 6, the Federal Food Administration of South Dakota (Aberdeen, S.D.: News Printing Co., 1918), folder "South Dakota," box 30, States Division, USFA Collection, Hoover Institution; "Rissoto [*sic*]" and polenta recipes, "War Recipes," 21 February 1918, folder "Cloverdale Courier News (OR)," box 570, RG 4, NARA; "Italian polenta," in "Corn," USFA leaflet, December 1917, folder "Publications," box 5, series 5H, USFA Collection, Hoover Institution; polenta recipe in "Consume Cornmeal," USFA Federal Food Board of New York, no. 3, 14 May 1918, loose items not in folder, box 15, series 6H, USFA Collection, Hoover Institution.

106. "Eat the Cheap Rooster," press release for women's pages of farm journals for week ending 2 February 1918, folder "Farm Journals Sections. Press Releases. 1918," box 41, series 12H, USFA Collection, Hoover Institution; recipes, folder "Cleveland Plaindealer News (OH)," box 567, RG 4, NARA; "War Recipes," 21 February 1918, folder "Cloverdale Courier News (OR)," box 570, RG 4, NARA.

107. USFA Potato Slip, Index E-27-5, April 1918, folder "Publications," box 5, series 5H, USFA Collection, Hoover Institution; *The Day's Food in War and Peace*, USFA and

the Woman's Committee, Council of National Defense, USDA, n.d., folder "Publications," box 5, series 5H, USFA Collection, Hoover Institution; Harrison and Clergue, *Allied Cookery*, 21; Nettleton, *One Hundred-Portion War Time Recipes*, 9; Ruth Kent, "Making a Little Meat Go as Far as Possible," 13 February 1918, folder "Philadelphia Telegraph News (PA)," box 569, RG 4, NARA; "War Time Recipes," 29 February 1918, folder "Rockland Courier Gazette News (ME)," box 556, RG 4, NARA; Mrs. M. A. Wilson, "How and What to Cook," 17 March 1918, folder "Philadelphia Public Ledger News. No. 1," box 569, RG 4, NARA.

108. "Meatless Recipes," February 1918, folder "Cleveland Press News (OH)," box 567, RG 4, NARA; Nettleton, *One Hundred-Portion War Time Recipes*, 12; Ruth Kent, "Making a Little Meat Go as Far as Possible," 13 February 1918, folder "Philadelphia Telegraph News (PA)," box 569, RG 4, NARA; "Household Hints," 21 January 1918, folder "Phoenix Gazette News (AZ)," box 550, RG 4, NARA.

109. Menu from Clyde Steamship Company, sent from George Edgcumbe, N.Y., to Ray Wilbur, 13 September 1917, folder "Clyde Steamship Company NYC," box 301, RG 4, NARA; "Household Hints," 21 January 1918, folder "Phoenix Gazette News (AZ)," box 550, RG 4, NARA; Nettleton, *One Hundred-Portion War Time Recipes*, 8; "Exploring for Sweets," press release to farm journals, 21 October 1917, folder "Press Releases, to Farm Journals," box 12, USFA Collection, Hoover Library.

110. See Inness, "Eating Ethnic," 4.

111. In 1910, one home economist had written, typically, "Spaghetti and macaroni, served with cheese [*sic*] are of course the familiar dishes of the Italians" (Williams, "Teaching Domestic Science," 272).

112. Both chili con carne and tamales were available in cans by the 1910s. *Mexican Cookery*.

113. "The Italian Method of Eating Macaroni Is a Surprise to Americans Seeing It for the First Time," *New-York Tribune*, 30 July 1905, B1, PQHN.

114. While cheap German and French restaurants gained moderate popularity, Italian restaurants took off among middle-class Americans. Haley, *Turning the Tables*, 94, 98–101.

115. Ibid., 101–6.

116. As Haley writes, "By the early twentieth century, an ethnic dinner at a restaurant was a commonplace experience for many urban middle-class Americans and a daring—but not too daring—adventure for midwestern tourists." Yet he is careful to point out that growing patronage of ethnic restaurants by no means necessarily meant growing support of immigration, or growing racial tolerance for that matter. Ibid., 115, 116, 94–95, 105.

117. Although "macaroni" in nineteenth-century cookbooks usually referred to the same tubular pasta that Americans think of today, nineteenth-century Americans sometimes used it as a generic term for any kind of pasta.

118. Among the many places spaghetti recipes appeared by the late nineteenth century was Fannie Farmer's authoritative tome on American cooking, *The Boston Cooking-School Cookbook*, where it was one of a relatively small number of "foreign" recipes. See page 91.

119. Skrabec, *H. J. Heinz*, 208, 198.

120. "Something You Want to Know," Van Camp canned spaghetti advertisement, *New York Times*, 29 March 1911, 4, PQHN. Chef Boyardee, a company started by the Italian American Hector Boiardi, started selling canned spaghetti in the 1930s. Gabaccia, *We Are What We Eat*, 150

121. Edwords, *Bohemian San Francisco*, 71; John Simpson, "Press Review: A Survey of Some Representative Articles on Food and Agriculture, Which Have Appeared in French Journals during the Last Few Days," 9 September 1918, typed booklet, Paris, folder "R 45–51 General Memoranda on France," France Division, box 115, USFA Collection, Hoover Institution.

122. For more on the canning industry, see Petrick, "Ambivalent Diet."

123. "Something You Want to Know," Van Camp canned spaghetti advertisement, *New York Times*, 29 March 1911, 4, PQHN.

124. See Diner, *Hungering for America*, 48–83, and Levenstein, "American Response to Italian Food."

125. Cuniberti, *Practical Italian Recipes*, 3; Gironci, *Italian Recipes*; letter from Rev. Victor Donati, Nesquehoning, Pa., to USFA, 29 October 1918, folder "D," box 405, RG 4, NARA; letter from Cuniberti, Janesville, Wisc., to Gertrude Lane, 5 December 1917, folder "F-G 84 Nov. 1," box 301, RG 4, NARA; recipes from Women's Italian Club, folder "Commercial Cookbooks & Recipes," box 329, RG 4, NARA.

126. "Housewives Like New Meat Substitute," 22 January 1918, folder "Boston Post News (MA)," box 557, RG 4, NARA.

127. Charles Cristadoro, "Macaroni the Oldest National Joke," typed article sent to USFA on 8 August 1917, folder "Macaroni," box 149, USFA Collection, Hoover Institution.

128. Untitled blurb, 14 March 1918, folder "Oklahoma City Times News (OK)," box 570, RG 4, NARA; "War Recipes," 21 February 1918, folder "Cloverdale Courier News (OR)," box 570, RG 4, NARA.

129. Cuniberti, *Practical Italian Recipes*, 6.

130. "Pale" was originally capitalized. Sheridan, *Stag Cook Book*, 146.

131. Putnam, *Tomorrow We Diet*, 82.

132. *Mendelssohn Club Cook Book*, 21; Hurlbut, *Stevenson Memorial Cook Book*, 59.

133. Captain Edward A. Salisbury, "Sauce for Spaghetti," in Sheridan, *Stag Cook Book*, 118.

134. Harding, *Twentieth Century Cook Book*, 52; Green, *How to Cook Vegetables*, 509–19.

135. Sheridan, *Stag Cook Book*, 169.

136. "The Italian Method of Eating Macaroni Is a Surprise to Americans Seeing It for the First Time," *New-York Tribune*, 30 July 1905, B1, PQHN.

137. Emma Rowe, "Spaghetti," *New York Observer*, 25 August 1898, 258, PQHN; Carleton and Chamberlain, "Commercial Status of Durum Wheat," 26; Hudson Maxim, "Spaghetti," in Sheridan, *Stag Cook Book*, 35; Gentile, *Italian Cook Book*, 27.

138. In response to government exhortations to eat cheap pasta, one wartime poem joked, "Take your troubles all to Hoover" when "spaghet' you can't maneuver" ("Helpful Herbert," folder "Poetry and Jingles," box 156, USFA Collection, Hoover Institution).

139. Edwords, *Bohemian San Francisco*, 71; Hoganson, *Consumers' Imperium*, 128.

140. "Canned Goods Are Going Up," advertisement for Foulds Macaroni and Spaghetti, *Atlanta Constitution*, 17 October 1911, 7; "Try This Dish Today," advertisement for Golden Age Macaroni, *[Baltimore] Sun*, 1 April 1920, 6, PQHN; "White Pearl Macaroni Products," advertisement for Tharinger Macaroni Co., Milwaukee, Wisc., back matter, in Kander, *Settlement Cook Book*, n.p.

141. For example, see Hamilton, *Primer of Cooking*.

142. "Mrs. Hoover's Cook Becomes an Ardent Hooverizer," 1 April 1918, folder "Muncie Press Edit (IN)," box 555, RG 4, NARA; Gentile, *Italian Cook Book*, 3.

143. Hamilton, *Primer of Cooking*, 140; "Start the Day Right with a Good Breakfast," U.S. Food Leaflet no. 1, USDA/USFA (Washington, D.C.: GPO, 1917), folder "Leaflets, inserts," box 8, USFA Collection, Hoover Library; Hudson Maxim, "Spaghetti," Sheridan, *Stag Cook Book*, 35.

144. S. M. R., "Macaroni à la Italy."

145. *Picayune Creole Cook Book*, 175.

146. S. M. R., "Macaroni à la Italy."

147. Wallace, *Rumford Complete Cook Book*; recipes, folder "Cleveland Plaindealer News (OH)," box 567, RG 4, NARA; *Castelar Crèche Cook Book*, 128; Cornforth, *Good Food*.

148. Letter from Mrs. E. Cramer, East Orange, N.J., to Hoover, March 1918, folder "D-E 83 Feb.1," box 301, RG 4, NARA. The term "Oriental" could apply to cuisine from the Far East or the Middle East, as used in Keoleian's *Oriental Cook*, although it increasingly meant East Asia as far as most Americans were concerned.

149. Bosse and Watanna, *Chinese-Japanese Cook Book*, 1.

150. For more on Chinese restaurants, see Haley, *Turning the Tables*; Hoganson, *Consumers' Imperium*, 118; and Coe, *Chop Suey*.

151. "Are Expert with Chopsticks: Americans Would Have Hard Time Manipulating Eating Implements of the Orientals," *Washington Post*, 30 May 1915, MS4, PQHN.

152. "Hooverizing Chop-Suey," 21 May 1918, folder "Baltimore Sun News (MD)," box 556, RG 4, NARA.

153. "'Meatless Chop Suey' Newest Chinese Dream," 8 November 1918, folder "Chicago Herald Edit (IL)," box 534, RG 4, NARA.

154. Farrar, "Oriental Recipes."

155. Emphasis added. Bosse and Watanna, *Chinese-Japanese Cook Book*, 1.

156. Ethel Moore Rock, preface to Moore, *Chinese Recipes*, x, viii.

157. Farrar, "Oriental Recipes," 518.

158. *College Woman's Cook Book*, 27; *Kitchen Klinic*, 78.

159. Spelling of "gefüllte" original. Levine, "Why We Should Be More Interested," 21.

160. "Strange Varieties of Food: People of Different Parts of Earth Are Shown to Have Decidedly Different Tastes," from *New York Sun*, 8 February 1918, folder "Hagerstown Globe News (MD)," box 557, RG 4, NARA; "The Shock to Food Habits," 11 September 1917, folder "Columbia State News (SC)," box 547, RG 4, NARA.

161. The recipe called for a teaspoon and a half of curry powder for a cup of raw rice and a cup of potatoes. Rombauer, *Joy of Cooking*, 47.

162. *Mandarin Chop Suey Cook Book*; *Ramona's Spanish-Mexican Cookery*; Kander, *Settlement Cook Book*; McGuire, *Old World Foods*. First published in 1901 and then

many times thereafter throughout the twentieth century, *The Settlement Cook Book* was originally created to raise money for the Jewish Settlement House in Milwaukee, and it was insistently pan-ethnic from the start. Besides long stretches on strudels, matzos, and Passover cookery, it also contained recipes for dishes like spaghetti, chili con carne, Waldorf salad, and canned peas with white sauce.

163. James Montgomery Flagg, "James Montgomery Suds," in Sheridan, *Stag Cook Book*, 54.

164. Brebner, *All-American Cook Book*.

165. The United States imported a growing variety of foods from a growing number of places around the world. Although Americans had relied on imported foods ranging from coffee to cinnamon for centuries, U.S. food imports had increased exponentially since the end of the Civil War, jumping from about $56 million worth of imported food in 1865 to more than $1.8 billion in 1920. Hoganson, *Consumers' Imperium*, 110–11.

166. Haley, *Turning the Tables*, 107–8.

167. For instance, as late as 1927, the nutritionist Charles Houston Goudiss gave a detailed description of broccoli for those not familiar with it, calling it "an Italian vegetable resembling green cauliflower" (Goudiss, *Eating Vitamines*, 78).

168. Frederick, *Selling Mrs. Consumer*, 123.

169. Brebner, *All-American Cook Book*, 50; Kander, *Settlement Cook Book*, 222; *Fashions in Foods*, 55.

170. *Dixie Cook Book*, 119.

171. Hoganson, *Consumers' Imperium*, 151.

172. *Castelar Crèche Cook Book*, 129.

173. *Fashions in Foods*, 52; *Kitchen Klinic*, 36.

174. Advertisement for Dromedary Cocoanut, in Allen, *Woman's World Calendar Cook Book*, 79.

175. "Heinz Cooks You a Spaghetti Supper!," advertisement, *Chicago Daily Tribune*, 16 March 1934, 20.

176. Hoganson, *Consumers' Imperium*, 134–35.

177. Gabaccia, *We Are What We Eat*, 99–100, 123.

178. Gabaccia argues that by the 1930s, Italian restaurants sold bohemianism and "Latin hedonism" as much as the food itself. Ibid., 101–2.

179. Cristadoro, "Macaroni the Oldest National Joke," typed article sent to USFA on 8 August 1917, folder "Macaroni," box 149, USFA Collection, Hoover Institution.

180. John Moroso, "Spaghetti-for-the-Gang," in Sheridan, *Stag Cook Book*, 147.

181. Horton, *Long Straight Road*, 18–19.

182. See Heldke, "Let's Cook Thai."

183. T. A. Dorgan, "Chili con Carne," in Sheridan, *Stag Cook Book*, 98.

184. Harry Carr, "Eating Native," in *Fashions in Foods*, 113.

185. *Fashions in Foods*.

186. For example, Nancy Caroll wrote, "I have heard many Americans remark that they do not care for foreign cooking," before she proceeded to offer her own recipe for "Hungarian Goulash." *Fashions in Foods*, 50.

187. Macleod, "Food Prices," 366.

188. Gabaccia, *We Are What We Eat*, 56; Levenstein, *Revolution at the Table*, 42.

189. Frederick, *Selling Mrs. Consumer*, 156.

190. Ibid., 122–23.

191. Hoganson, *Consumers' Imperium*, 115; *Mexican Cookery*, 9.

192. Frederick, *Selling Mrs. Consumer*, 121–22. See also Deutsch, *Building a House-wife's Paradise*.

193. "The Old-Time Vittles," *Atlanta Constitution*, 16 May 1926, C2, PQHN.

194. Some of the many southern-themed cookbooks published between the 1910s and the 1930s include Martha McCulloch-Williams, *Dishes & Beverages of the Old South* (New York: McBride, Nast, 1913); *Echoes of Southern Kitchens*, United Daughters of the Confederacy, California Division, Robert E. Lee Chapter, no. 278 (Los Angeles: n.p., 1916); Kate Brew Vaughn, *Culinary Echoes from Dixie* (Cincinnati: McDonald Press, 1917); *Dixie Cook Book*; *Virginia Cookery Book*; Emma McKinney, *Aunt Caroline's Dixieland Recipes* (Chicago: Gold Seal, 1922); Queenie Washington, *The Sewanee Cook Book: A Collection of Autographed Recipes from Southern Homes and Plantations* (Nashville: Baird-Ward, 1926); Katharin Bell, *Mammy's Cook Book* (New York: H. Holt, 1928), MSU Special Collections; Natalie Vivian Scott, *Mirations and Miracles of Mandy* (New Orleans: R. H. True, 1929); *Southern Recipes from Old Green Hill Plantation House* (Columbia, S.C.: R. L. Bryan, 1929); Mary Denson Pretlow, *Old Southern Receipts* (New York: R. M. McBride, 1930); Blanche Rhett, *200 Years of Charleston Cooking*, edited by Lettie Gay (New York: Random House, 1934); Bessie Murphy, *A Hundred Recipes from The Old South, Selected and Compiled for the Housewives of America* (Columbus, Ohio: National Association of Margarine Manufactures, 1938); and Eleanor Ott, *Plantation Cookery of Old Louisiana* (New Orleans: Harmanson, 1938).

195. Brebner, *All-American Cook Book*, 52.

196. Sheridan, *Stag Cook Book*, 48.

197. America Eats Papers, boxes A829–A833, Records of the U.S. Work Projects Administration, LOC.

198. Recipes and advertisements for Boston Baked Beans continually alluded to their status as a historical food item. For instance, "Boston Baked Beans," *Hall's Journal of Health* 37, no. 9 (September 1890), 212; and "Bond's Boston Brown Bread Meal," *Good Housekeeping*, 26 December 1885, ii.

199. *Kitchen Klinic*, 89.

200. Gabaccia, *We Are What We Eat*, 57, 62.

201. "How to Cook Frijoles," press release for farm journals, [ca. 1917], folder "Farm Journals Section. Press Releases. Undated," box 41, series 12H, USFA Collection, Hoover Institution; press release no. 552, 23 December 1917, Public Information Division, folder "Press Releases, #500–599," box 11, USFA Collection, Hoover Library.

202. Packman, *Early California Hospitality*; Callahan, *Sunset All-Western Cook Book*.

203. *Recipes from Many Lands*.

204. Man, ed., *Chinese Cook Book*; *'Round the World Cookery*; *New England Cook Book*; Morrow, *Southern Cook Book*; Morrow, *Culinary Arts*; *Pennsylvania Dutch Cook Book*.

205. Like the new visions of Indian cuisine in the 1980s that the anthropologist Arjun Appadurai describes, the emerging cuisine of the United States in the interwar

period was also one "in which regional cuisines play an important role, and the national cuisine does not seek to hide its regional or ethnic roots" (Appadurai, "How to Make a National Cuisine," 3, 5).

206. Frederick, *Selling Mrs. Consumer*, 122.

207. Writing about the period from the end of the Civil War through 1920, Kristin Hoganson writes that by cooking and eating foreign foods, middle-class women "could profit from the immigrants who in other contexts appeared so threatening in their difference. . . . To consume novel foods was to become the woman in the advertisement—the beneficiary of global networks of wealth, power, and labor" (Hoganson, *Consumers' Imperium*, 120).

208. In 1921, the linguist H. L. Mencken discussed the Americanization of foreign foods, by which he meant how they came to be commonly consumed and talked about among Americans. He discussed newly common terms like "paprika," "goulash," "spaghetti," and "chianti." Mencken, *American Language*, 199.

209. *Fashions in Foods*, 60; "Americanized Chop Suey," *American Home Magazine* 12 (1934): 425; "Americanized Smörgåsbord," *Woman's Home Companion* 64, no. 9 (1937).

210. The *OED* attributes the use of "melting pot" in this sense to Israel Zangwill, who wrote in 1909, "America is God's Crucible, the great Melting-Pot where all the races of Europe are melting and reforming" (*Oxford English Dictionary*, s.v. "melting pot, n.").

211. The statistician Raymond Pearl's 1920 *Nation's Food* was the first definitive study of Americans' changing levels of commodity consumption.

212. *Food Questions Answered*, USFA, October 1918, folder "FA-II/Food Conservation, General," box 8, USFA Collection, Hoover Library; Hoover, "Food and the War," *The Day's Food in War and Peace*, bound folder "Addresses, Letters, Magazine Articles, Press Statements, Etc. Inclusive Dates: February 1, 1917–April 6, 1918," vol. I, part 1, box 93, Hoover Collection, Hoover Institution; Frances Marshall, "Kitchen Tips," 9 March 1918, folder "Oklahoma City News (OK)," box 570, RG 4, NARA.

213. Haley, *Turning the Tables*, 116, 95.

CHAPTER SEVEN

1. Putnam, *Tomorrow We Diet*, 7–8, 30, 34–35, 42–48, 52, 70–72.

2. Ibid., 79–80, 66, 74–75, 90.

3. See Vester, "Regime Change," 39.

4. For more on the history of diet, weight reduction, and the thin ideal, see Schwartz, *Never Satisfied*; Vester, "Regime Change"; Bargielowska, "Culture of the Abdomen"; Forth and Carden-Coyne, *Cultures of the Abdomen*; Jou, *Controlling Consumption*; Stearns, *Fat History*; Seid, *Never Too Thin*; Gilman, *Fat*; and Lowe, "From Robust Appetite to Calorie Counting."

5. See Cullather, "Foreign Policy of the Calorie."

6. Vester, "Regime Change," 42.

7. See Stearns, *Fat History*.

8. "Feel Better, Look Better!," 9 February 1918, folder "New York City Tribune Edit (NY)," box 566, RG 4, NARA; "War Foods Healthful as Well as Patriotic," 9 July 1918,

folder "Wapakoneta News News (OH)," box 567, RG 4, NARA; "Food and Health," 26 February 1918, folder "Clinton Chronicle News (OK)," box 570, RG 4, NARA; "People *Benefit Physically* Now by Eating Less Meat," 10 May 1918, "Philadelphia Inquirer News (PA)," box 568, RG 4, NARA; "Saving of Food Help to Health," 11 July 1917, folder "Alameda Times-Star News (CA)," box 530, RG 4, NARA; "War*Time*Cook*Book," press release to farm journals, 1 December 1917, folder "Press Releases, to Farm Journals," box 12, USFA Collection, Hoover Library.

9. "Sweetbread for Economy," 3 January 1918, folder "Columbus State Journal News (OH)," box 567, RG 4, NARA; L. Harper Leech, "War Diet Real Health Saver," 20[?] October 1917, folder "Waterloo Times Tribune News (IA)," box 535, RG 4, NARA; "Exit the Double Chin," 10 July 1917, folder "Hackensack Record Edit (NJ)," box 540, RG 4, NARA.

10. "Eat Less Sugar, Be Sylphlike, Cooke's Advice to Young Women," 9 May 1918, folder "Philadelphia North American News (PA)," box 568, RG 4, NARA; "Reducing Excess Weight," 13 December 1917, folder "Merced Sun Edit (CA)," box 530, RG 4, NARA; untitled blurb, 1 December 1917, folder "Anderson Bulletin (IN)," box 534, RG 4, NARA.

11. Schwartz, *Never Satisfied*, 175.

12. "What Ohio's War Board Says Today," 11 January 1918, folder "Dayton News Edit (OH), box 567, RG 4, NARA; "Food Saving Means 'Defeatless Days,'" 3 January 1918, folder "Columbus State Journal Edit (OH)," box 567, RG 4, NARA; letter from the teachers and pupils of Bremestead School, Diamond Point, Lake George, N.Y., to Hoover, 28 May 1918, folder "58 Bremestead School," box 300, RG 4, NARA; letter from Mrs. Cardine Wardle, West Coxsackie, N.Y., 7 August 1918, folder illegible, box 296, RG 4, NARA.

13. "Cannot Be Fat and Be Patriotic," 18 March 1918, folder "Boston Post News (MA)," box 557, RG 4, NARA.

14. Hoover, quoted in an originally anonymous interview with Will Irwin, typed text of "First Aid to America: How Civilians Must Get Together and Get Behind Strong Leaders," *Saturday Evening Post*, 24 March 1917, bound folder "Addresses, Letters, Magazine Articles, Press Statements, Etc. Inclusive Dates: February 1, 1917–April 6, 1918," vol. I, part 1, box 93, Hoover Collection, Hoover Institution.

15. Frederic J. Haskin, "Lean Europe and Fat America," 1 June 1917, folder "Lexington Herald Edit (KY)," box 535, RG 4, NARA.

16. This was not necessarily the case with second-generation immigrants, however. By the late 1920s, Christine Frederick reported that even in immigrant communities, the "young women, traditionally buxom, now want the slim American figure" (Frederick, *Selling Mrs. Consumer*, 75).

17. Stearns, *Fat History*, 30.

18. "Your Fuel Need," n.d., typed document, folder 8, "Dr. Ray Lyman Wilbur. 17 May–24 November 1917," box 1, series 5H, USFA Collection, Hoover Institution.

19. Rose, *Everyday Foods in War Time*, 62.

20. The historian Harvey Levenstein argues that it was in the late 1910s that "overweight and underweight reach[ed] a kind of balance in public concern" (*Revolution at the Table*, 166).

21. *Oxford English Dictionary*, s.vv. "overweight, adj.," "underweight, adj." For more on hardening concepts of "average" and "normal," see Igo, *Averaged American*.

22. For instance, the health and beauty lecturer Susanna Cocroft stressed that she had helped equal numbers of women gain weight and lose weight. "Reduce Your Weight," Susanna Cocroft advertisement, *Union Signal* 43, no. 9 (1 March 1917): 16; "Why Be Thin?," Susanna Cocroft advertisement, *Union Signal* 43, no. 7 (15 February 1917): 15; Blythe, *Fun of Getting Thin*, 11; Antoinette Donnelly, "Watch Your Weight! Says Lulu Hunt Peters, A.B., M.D.," *Chicago Daily Tribune*, 15 September 1915, B4, PQHN.

23. While Americans were growing somewhat heavier, Schwartz argues that their modest weight gains alone cannot nearly account for growing rejection of fat. Schwartz, *Never Satisfied*, 157.

24. Christian, "Three Great Laws that Govern Life," 6; Donahey, *Calorie Cook Book*, 13; McFadden, *Eating for Health and Strength*, 210; Rorer, "Food," 19.

25. Purdy, *Food and Freedom*, 35–36.

26. *The Day's Food in War and Peace*, USFA booklet, AAFCSR, #6578, DRMC; Reverend Lloyd H. Miller, at Woodward Avenue Christian Church in Detroit, quoted in "Heavy Eater Is a Traitor," 29 October 1917, folder "Detroit Free Press News (MI)," box 537, RG 4, NARA.

27. "Anyway, We Eat Too Much," 8 December 1917, folder "San Pedro News Editorial (CA)," box 530, RG 4, NARA.

28. Cocroft, *What to Eat and When*, x.

29. Goudiss and Goudiss, *Foods That Will Win the War*, 74.

30. Blythe, *Fun of Getting Thin*, 9–10.

31. Dr. T. J. Allen, "Daily Diet Hints: Longevity Favored by Reducing Weight," *Washington Post*, 26 February 1910, 7, PQHN; C. M. Cartwright, "Risk Firms Find Mortality High Among Fat Men," *Chicago Daily Tribune*, 1 May 1916, 12, PQHN; Dr. W. A. Evans, "How to Keep Well: Insurance and Health," *Chicago Daily Tribune*, 18 January 1918, 8, PQHN.

32. "Your Weight and Health: Better Be Over the Average When Young and Under When Old, Say Insurance Men," *Pittsburgh Courier*, 29 November 1912, 8, PQHN; "Your Weight and Health: People Past Thirty Years of Age Should Combat Any Increase of Adipose Tissue," *Los Angeles Times*, 4 July 1915, I6, PQHN.

33. Schwartz, *Never Satisfied*, 155.

34. McCollum and Simmonds, *American Home Diet*, 111.

35. "The Prevention of Diseases of Heart, Blood Vessels and Kidneys," Life Extension Institute advertisement, display ad 139, *New York Times*, 5 September 1920, BRM17, PQHN.

36. Peters, *Diet and Health*, 80.

37. Harvey Wiley, "Dr. Wiley's Question Box," *Good Housekeeping*, September 1918, 88; Harvey Wiley, "Dr. Wiley's Question-Box," *Good Housekeeping*, January 1918, 55–56, 93.

38. Untitled blurb, 16 January 1918, folder "Chicago News Edit (IL)," box 554, RG 4, NARA; "Dr Wiley Would Put Nation on Rations—Not as War Measure, but in Interest of Health," *Boston Daily Globe*, 28 January 1918, 5, PQHN.

39. "To Find Out How Much We Over-Eat," 7 October 1917, folder "Boston Herald News (MA)," box 536, RG 4, NARA; "Less Food, Better Health," 19 June 1917, folder "DC Washington Post Editorials," box 532, RG 4, NARA; "How to Be Healthy," 19 January 1918, folder "Idaho Boise News Editorials," box 533, RG 4, NARA.

40. "Become Disciple of Hoover and Live Longer, New War Food Maxim," 19 November 1917, folder "Boston Traveler Edit (MA)," box 537, RG 4, NARA.

41. "Hooverize for Health," 4 October 1917, folder "East Ellsworth Record News (WI)," box 549, RG 4, NARA.

42. "Eat by 'Calories,' Slogan of Fatless League Campaign," 11 January 1918, folder "Los Angeles Record News (CA)," box 551, RG 4, NARA; "Fat Men Plan to Save Food by Reducing at Waist," 25 October 1917, folder "Los Angeles Herald News (CA)," box 530, RG 4, NARA; Peters, *Diet and Health*, 79.

43. Irwin, "The Autocrat of the Dinner Table," *Saturday Evening Post*, 23 June 1917, 57–58, folder "Writings about Hoover," box 219, Hoover Collection, Hoover Institution.

44. "Ways of the World," 11 December 1917, folder "San Francisco Bulletin Edit (CA)," box 531, RG 4, NARA; Irwin, "The Autocrat of the Dinner Table," *Saturday Evening Post*, 23 June 1917, 57–58, folder "Writings about Hoover," box 219, Hoover Collection, Hoover Institution; "Here's the Food Boss of America 'Snapped' on Visit to Chicago," August 1917, folder "Chicago Herald News (IL)," box 533, RG 4, NARA; Donald Wilhelm, "Herbert Hoover: The Man Who Fed Twenty-one Nations," in "If He Were President: The Independent Series of Articles on Some Likely Candidates for 1920s, Presenting the Views of Leading Republicans and Democrats on the Vital Issues of Today," *The Independent*, 13 December 1919, folder "Writings about Hoover," box 219, Hoover Collection, Hoover Institution; "Herbert C. Hoover—How He Made His Millions," 3 June 1917, folder "San Francisco Examiner Edit (CA)," box 530, RG 4, NARA; William C. Edgar, "Two American Heroes," *The Bellman* 19, no. 468, 3 July 1915, folder "Writings about Hoover," box 219, Hoover Collection, Hoover Institution.

45. "Hoover—the Man and the Moral," 27 January 1918, folder "New York City Tribune Edit (NY)," box 566, RG 4, NARA; Ernest Poole, "Hoover of Belgium," *Saturday Evening Post*, 26 May 1917, folder "Writings about Hoover," box 219, Hoover Collection, Hoover Institution.

46. Joe Toye, "Who's Hoover?," 27 May 1917, *Boston Sunday Post*, folder "May 27–June 17, 1917, Hoover's Genius," box 12, Hoover Library; "Here's the Food Boss of America 'Snapped' on Visit to Chicago," August 1917, folder "Chicago Herald News (IL)," box 533, RG 4, NARA.

47. Ben Allen, interoffice memo to Gertrude Lane, 13 September 1918, folder "Home Card, Oct. 1917–1918," box 3, series 5H, USFA Collection, Hoover Institution; Kellogg, "Herbert Hoover, as Individual and Type," *The Atlantic*, March 1918, folder "Writings about Hoover," box 219, Hoover Collection, Hoover Institution.

48. William Jennings Bryan, "Bryan Gets after Food Profiteers: Greedy Few Must Not Fatten on Nation's Sufferings," 6 January 1918, folder "Boston American News (MA)," box 557, RG 4, NARA.

49. Cartoon, 5 June 1917, folder "Jersey City Journal Edit (NJ)," box 540, RG 4, NARA.

50. Cartoon, 22 October 1918, folder "New York City World News No. 3 (NY)," box 566, RG 4, NARA.

51. Cartoons, 17 November 1917, folder "Literary Digest Edit (NY)," box 541, RG 4, NARA; "The Farmer or the Profiteer—Which Should the Nation Help?," 4 April 1918, folder "Washington Herald Edit (DC)," box 552, RG 4, NARA.

52. Cartoon, *Literary Digest*, 1 September 1917, n.p., folder "September 1, 1917. Our national wheat corporation," box 13, Hoover Library.

53. Antoinette Donnelly, "Watch Your Weight! Says Lulu Hunt Peters, A.B., M.D.," *Chicago Daily Tribune*, 15 September 1915, B4, PQHN.

54. Ibid. "Watching the Fat Man," 4 November 1917, folder "Charlotte Chronicle Edit (NC)," box 544, RG 4, NARA.

55. "Are You a Fat Hoarder? Food Speculators No Worse Than Over Weight Individual—He Carries Food Value," 17 January 1918, folder "Piqua Call News (OH)," box 567, RG 4, NARA; Antoinette Donnelly, "Watch Your Weight! Says Lulu Hunt Peters, A.B., M.D.," *Chicago Daily Tribune*, 15 September 1915, B4, PQHN.

56. Calculations of *Popular Science Monthly* noted in "Are You Over Weight?," 13 December 1917, folder "Los Angeles Tribune News Edit (CA)," box 530, RG 4, NARA.

•57. "Potato Pointers: Keep Your Figure," n.d., typed document, USDA, American Home Economics Association collection, AAFCSR, #6578, DRMC.

58. "Exit the Double Chin," 10 July 1917, folder "Hackensack Record Edit (NJ)," box 540, RG 4, NARA.

59. Letter from Tom Flinty, Dallas, Tex., to Honorable Clarence Ousley at USDA, 13 July 1917, folder illegible, box 290, RG 4, NARA.

60. "Cannot Be Fat and Be Patriotic," 18 March 1918, folder "Boston Post News (MA)," box 557, RG 4, NARA.

61. The author originally wrote "theiy [*sic*] are doing their bit." "Fat Persons Not Patriots, She Says," 9 November 1917, folder "Los Angeles Record Edit (CA)," box 530, RG 4, NARA.

62. "Are You Over Weight?," 13 December 1917, folder "Los Angeles Tribune News Edit (CA)," box 530, RG 4, NARA.

63. "Fat Persons Not Patriots, She Says," 9 November 1917, folder "Los Angeles Record Edit (CA)," box 530, RG 4, NARA.

64. Frederick, *Selling Mrs. Consumer*, 131, 26.

65. Frederick, "Mrs. Consumer Speaks Up!," 1, typewritten remarks given to New York Rotary Club, 19 March 1938, folder 10[?], box 1, Christine Frederick Papers, 1887–1970, Schlesinger.

66. Eunice Fuller Barnard, "Our Quest for the Fountain of Youth," *New York Times*, 15 November 1930, SM3, PQHN.

67. "What Thos. E. Young Says," *Atlanta Daily World*, 4 December 1931, 4, PQHN.

68. Rombauer, *Joy of Cooking*, unnumbered prefatory material.

69. Blythe, *Fun of Getting Thin*, 43, 10.

70. Putnam, *Tomorrow We Diet*, 7–8; Axtell, *Grow Thin on Good Food*, 3; Schwartz, *Never Satisfied*, 157.

71. Peters, *Diet and Health*, 13.

72. Blythe, *Fun of Getting Thin*, 14, 55–57, 13, 68.

73. Axtell was a doctor, and after she lost weight and kept it off, she began to treat overweight patients. Axtell, *Grow Thin on Good Food*, 3–4.

74. Donahey, *Calorie Cook Book*, 11; McFadden, *Eating for Health and Strength*, 210.

75. Harvey Wiley, "The Eternal Svelte," *Good Housekeeping*, December 1917, folder "Dec. 1917," box 163, Harvey Wiley Papers, LOC; Donahey, *Calorie Cook Book*, 26, 29.

76. Sylvia of Hollywood, *"No More Alibis!"*; Ullback, *Pull Yourself Together, Baby!*; "Sylvia, Beauty Adviser, Weds," *Los Angeles Times*, 6 July 1932, 7, PQHN; Frances Mangum, "Beauty Is Community Property, Says Hollywood's Mme. Sylvia," *Washington Post*, 17 August 1934, 12, PQHN.

77. Emphasis original. Sylvia of Hollywood, *"No More Alibis!,"* 12–13.

78. Ibid., 22–29.

79. Peters, *Diet and Health*, 81.

80. Spelling original. Diary of Yvonne Blue Skinner, 18 April 1925 [or 1926], 48, Yvonne Blue Skinner Collection, microfilm, Schlesinger.

81. Ibid., 3 July 1925 [or 1926], 69, and 10 July 1925 [or 1926], 72.

82. Ibid., 1 August 1925 [or 1926], 78.

83. "Will power" was originally capitalized. Rosalind Shaffer, "Follows Her Own Rules for Diet: Iron Will Is Needed for Process," *Chicago Daily Tribune*, 22 December 1935, E10, PQHN.

84. Thompson and Thompson, *Health Recipe Cook Book*, 55; W. H. Shackleford, "Maybe So and Maybe Not: Attention! Heavyweight Sisters!," *Atlanta Daily World*, 31 August 1934, 6, PQHN; Madame Qui Vive, "Beauty Hints: Take Your Time, Girls, When Reducing," *Atlanta Daily World*, 6 September 1932, 3, PQHN; "How Film Stars Keep Slim," *Washington Post*, 18 October 1925, SM8, PQHN.

85. First published in 1936, it sold a million and a half copies in the next ten years. Lindlahr, *7-DAY Reducing Diet*.

86. Donahey, *Calorie Cook Book*, 25. Ullback likewise advised pityingly that even after they had lost weight, "You fat babies must always watch your diet" (Sylvia of Hollywood, *"No More Alibis!,"* 75).

87. Peters, *Diet and Health*, 18.

88. Schwartz argues that Peters helped make dieting "a quality of personality" rather than a mere act. Schwartz, *Never Satisfied*, 175–76.

89. Blythe, *Fun of Getting Thin*, 37.

90. Peters, *Diet and Health*, 13.

91. Fisher and Fisk, *How to Live*, 257. During the 1920s, the makers of weight tables were no longer allowing for weight gain as people aged, and new tables, instead, began to shave pounds off the ideal weights listed for older people. Schwartz, *Never Satisfied*, 157.

92. Schwartz, *Never Satisfied*, 193.

93. Peters, *Diet and Health*, 25; McFadden, *Eating for Health and Strength*, 210–11; Fisk, "Possible Extension of the Human Life Cycle," 185.

94. "Now Is Good Time to Reduce Flesh," 19 October 1917, folder "Eugene Guard News (OR)," box 546, RG 4, NARA.

95. "Watching the Fat Man," 4 November 1917, folder "Charlotte Chronicle Edit (NC)," box 544, RG 4, NARA; Donahey, *Calorie Cook Book*, 11.

96. Peters, *Diet and Health*, 77; Peters, "Diet and Health," *Los Angeles Times*, 17 April 1924, A6, PQHN.

97. *Oxford English Dictionary*, s.v. "will-power, n."

98. Payot, *Education of the Will*; Haddock, *Power of Will*. The genre also included books like J. Milner Fothergill, *Will Power; Its Range in Action* (London: Hodder and Stoughton, 1885); Horace Fletcher, *Menticulture; or, The A-B-C of True Living* (Chicago: A. C. McClurg, 1895); Thomas Sharper Knowlson, *The Education of the Will: A Popular Study* (London: T. W. Laurie, 1909); Sophia Shaler, *The Masters of Fate: The Power of the Will* (1906; New York: Duffield and Company, 1913); James Walsh, *Health through Will Power* (Boston: Little, Brown, 1919); Paul Émile Lévy, *The Rational Education of the Will: Its Therapeutic Value* (Philadelphia: McKay, 1920); Henry Hazlitt, *The Way to Will-Power* (New York: E. P. Dutton, 1922); and June Downey, *The Will-Temperament and Its Testing* (Yonkers-on-Hudson, N.Y.: World Book, 1923).

99. Finck, *Girth Control*, 16.

100. Axtell, *Grow Thin on Good Food*, 9; Donahey, *Calorie Cook Book*, 29.

101. "How Much Are You Worth?," Life Extension Institute ad, display ad 195, *New York Times*, 7 May 1922, 65.

102. Nissenbaum, *Sex, Diet, and Debility*; Whorton, *Crusaders for Fitness*, 271.

103. "Human Body Like Machine or Watch," *Hartford Courant*, 10 December 1914, 5, PQHN; Rapeer, "Health as a Means to Happiness," 67, 97. For more on physical fitness and physical culture, see Whorton, *Crusaders for Fitness*; Budd, *Sculpture Machine*; Todd, *Physical Culture*; Kasson, *Houdini, Tarzan*; Stewart, *For Health and Beauty*; Verbrugge, "Gender, Science & Fitness"; and Dworkin and Wachs, *Body Panic*.

104. Whorton, *Crusaders for Fitness*, 284.

105. Finck, *Girth Control*, 22–23.

106. Frederick, *Selling Mrs. Consumer*, 117–18; Hamilton, *Primer of Cooking*, 20–21.

107. Frederick, *Selling Mrs. Consumer*, 116.

108. "Number of Fat Women is Appalling!," *Washington Post*, 25 April 1915, 14, PQHN.

109. Dorothy Dix, "Housework for Exercise," Dorothy Dix Talks, *Boston Daily Globe*, 12 November 1917, 10, PQHN.

110. Marjorie Stewart Joyner, "Irresistible Charm: Fat Under Arm," *Chicago Defender*, 16 July 1932, 15, PQHN.

111. "Don't Be a Machine," 10 February 1918, folder "Augusta Herald News (GA)," box 553, RG 4, NARA.

112. Cocks, *Etiquette of Beauty*, 42.

113. Ibid., 40; Marjorie Stewart Joyner, "Irresistible Charm: Fat Under Arm," *Chicago Defender*, 16 July 1932, 15, PQHN; Antoinette Donnelly, "Merry Warriors in War on Fat Hike, Hike, Hike," *Chicago Daily Tribune*, 3 May 1920, 3, PQHN.

114. "She Found a Pleasant Way to Reduce Her Fat," Marmola Company advertisement, *Chicago Defender*, 2 February 1924, A5, PQHN; "Love Scenes Show No Fat," advertisement for Marmola Prescription Tablets, *Chicago Defender*, 19 November 1927, 3, PQHN.

115. McFadden, *Eating for Health and Strength*, 210; Buckstein, *Food, Fitness and Figure*, 143; "Free Fat Reducer," advertisement for Reliable Drug Co., *Chicago Defender*,

22 February 1919, 7, PQHN; "Get Rid of Your Fat," advertisement for Dr. Newman's diet compound, *Chicago Defender*, 2 October 1926, A5, PQHN.

116. *Reducing Diets and Recipes*, 4; *Sunny Side of Life Book*.

117. "Lorenz Turkish Baths," advertisement, *New York Amsterdam News*, 2 December 1931, 4, PQHN; "How to Safely Lose Fat," advertisement for Sleepy Water Company bath salts, *Atlanta Daily World*, 16 January 1935, 6, PQHN; "Bathe Your Way to Health," advertisement for Brooks Health Baths, *Los Angeles Sentinel*, 24 May 1934, 5, PQHN; "How One Woman Lost 47 Lbs," advertisement for Kruschen Salts, *New York Amsterdam News*, 27 July 1932, 3, PQHN; Putnam, *Tomorrow We Diet*, 57; "Stenographer Keeps in Trim: Shimmying Chair Helps Girls to Retain Figures," *Los Angeles Times*, 1 February 1935, A3, PQHN.

118. "Remove Your Fat and Be Happy," advertisement for Wayne's Reducing Soap, *Chicago Defender*, 29 November 1924, A5, PQHN.

119. Schwartz, *Never Satisfied*, 191–92.

120. Hamlin, "Bathing Suits and Backlash," 32.

121. Ibid., 29, 32, 40–41; Schwartz, *Never Satisfied*, 177.

122. Sylvia of Hollywood, *"No More Alibis!,"* 13; *7-DAY Reducing Diet*, inside front cover; Schwartz, *Never Satisfied*, 170; Booher, *Scientific Weight Control*, 4.

123. Putnam, *Tomorrow We Diet*, 74–75.

124. Thompson, *Eat and Grow Thin*, 25.

125. "Health Officer Warns 'Flappers,'" *Boston Daily Globe*, 17 February 1922, 6, PQHN; "Scanty Dress + Boyish Figure = HIGHER DEATH RATE," *Washington Post*, 8 April 1928, MS2, PQHN.

126. Leonard Hill, "Man Advised to Wear Much Less Clothing," *New York Times*, 13 September 1925, 26, PQHN; Antoinette Donnelly, "Shorter Skirts Make Slender Legs Necessity," *Chicago Daily Tribune*, 23 November 1935, 18, PQHN; Schwartz, *Never Satisfied*, 162.

127. Lucrezia Bori, "How to Exercise to Win More Beautiful Hip Lines," *Washington Post*, 25 August 1922, 5, PQHN.

128. Sylvia of Hollywood, *"No More Alibis!,"* 16.

129. "Beauty Hints: Dressing the Plump Figure," *Atlanta Daily World*, 14 September 1934, 2, PQHN.

130. "Salem Tutt Whitney," *Chicago Defender*, 16 June 1928, 7, PQHN.

131. "Love Scenes Show No Fat," advertisement for Marmola Prescription Tablets, *Chicago Defender*, 19 November 1927, 3, PQHN.

132. "How Film Stars Keep Slim," *Washington Post*, 18 October 1925, SM8, PQHN.

133. "Romance and Fat Won't Mix on Screen," *Washington Post*, 29 November 1925, SM3, PQHN.

134. "How Film Stars Keep Slim," *Washington Post*, 18 October 1925, SM8, PQHN.

135. *Milady's Style Parade and Recipe Book for 1935*; W. H. Shackleford, "Maybe So and Maybe Not: Attention! Heavyweight Sisters!," *Atlanta Daily World*, 31 August 1934, 6, PQHN; Madame Qui Vive, "Beauty Hints: Take Your Time, Girls, When Reducing," *Atlanta Daily World*, 6 September 1932, 3, PQHN; "Hollywood Diet Given 'Knockout,'" *Los Angeles Times*, 1 August 1929, 20, PQHN.

136. "'Hollywood Diet' Wins: New York Faddists Start Grapefruit Regimen," *Los Angeles Times*, 18 June 1929, 11, PQHN.

137. "Tels corps, telles âmes!," Harrison and Clergue, *Cuisine des Alliés*, iii.

138. *Funny Bone, Laugh and Grow Fat: A Collection of Puns and Jokes* (Hannibal, Mo.: Hannibal Printing Company, 1880), Beinecke Library, Yale University, New Haven, Conn.

139. These associations would only harden in the decades that followed. Schwartz argues that Americans in the twentieth century increasingly saw fat people as searching for love and comfort. Schwartz, *Never Satisfied*, 195. By the mid-twentieth century, doctors would generally agree that obese people—and especially obese women—were repressed, unfocused, anxious, unable to achieve goals, and prone to depression. In 1944, for example, the dieting and anti-aging celebrity Gaylord Hauser wrote that many people were overweight "because they are bored, troubled, or emotionally upset. They gorge themselves as an escape mechanism in the same way that an alcoholic drinks to forget his difficulties" (Hauser, *Diet Does It* [New York: Coward-McCann, Inc., 1944], 86, MSU Special Collections). See also Miriam Lincoln, *Danger! Curves Ahead: How to Prevent and Correct Overweight* (New York: MacMillan, 1948), photo insert between 44 and 45; and Leonid Kotkin, *Eat, Think and Be Slender* (New York: Hawthorn Books, 1954), 41, MSU Special Collections.

140. Thompson, *Eat and Grow Thin*, 23.

141. Abstract of letter sent from Mrs. Marie Sheldon, Lexington, Mich., to USFA, 19 February 1918, box 328, RG 4, NARA; William Brady, "Is Reduction Healthful?," Health Talks, *Atlanta Constitution*, 20 August 1923, 4, PQHN.

142. "Number of Fat Women is Appalling!," *Washington Post*, 25 April 1915, 14, PQHN; Lora Kelly, "Through the Periscope," folder "Cleveland Plaindealer News (OH)," box 567, NARA.

143. "The Frugal Life," 4 December 1917, folder "Birmingham News News (AL)," box 529, RG 4, NARA.

144. Dana, "Your Weight and Your Nerves," 85.

145. Peters, *Diet and Health*, 13–14.

146. Finck, *Girth Control*, 12; McFadden, *Eating for Health and Strength*, 189–90. Hamilton wrote that eating a heavy breakfast made people "stupid all day" (*Primer of Cooking*, 20–21). Harvey Wiley, "Lecture on Diet of a Normal Man," 3, lecture no. 10, The United Schools of Physical Culture, 1909, MSU Special Collections.

147. Dana, "Your Weight and Your Nerves," 85.

148. Finck, *Girth Control*, 13.

149. Bragg, *Paul C. Bragg's Personal Health Food Cook Book and Menus*, 12; Sylvia of Hollywood, *"No More Alibis!*," 53; Peters, *Diet and Health*, 60.

150. McFadden, *Eating for Health and Strength*, 189–90.

151. Dana, "Your Weight and Your Nerves," 85–86.

152. Fisk, "Life Insurance," 339.

153. Blythe, *Fun of Getting Thin*, 58–59. After Mr. and Mrs. Thomas Edison cut their meals almost in half in order to lose weight in the early 1910s, Mrs. Edison reported that she could think more clearly than ever before. "Eat Less and Be Happy," *Chicago Defender*, 21 March 1914, 3, PQHN.

154. Donahey, *Calorie Cook Book*, 10.

155. Sylvia of Hollywood, *"No More Alibis!,"* 13.

156. Axtell, *Grow Thin on Good Food*, 201.

157. Peters, *Diet and Health*, 19.

158. See Vester, "Regime Change"; Kasson, *Houdini, Tarzan*; and Griffith, *Born Again Bodies*.

159. Vester also claims that it was "women's rights activists who started to encourage their followers to control their food intake, arguing that women had mastery over their bodies, too" ("Regime Change," 39–40).

160. "Eat Less—Hoe More," 31 July 1917, "Elmira Gazette Edit (NY)," box 543, RG 4, NARA; "Feel Better, Look Better!," 9 February 1918, folder "New York City Tribune Edit (NY)," box 566, RG 4, NARA.

161. "Fat Men Plan to Save Food by Reducing at Waist," 25 October 1917, folder "Los Angeles Herald News (CA)," box 530, RG 4, NARA.

162. Putnam, *Tomorrow We Diet*, 32; Sylvia of Hollywood, *"No More Alibis!,"* 21; Blythe, *Fun of Getting Thin*.

163. Putnam, *Tomorrow We Diet*, 31.

164. Lydia Lane, "Beauty Needs Slender Lines: Overweight Avoidable through Exercise," *Los Angeles Times*, 4 January 1935, A7, PQHN; Ullback, quoted in Frances Mangum, "Beauty Is Community Property, Says Hollywood's Mme. Sylvia," *Washington Post*, 17 August 1934, 12, PQHN.

165. Thompson, *Eat and Grow Thin*, 4; "Romance and Fat Won't Mix on Screen," *Washington Post*, 29 November 1925, SM3, PQHN.

166. Finck, *Girth Control*, 9–10.

167. Hastings, *Physical Culture Food Directory*, 62–63.

168. David Arlen, "Achieving Camera Beauty," *New York Amsterdam News*, 31 May 1933, 8, PQHN.

169. Walter B. Pitkin quoted in William Feather, "Effect of Dieting," *Pittsburgh Courier*, 27 April 1935, 5, PQHN.

170. Bragg, *Paul C. Bragg's Personal Health Food Cook Book and Menus*, 12.

171. Smith, *Official Cook Book*, 393.

172. Frederick, *Selling Mrs. Consumer*, 131–32.

173. Axtell, *Grow Thin on Good Food*, 10.

174. *Sunny Side of Life Book*, 28; Rosalind Shaffer, "Danish Sylvia Gives Lowdown on Hollywood: Cinema Stars Amused by Exposé," *Chicago Daily Tribune*, 6 September 1931, D8, PQHN.

175. Finck, *Girth Control*, 10; Thompson, in *Eat and Grow Thin*, 13.

176. Doris Blake, "It's the Wise Wife Who Refuses to Age Before She Has To," *Chicago Daily Tribune*, 13 September 1928, 30, PQHN.

177. Writers occasionally enticed men into dieting by promising it would make them more attractive, too. Axtell, *Grow Thin on Good Food*, 202.

178. Putnam, *Tomorrow We Diet*, 30.

179. Dix, "Dorothy Dix's Letter Box," *Hartford Courant*, 23 June 1928, 10, PQHN.

180. Peters, *Diet and Health*, 18–19; Peters, "Diet and Health," *Los Angeles Times*, 20 September 1923, I16, PQHN.

181. Sylvia of Hollywood, *"No More Alibis!,"* 21.

182. "Sylvia, Beauty Adviser, Weds," *Los Angeles Times*, 6 July 1932, 7, PQHN; "Wives Are Told to Keep Figure, Sense of Humor: Right Diet, Systematic Exercise Advised by Mme. Sylvia," *Washington Post*, 27 November 1935, 15, PQHN.

183. W. H. Shackleford, "Maybe So and Maybe Not: Attention! Heavyweight Sisters!," *Atlanta Daily World*, 31 August 1934, 6, PQHN.

184. Egypsy Ann, "Confidences: Questions and Answers," *New York Amsterdam News*, 19 June 1929, 7, PQHN.

185. "Electric Treatment for Reducing Weight," advertisement, *New York Amsterdam News*, 16 April 1930, 8, PQHN. Other examples include "Eat Less and Be Happy," *Chicago Defender*, 21 Mar 1914, 3, PQHN; "Free Fat Reducer," advertisement for Reliable Drug Co., *Chicago Defender*, 22 February 1919, 7, PQHN; "She Found a Pleasant Way to Reduce Her Fat," Marmola Company advertisement, *Chicago Defender*, 2 February 1924, A5, PQHN; display ad 117, *Chicago Defender*, 1 March 1924, A10, PQHN; "Lorenz Turkish Baths," advertisement, *New York Amsterdam News*, 2 December 1931, 4, PQHN; Betty Barclay, "Recipes for Reducers," *New York Amsterdam News*, 11 May 1932, 5, PQHN; "How One Woman Lost 47 Lbs," advertisement for Kruschen Salts, *New York Amsterdam News*, 27 July 1932, 3, PQHN; "Bathe Your Way to Health," advertisement for Brooks Health Baths, *Los Angeles Sentinel*, 24 May 1934, 5, PQHN; "How to Safely Lose Fat," advertisement for Sleepy Water Company bath salts, *Atlanta Daily World*, 16 January 1935, 6, PQHN.

186. Leila Hubbard, "Beauty Hints," *Chicago Defender*, 20 December 1919, 12, PQHN; "To Reduce Weight," *Chicago Defender*, 6 March 1915, 6, PQHN; Marjorie Stewart Joyner, "Irresistible Charm: Fat Under Arm," *Chicago Defender*, 16 July 1932, 15, PQHN; Helen Jameson, "Beauty Hints," *Atlanta Daily World*, 21 October 1935, 2, PQHN.

187. "Problems of Everyday Life," *Atlanta Daily World*, 22 September 1932, 3, PQHN.

188. For instance, in 1917 one writer imagined the contemporary "fat black cook" of the South, "waddl[ing] homeward with a basketful of grub from the white folks' table" (Harris Dickson, "Save and Serve with Hoover: What Will Feed Three Will Feed Four," *Collier's: The National Weekly*, ed. Mark Sullivan, 11 August 1917, folder "Writings about Hoover," box 219, Hoover Collection, Hoover Institution). Vester argues that "the racial and ethnic other was imagined as overweight, and thus as less disciplined, more sensual, and unfit to exercise social power" ("Regime Change," 40). See also McElya, *Clinging to Mammy*.

189. Ullback, quoted in "Wives Are Told to Keep Figure, Sense of Humor: Right Diet, Systematic Exercise Advised by Mme. Sylvia," *Washington Post*, 27 November 1935, 15, PQHN.

EPILOGUE

1. Emphasis added. Frederick, *Selling Mrs. Consumer*, 130–33.

2. Dr. William Brady, "Eat and Grow Young," *Atlanta Constitution*, 25 January 1930, 6, PQHN.

3. Eunice Fuller Barnard, "Our Quest for the Fountain of Youth," *New York Times*, 15 November 1930, SM3, PQHN.

4. Bennett, *World's Food*, 167, 164, 180, 173–74; DuPuis, *Nature's Perfect Food*, 114. Another way to measure the quality of nutrition over time is to look at average heights. Good diets tend to result in heights that rise or remain stable over time, so the heights of populations can serve as surrogates for nutrition levels. In the United States in the 1910s, children from wealthy families grew up to be significantly taller on average than children from poorer families. In the 1930s, for example, boys who applied to Harvard from private high schools—and were thus likely to come from financially comfortable families—had reached an average height of five feet eleven, while applicants to Harvard from public high schools were significantly shorter. Yet during the next two decades, the average height of private school applicants did not change, whereas the average height of public school applicants rose steadily. This not only suggests that there was a marked difference in the quality of diets between wealthy and nonwealthy people in the 1910s and 1920s—when those Harvard applicants would have been children—but it also suggests that in the three decades that followed, other Americans caught up. See Riley, "Height, Nutrition, and Mortality Risk," 486. For more on anthropometric history, see Komlos and Cuff, *Classics in Anthropometric History*; Komlos, *Stature, Living Standards*; Komlos, *Biological Standard of Living*; and Scott and Duncan, *Demography and Nutrition*.

5. Freidberg, *Fresh*.

6. Craig, Goodwin, and Grennes, "Effect of Mechanical Refrigeration"; Flour et al., *Changing Body*, 311; Petrick, "'Like Ribbons of Green and Gold.'"

7. See Fitzgerald, *Every Farm a Factory*; Deutsch, *Building a Housewife's Paradise*.

8. Aaron Bobrow-Strain defines industrial food as "the products of capital-intensive agriculture, processed into homogenous, standardized edibles designed to maximize efficiency and profit over other values such as taste or sustainability" (Bobrow-Strain, *White Bread*, 8).

9. See Neuhaus, *Manly Meals*, 191–218.

10. See Guthman, *Weighing In*, and Johnston and Baumann, *Foodies*.

11. As a result, as scholars like Josée Johnston and Shyon Baumann have argued, it is a powerful way to assert standing and prestige. Johnston and Baumann, *Foodies*.

12. "How Obesity Harms a Child's Body," *Washington Post*, 18 May 2008, A13.

13. "Cannot Be Fat and Be Patriotic," 18 March 1918, folder "Boston Post News (MA)," box 557, RG 4, NARA; Biltekoff, "Terror Within," 42.

14. "If" was capitalized in Guthman's original wording. Guthman, "Can't Stomach It," 78. She calls anti-obesity rhetoric "a self-serving, self-congratulatory discourse that exalts certain ways of being and disparages others, and places blame in many of the wrong places" (Guthman, *Weighing In*, 6). Anna Kirkland argues that environmental explanations for obesity suggest that "some people are impervious to bad environments (the elites, who still manage their bodies properly) while others are more fully constructed by their environments (poor fat people). Members of one group move powerfully through the world determining their body sizes and health statuses; others are pitiably stuck within and determined by the environment" (Kirkland, "Environmental Account of Obesity," 476–77, 466).

15. Given the class and racial dimension of obesity, scholars have argued that it has become a new crucible for concerns about poverty and minorities. Kirkland suggests that the focus on environmental causes of obesity may simply be "a more palatable way" for elites "to express their disgust at fat people, the tacky, low-class food they eat, and the indolent ways they spend their time" (Kirkland, "Environmental Account of Obesity," 474–75). See also Biltekoff, "Terror Within," 42.

BIBLIOGRAPHY

ARCHIVES

Archives Départementales de l'Aisne, Laon, France
Archives Départementales de la Marne, Châlons en Champagne, France
Archives Départementales de la Somme, Amiens, France
Beinecke Library, Yale University, New Haven, Connecticut
Biblioteca Nacional de España, Madrid, Spain
Bibliothèque Nationale de France, Paris, France
Division of Rare and Manuscript Collections, Cornell University, Ithaca, New York
Hoover Institution on War, Revolution, and Peace, Stanford, California
Hoover Presidential Library, West Branch, Iowa
Michigan State University Special Collections, East Lansing, Michigan
Schlesinger Library, Radcliffe Institute, Harvard University, Cambridge,
    Massachusetts
United States Library of Congress, Washington, D.C.
United States National Archives and Records Administration, College Park, Maryland
Widener Library, Harvard University, Cambridge, Massachusetts

SELECTED PUBLISHED PRIMARY SOURCES

Adair, A. H. *Dinners, Long and Short*. New York: Knopf, 1929.
Alcalá Galiano y Osma, Alvaro. *El fin de la tragedia: La "entente" victoriosa y España neutral*. Madrid: Pueyo, 1919. Biblioteca Nacional de España, Madrid, Spain.
Alcott, William. *Young Housekeeper; or, Thoughts on Food and Cookery*. 6th ed. Boston: Waite, Peirce, 1846.
Allen, Ida Bailey. *Mrs. Allen's Book of Sugar Substitutes*. Boston: Small, Maynard, 1918. Division of Rare and Manuscript Collections, Cornell University, Ithaca, N.Y.
———. *Woman's World Calendar Cook Book*. Chicago: Woman's World Magazine, 1922.
Allen, Lucy Grace. *Choice Recipes for Clever Cooks*. Boston: Little, Brown, 1924.
Armitage, Francis Paul. *Diet and Race: Anthropological Essays*. New York: Longmans, Green, 1922.
Atkinson, Edward. *The Science of Nutrition: Treatise upon the Science of Nutrition*. Boston: Damrell and Upham, 1896.
Atwater, Helen. "A Guide to the Nation's Dietary Needs." *World's Food* 74 (November 1917): 108–18.
Augé-Laribé, Michel. *Agriculture and Food Supply in France during the War: Agriculture*. New Haven: Yale University Press, 1927.

Austin, Bertha. *Domestic Science*. Chicago: Lyons and Carnahan, 1914.

Axtell, Luella. *Grow Thin on Good Food*. New York: Funk & Wagnalls, 1930. Schlesinger Library, Radcliffe Institute, Harvard University, Cambridge, Mass.

Balderston, Lydia. *Housewifery: A Manual and Text Book of Practical Housekeeping*. Philadelphia: Lippincott, 1919.

Ballesteros, Lázaro. *La guerra Europea y la neutralidad española*. Madrid: Jaime Ratés, 1917. Biblioteca Nacional de España, Madrid, Spain.

Barker, Clara. *Wanted, a Young Woman to Do Housework: Business Principles Applied to Housework*. New York: Moffat, Yard, 1915.

Beecher, Catharine. *A Treatise on Domestic Economy, for the Use of Young Ladies at Home, and at School*. Rev. ed. Boston: T. H. Webb, 1842.

Behnke, Kate Emil, and E. Colin Henslowe. *The Broadlands Cookery-Book: A Comprehensive Guide to the Principles and Practice of Food Reform*. London: G. Bell, 1910. Division of Rare and Manuscript Collections, Cornell University, Ithaca, N.Y.

Bellamy, Edward. *Looking Backward, 2000–1887*. Oxford: Oxford University Press, 2007.

Benton, Caroline French. *Gala-Day Luncheons; A Little Book of Suggestions*. New York: Dodd, Mead, 1903.

——. "A Poverty Luncheon Club." *Good Housekeeping*, April 1906, 445–47.

Bitting, Arvil Wayne. *Canning and How to Use Canned Foods*. Washington, D.C.: National Canning Association, 1916.

Blythe, Samuel. *The Fun of Getting Thin: How to Be Happy and Reduce the Waist Line*. Chicago: Forbes, 1912.

Bomberger, Maude. *Colonial Recipes, from Old Virginia and Maryland Manors, with Numerous Legends and Traditions Interwoven*. New York: Neale, 1907.

Booher, James M., ed. *Scientific Weight Control: An Improved System for Reducing or Increasing Weight*. Chicago: Continental Scale Works, 1925.

Bosse, Sara, and Onoto Watanna [pseud.]. *Chinese-Japanese Cook Book*. Chicago: Rand McNally, 1914.

Bradley, Mrs. Robert S. *Cook Book: Helpful Recipes for War Time*. Manchester-by-the-Sea, Mass.: North Shore Breeze, 1917. Division of Rare and Manuscript Collections, Cornell University, Ithaca, New York.

Bragg, Paul. *Paul C. Bragg's Personal Health Food Cook Book and Menus*. 2d ed. Burbank, Calif.: Aetna, 1935.

Brebner, Mrs. Gertrude Frelove. *The All-American Cook Book*. Chicago: Judy, 1922.

Brewster, Edwin, and Lilian Brewster. *The Nutrition of a Household*. Boston: Houghton Mifflin, 1915.

Bruntz, George. *Allied Propaganda and the Collapse of the German Empire in 1918*. Hoover War Library Publications, no. 13. Stanford University, Calif.: Stanford University Press, 1938.

Bryce, Alexander. *Modern Theories of Diet and Their Bearing upon Practical Dietetics*. New York: Longmans, Green, 1912.

Buckstein, Jacob. *Food, Fitness and Figure*. New York: Emerson Books, 1936. Michigan State University Special Collections, East Lansing, Michigan.

Buell, Mrs. C. S. "Household Adjustment to Changing Industrial Conditions."
    Proceedings of Lake Placid Conference on Home Economics, Essex Co., N.Y. (1–6
    July 1907): 93–99.
Buttner, Jacques. *A Fleshless Diet: Vegetarianism as a Rational Dietary.* New York,
    F. A. Stokes, 1910. Michigan State University Special Collections, East Lansing,
    Michigan.
Callahan, Genevieve. *Sunset All-Western Cook Book: How to Select, Prepare, Cook, and
    Serve All Typically Western Food Products.* Palo Alto, Calif.: Stanford University
    Press, 1933.
Cambell, Mrs. Sylvia. *The Practical Cook Book: Containing Recipes, Directions, &c.,
    for Plain and Fancy Cooking.* Albany: Munsell & Rowland, 1860.
Carleton, Mark, and Joseph Chamberlain. "The Commercial Status of Durum
    Wheat." Bureau of Plant Industry Bulletin 70, U.S. Department of Agriculture.
    Washington, D.C.: Government Printing Office, 1904.
Carrington, Hereward. *Vitality, Fasting and Nutrition: A Physiological Study of the
    Curative Power of Fasting, Together with a New Theory of the Relation of Food to
    Human Vitality.* New York: Rebman, 1908.
Castelar Crèche Cook Book, ed. and comp. by the Board of Directors for the benefit of
    the Castelar Crèche. Los Angeles: Los Angeles Times-Mirror, 1922.
Chahraberty, Chandra. *Food and Health.* Calcutta: Ramchandra Chakraberty, 1922.
Chittenden, Alice. "Foreign Lenten Dishes." *Good Housekeeping*, March 1904, 287.
Christian, Eugene. "Emaciation, Its Cause and Cure—with Sample Menus." *Little
    Lessons in Scientific Eating.* Lesson 12. Maywood, N.J.: Corrective Eating Society,
    1916. Michigan State University Special Collections, East Lansing, Michigan.
———. "Food and Morality." *Little Lessons in Scientific Eating.* Lesson 15. Maywood,
    N.J.: Corrective Eating Society, 1916. Michigan State University Special
    Collections, East Lansing, Michigan.
———. "The Three Great Laws that Govern Life—Human Nutrition—Corrective
    Eating." *Little Lessons in Scientific Eating.* Lesson 1. Maywood, N.J.: Corrective
    Eating Society, 1916. Michigan State University Special Collections, East Lansing,
    Michigan.
———. "What Food Is and Its True Purpose." *Little Lessons in Scientific Eating.* Lesson
    2. Maywood, N.J.: Corrective Eating Society, 1916. Michigan State University
    Special Collections, East Lansing, Michigan.
Claire, Mabel. *Short Cut Cookery.* New York: Greenberg, 1927.
Clarke, Helen Carroll. *The Cook Book of Left-Overs; A Collection of 400 Reliable
    Recipes for the Practical Housekeeper.* New York: Harper & Brothers, 1911.
Cocks, Dorothy. *The Etiquette of Beauty.* New York: George H. Doran, 1927.
Cocroft, Susanna. *Let's Be Healthy in Mind and Body: How to Build and Retain
    Health.* New York: G. P. Putnam's Sons, 1916.
———. *Self-Sufficiency: Mental Poise.* Chicago: Physical Culture Extension Society,
    1908.
———. *What to Eat and When.* 4th ed. New York: G. P. Putnam's Sons, 1916.
The College Woman's Cook Book. 2d ed. New York: Alpha Gamma Delta Fraternity,
    1934. Michigan State University Special Collections, East Lansing, Michigan.

Conrad, Jessie. *A Handbook of Cookery for a Small House*. London: W. Heinemann, 1923.

Cooke, Maud C. *Breakfast, Dinner and Supper; or, What to Eat and How to Prepare It*. Philadelphia: National Publishing, 1897.

Cooper, Lenna F. *The New Cookery*. 3d ed. Battle Creek, Mich.: Good Health, 1916.

Cornforth, George. *Good Food, How to Prepare It*. Washington, D.C.: Review and Herald, 1920.

Craig, Hazel Thompson. *The History of Home Economics*. New York: Practical Home Economics, 1946.

Cramp, Helen. *The Institute Cook Book, Planned for a Family of Four*. Philadelphia: Department of Domestic Science, 1913.

Cuniberti, Julia Lovejoy. *Practical Italian Recipes for American Kitchens*. Washington, D.C., 1918.

Curtis, Isabel Gordon. *Mrs. Curtis's Cook Book; a Manual of Instruction in the Art of Everyday Cookery*. New York: Success, 1909.

Dana, Charles L. "Your Weight and Your Nerves." In *Your Weight and How to Control It: A Scientific Guide by Medical Specialists and Dieticians*. New York: George H. Doran, 1927. Schlesinger Library. Radcliffe Institute. Harvard University, Cambridge, Mass.

Dewey, Edward Hooker. *A New Era for Woman: Health without Drugs*. Norwich, Conn.: Henry Bill, 1896.

Dickey, Ellen Rose. *Economy in the Kitchen*. New York: E. J. Clode, 1928.

Dickson, Maxcy Robson, and American Council on Public Affairs. *The Food Front in World War I*. Washington, D.C.: American Council on Public Affairs, 1944.

Dixie Cook Book: 440 Tried and Tested Recipes. Kansas City, Mo.: Kansas City Business Woman's Club, 1921. Michigan State University Special Collections, East Lansing, Michigan

Donahey, Mary Dickerson. *The Calorie Cook Book*. Chicago: Reilly and Lee, 1923. Michigan State University Special Collections, East Lansing, Michigan.

Donham, S. Agnes, *Marketing and Housework Manual*. Boston: Little, Brown, 1918.

Dumas, Alexandre. *Grand dictionnaire de cuisine*. Paris: Éditions Phébus, 2001.

Eaves, Lucile. *The Food of Working Women in Boston*. An Investigation by the Department of Research Women's Educational and Industrial Union, Boston, in Co-operation with the State Department of Health. Boston: Wright and Potter, State Printers, 1917.

Edwords, Clarence E. *Bohemian San Francisco, Its Restaurants and Their Most Famous Recipes: The Elegant Art of Dining*. San Francisco: Paul Elder, 1914.

Esther C. Mack Industrial School. *What Salem Dames Cooked*. Salem, Mass.: Stetson Press of Boston for the Esther C. Mack Industrial School, 1910.

Eustis, Célestin. *Cooking in Old Créole Days. La cuisine Créole à l'usage des petits ménages*. New York: R. H. Russell, 1903.

Farmer, A. N., and Janet Rankin Huntington. *Food Problems: To Illustrate the Meaning of Food Waste and What May Be Accomplished by Economy and Intelligent Substitution*. Boston: Ginn, 1918.

Farmer, Fannie. *The Boston Cooking-School Cook Book*. Boston: Little, Brown, 1896.

————. *Catering for Special Occasions, with Menus and Recipes.* Philadelphia: D. McKay, 1911.

Farrar, Addie. "Oriental Recipes that are Worth the Making." *American Cookery* 23, no. 7 (February 1919): 518–20.

Fashions in Foods in Beverly Hills. Beverly Hills, Calif.: Beverly Hills Citizen, 1931. Michigan State University Special Collections, East Lansing, Michigan.

Finck, Henry Theophilus. *Girth Control, for Womanly Beauty, Manly Strength, Health and a Long Life for Everybody.* New York: Harper & Brothers, 1923. Michigan State University Special Collections, East Lansing, Michigan.

Fisher, Irving. "Impending Problems of Eugenics." *Scientific Monthly,* September 1921, 214–31.

Fisher, Irving, and Eugene Lyman Fisk. *How to Live: Rules for Healthful Living Based on Modern Science.* Authorized by Hygiene Reference Board of the Life Extension Institute. 15th ed. New York: Funk & Wagnalls, 1919.

Fisher, Marian Cole. *Twenty Lessons in Domestic Science: A Condensed Home Study Course.* M. C. Fisher, 1916.

Fisher, Marian Cole. *Twenty Lessons in Domestic Science.* S.L.: S.N., 1916.

Fisk, Eugene. "Life Insurance and Life Conservation." *Scientific Monthly* 4, no. 4 (April 1917): 330–42.

————. "Possible Extension of the Human Life Cycle." *Annals of the American Academy of Political Social Science* 145 (September 1929): 153–201.

Flagg, Etta Proctor. *A Handbook of Home Economics.* Boston: Little, Brown, 1912.

Fletcher-Berry, Riley M. *Fruit Recipes.* New York: Doubleday, Page, 1907.

"Food and Diet in the United States." U.S. Department of Agriculture. *Yearbook.* Washington, D.C.: Government Printing Office, 1907.

Food Saving and Sharing: Telling How the Older Children of America May Help Save from Famine Their Comrades in Allied Lands Across the Sea. Prepared under the direction of the United States Food Administration. Garden City, N.Y.: Doubleday, Page, 1918. Division of Rare and Manuscript Collections, Cornell University, Ithaca, New York.

Ford, Allyn K. *Home Laundry Hints: A Book of Laundry Information for Housewives, Laundresses, Students in Domestic Science, and All Others Interested in the Best Laundry Work.* 3d ed. Minneapolis: Luther Ford, 1914.

Frederick, Christine. *Selling Mrs. Consumer.* New York: Business Bourse, 1929.

Fullerton, H. B. "The Long Island Home Hamper." *Annals of the American Academy of Political and Social Science* 50, Reducing the Cost of Food Distribution (November 1913): 166–70. Bibliothèque Nationale de France, Paris.

Gentile, Mrs. Maria. *The Italian Cook Book: The Art of Eating Well, Practical Recipes of the Italian Cuisine.* New York: Italian Book, 1919.

Gillett, Lucy. *Food Primer for the Home.* New York: New York Association for Improving the Condition of the Poor, 1918.

Gilman, Charlotte Perkins. "The Housekeeper and the Food Problem." *World's Food* 74 (November 1917): 123–30.

Gironci, Maria. *Italian Recipes for Food Reformers.* 3d ed. London: G. Bell & Sons, 1917.

Goudiss, C. Houston. *Eating Vitamines: How to Know and Prepare the Foods that Supply These Invisible Life-Guards*. New York: Funk & Wagnalls, 1922.

Goudiss, C. Houston, and Alberta M. Goudiss. *Foods That Will Win the War and How to Cook Them*. New York: Forecast, 1918.

Green, Lilian Bayliss. *The Effective Small Home*. New York: Robert M. McBride, 1917.

Green, Olive. *How to Cook Vegetables*. New York: G. P. Putnam's Sons, 1909.

Greer, Edith. *Food: What It Is and Does*. Boston: Ginn and Co., 1915.

Gridley, Mary Twining. *The Elm City Free Kindergarten Receipt Book*. New Haven: Tuttle, Morehouse & Taylor, 1909.

Guerrier, Edith. *We Pledged Allegiance: A Librarian's Intimate Story of the United States Food Administration*. Stanford University, Calif.: Stanford University Press, 1941.

Haddock, Frank. *Power of Will*. Meriden, Conn.: Pelton, 1916.

Hall, Florence Howe. *A Handbook of Hospitality for Town and Country*. Boston: Dana Estes, 1909.

Hamilton, Dorothy M. *A Primer of Cooking*. New York: Century, 1921.

Harding, Florence. *Twentieth Century Cook Book: An Up-to-Date and Skillful Preparation on the Art of Cooking and Modern Candy Making Simplified*. Chicago: Geographical, 1921.

Harrison, Grace Clergue, and Gertrude Clergue. *Allied Cookery, British, French, Italian, Belgian, Russian*. New York: G. P. Putnam's Sons, 1916.

——. *Cuisine des Alliés*. Paris: Édition Française Illustrée, 1918.

Harrow, Benjamin. *Eminent Chemists of Our Time*. D. Van Nostrand, 1920.

Hastings, Milo. *Physical Culture Food Directory*. New York: McFadden, 1927. Michigan State University Special Collections, East Lansing, Michigan.

Hazlitt, William Carew. *Old Cookery Books and Ancient Cuisine*. London: E. Stock, 1902.

Heath, Mrs. Julian. "Work of the Housewives League." *Annals of the American Academy of Political and Social Science* 48, The Cost of Living (July 1913): 121–26.

Heywood, Margaret Weimer. *The International Cook Book*. Boston: Merchandisers, 1929.

Hiscox, Gardner Dexter. *Henley's Twentieth-Century Formulas, Recipes and Processes*. New York: Henley, 1919.

Hitchcock, Nevada Davis. "The Relation of the Housewife to the Food Problem." *World's Food* 74 (November 1917): 130–40.

Holbrook, Sara. "The Home Environment as Affecting the Physical and Mental Growth of School Children." *Journal of Home Economics* 5, no. 3 (June 1913): 211–17.

Holt, Emily. *The Complete Housekeeper*. Garden City, N.Y.: Doubleday, Page, 1917.

Hoover, Herbert. *An American Epic, Introduction: The Relief of Belgium and Northern France, 1914–1930*, Chicago: H. Regnery, 1959.

——. *The Memoirs of Herbert Hoover, Years of Adventure 1874–1920*. New York: Macmillan, 1951.

Horton, George. *The Long Straight Road*. Indianapolis: Bowen-Merrill, 1922.

Hurlbut, Mrs. William D., ed. *Stevenson Memorial Cook Book.* Chicago: Sarah Hackett Stevenson Memorial Lodging House Association, 1919.

"Interesting Westerners: The Americans of the Hour in Europe." *Sunset Magazine,* June 1915, 1175–79.

Irwin, Wallace. "Togo Wrestles with the Food Shortage." *Good Housekeeping,* July 1917, 58.

Irwin, Will. "The Babes of Belgium." *The Need of Belgium.* 3d ed. New York: Commission for Relief in Belgium, n.d.

Isaacs, Nathan. "In the Hope of the New Diaspora." *Menorah Journal* 5, no. 4 (August 1919): 185–95.

James, William. *The Moral Equivalent of War.* New York: American Association for International Conciliation, 1910.

Kander, Mrs. Simon. *The Settlement Cook Book.* 10th ed. Milwaukee: Settlement Cook Book Co., 1920.

Kellogg, E. E. *Science in the Kitchen.* Battle Creek, Mich.: Modern Medicine, 1904.

Keoleian, Ardashes. *The Oriental Cook Book: Wholesome, Dainty and Economical Dishes of the Orient, Especially Adapted to American Tastes and Methods of Preparation.* New York: Sully & Kleinteich, 1913.

Kingsland, Florence. "If You Are Well Bred." *Success Magazine,* December 1905, 840.

———. *In and Out Door Games: With Suggestions for Entertainments.* New York: Sully & Kleintech, 1913.

Kinne, Helen. *Food and Health; an Elementary Textbook of Home Making.* New York: Macmillan, 1918.

———. *Foods and Household Management: A Textbook of the Household Arts.* New York: Macmillan, 1918.

Kitchen Klinic. Compiled by the Women's Club of St. Vincent Charity Hospital. Cleveland: n.p., 1936.

Kittredge, Mabel Hyde, and American Home Economics Association. *Practical Homemaking: A Textbook for Young Housekeepers.* New York: Century, 1914.

Landis, H. R. M. "Dietary Habits and their Improvement: Some Results of the Work of the Phipps Institute." *World's Food* 74 (November 1917): 103–8.

Langworthy, Charles. *Food Customs and Diet in American Homes.* U.S. Department of Agriculture. Washington, D.C.: Government Printing Office, 1911.

Langworthy, Charles, and R. D. Milner. *Investigations on the Nutrition of Man in the United States.* USDA Office of Experiment Stations. Washington, D.C.: Government Printing Office, 1904.

Lansing, Marion Florence, and Luther Gulick. *Food and Life.* Boston: Ginn, 1920.

Legendre, R. *Alimentation et ravitaillement.* Paris: Masson, 1920.

Levine, Victor E. "Why We Should Be More Interested in Nutrition." *Scientific Monthly,* January 1926, 19–24.

The Library of Home Economics: A Complete Home-Study Course on the New Profession of Home-Making and Art of Right Living. Chicago: American School of Home Economics, 1907.

Lindlahr, Victor H. *7-DAY Reducing Diet.* Serutan, 1946. Michigan State University Special Collections, East Lansing, Michigan.

Lorain Cooking. 7th ed. St. Louis: American Stove, 1929.

Lorand, Arnold. *Health through Rational Diet: Practical Hints in Regard to Food and the Usefulness or Harmful Effects of the Various Articles of the Diet.* Philadelphia: F. A. Davis, 1913.

Love, Albert, and Charles Davenport. *Defects Found in Drafted Men.* Washington, D.C., 1920.

Luff, Arthur Pearson. *Gout: Its Pathology, Forms, Diagnosis and Treatment.* 3d ed. New York: William Wood, 1907.

Lyman, Joseph, and Laura Lyman. *The Philosophy of House-Keeping: A Scientific and Practical Manual.* Hartford: Goodwin and Bets, 1867.

MacLeod, Sarah Josephine. *The Housekeeper's Handbook of Cleaning.* New York: Harper & Brothers, 1915.

Maddocks, Mildred, ed. *The Pure Food Cook Book: The Good Housekeeping Recipes Just How to Buy—Just How to Cook.* New York: Hearst's International Library, 1915.

The Malone Cook Book. Malone, N.Y.: Woman's Aid Society of the First Congregation Church, 1917.

Man, Sing Au, ed. *The Chinese Cook Book: Covering the Entire Field of Chinese Cookery in the Chinese Order of Serving.* Reading, Pa.: Culinary Arts Press, 1936.

Mandarin Chop Suey Cook Book. Chicago: Pacific Trading, 1928.

Marguey, M. Introduction to *La cuisine et la table moderne.* Paris: Librairie Larousse, 1923.

McCann, Alfred. *Thirty Cent Bread: How to Escape a Higher Cost of Living.* New York: George H. Doran, 1917.

———. *This Famishing World.* New York: George H. Doran, 1918.

McCollum, E. V. *The Newer Knowledge of Nutrition: The Use of Food for the Preservation of Vitality and Health.* New York: Macmillan, 1918.

———. "Some Essentials to a Safe Diet." *World's Food* 74 (November 1917): 95–102.

McCollum, E. V., and Nina Simmonds. *The American Home Diet: An Answer to the Ever Present Question, What Shall We Have for Dinner.* Detroit: Frederick C. Matthews, 1923. Michigan State University Special Collections, East Lansing, Michigan.

McFadden, Bernarr. *Eating for Health and Strength.* New York: Macfadden, 1923. Michigan State University Special Collections, East Lansing, Michigan.

Mencken, Henry Louis. *The American Language: An Inquiry into the Development of English in the United States.* 2d ed. New York: Knopf, 1921.

Mendel, Lafayette. *Changes in the Food Supply and their Relation to Nutrition.* New Haven: Yale University Press, 1916.

The Mendelssohn Club Cook Book. Rockfield, Ill.: Horton Printing, 1909.

Mexican Cookery for American Homes. San Antonio, Tex.: Gebhardt, 1923. Michigan State University Special Collections, East Lansing, Michigan.

Milady's Style Parade and Recipe Book for 1935, with Photos of Favorite Movie Stars. Chicago: New Regent Theatre, 1935.

Moore, Alice. *Chinese Recipes: Letters from Alice Moore to Ethel Moore Rook.* Garden City, N.Y.: Doubleday, Page, 1923.

Moore, Helen. *Camouflage Cookery: A Book of Mock Dishes.* New York: Duffield, 1918.

Morehead, Willie Carhart. "Better Mothers." *American Journal of Nursing* 19, no. 8 (May 1919): 602–4.

Morse, Sidney. *Household Discoveries; An Encyclopaedia of Practical Recipes and Processes.* New York: Success, 1909.

Mullendore, William Clinton. *History of the United States Food Administration, 1917–1919.* Stanford University, Calif.: Stanford University Press, 1941.

Murray, J. Alan. *Economy of Food: A Popular Treatise on Nutrition, Food and Diet.* New York: Appleton, 1911.

Myerson, Abraham. *The Nervous Housewife.* Boston: Little, Brown, 1920.

N. W. Ayer & Son's American Newspaper Annual and Directory. Philadelphia: N. W. Ayer & Son, n.d.

Neil, Marion Harris. *How to Cook in Casserole Dishes.* Philadelphia: David McKay, 1912.

Nesbitt, Florence. *Low Cost Cooking.* Chicago: American School of Home Economics, 1915.

Nettleton, Bertha E. *One Hundred–Portion War Time Recipes: Wheatless, Economical, Tested.* Philadelphia: J. B. Lippincott, 1918.

The New England Cook Book of Fine Old Recipes. Reading, Pa.: Culinary Arts Press, 1936.

Norton, Jeanette Young. *Mrs. Norton's Cook-Book; Selecting, Cooking, and Serving for the Home Table.* New York: G. P. Putnam's Sons, 1917. Division of Rare and Manuscript Collections, Cornell University, Ithaca, New York.

McGuire, Lelia M. *Old World Foods for New World Families: A Handbook.* Edited by Dorothy Tyler. Detroit: Merrill-Palmer Motherhood and Home Training School, 1931.

Morrow, Kay. *Culinary Arts: Western Cookery.* Reading, Pa.: Culinary Arts Press, 1936.

———. *The Southern Cook Book of Fine Old Recipes.* Edited by Lillie Lustig. Reading, Pa.: Culinary Arts Press, 1935.

Pack, Charles Lathrop. *The War Garden Victorious.* Philadelphia: J. P. Lippincott, 1919.

Pattison, Mrs. Frank A. "Scientific Management in Home-Making." *Annals of the American Academy of Political and Social Science* 48, The Cost of Living (July 1913): 96–103.

Pattison, Mary. *Principles of Domestic Engineering; or, The What, Why and How of a Home.* New York: Trow Press, 1915.

Payot, Jules. *The Education of the Will: The Theory and Practice of Self-Culture.* Translated from 30th French edition. New York: Funk & Wagnalls, 1909.

Pearl, Raymond. *The Nation's Food: A Statistical Study of a Physiological and Social Problem.* Philadelphia: W. B. Saunders, 1920.

Pearl, Raymond, and Esther Pearl Matchett. *Reference Handbook of Food Statistics in Relation to the War.* Washington, D.C.: Government Printing Office, 1918.

Pennsylvania Dutch Cook Book of Fine Old Recipes. Reading, Pa.: Culinary Arts Press, 1936.

Pennybacker, Mrs. Percy V. "What Our Country Asks of Its Young Women." Address at Speakers' Training Camp. Chautauqua, N.Y., July 6 1917. Patriotism Through Education Series 3. New York: National Security League, 1917.

Peters, Lulu Hunt. *Diet and Health with Key to the Calories.* Chicago: Reilly and Lee, 1918. Michigan State University Special Collections, East Lansing, Michigan.

The Picayune Creole Cook Book. 6th ed. New Orleans: Times-Picayune, 1922.

Pietkiewicz, Dr. "La mastication; son utilité pour l'individu et pour l'espèce." *Bulletin de la Société scientifique d'hygiène alimentaire et d'alimentation rationnelle de l'homme* 3, no. 2 (23 February 1913): 174.

Popenoe, Paul. *Applied Eugenics.* New York: Macmillan, 1918.

The Proceedings of the Second Pan American Scientific Congress. 27 December 1915–8 January 1916. Edited by Glen Levin Swiggett. Washington, D.C.: Government Printing Office, 1917.

Purdy, Mabel Dulon. *Food and Freedom: A Household Book.* New York: Harper & Brothers, 1918. Division of Rare and Manuscript Collections, Cornell University, Ithaca, New York.

Putnam, Nina Wilcox. *Tomorrow We Diet.* New York: George H. Doran, 1922. Michigan State University Special Collections, East Lansing, Michigan.

Quinn, Mary Josephine. *Planning and Furnishing the Home: Practical and Economical Suggestions for the Homemaker.* New York: Harper & Brothers, 1914.

R., S. M. "Macaroni à la Italy." *American Cookery* 19, no. 8 (March 1915): 628.

Ramona's Spanish-Mexican Cookery: The First Complete and Authentic Spanish-Mexican Cook Book in English. Los Angeles: West Coast, 1929.

Rapeer, Louis W. "Health as a Means to Happiness, Efficiency and Service." *Annals of the American Academy of Political and Social Science* 67, New Possibilities in Education (September 1916): 97–106.

Recipes from Many Lands. Furnished by North Dakota Homemakers' Clubs. Compiled by Dorothy Ayers Loudon. Fargo, N.D.: Agricultural Extension Division, North Dakota Agricultural College, 1927.

Reducing Diets and Recipes. 2d ed. Johnstown, N.Y.: Knox Gelatine Laboratories, 1935. Michigan State University Special Collections, East Lansing, Michigan.

Rich, Jessie Pinning, and University of Texas. *Simple Cooking of Wholesome Food for the Farm Home.* Austin: University of Texas, 1913.

Richards, Ellen. *The Cost of Food: A Study in Dietaries.* New York: John Wiley & Sons, 1901.

Richards, Ellen H., and John F. Norton. *The Cost of Food: A Study in Dietetics.* 3d ed. New York: John Wiley & Sons, 1917.

Rombauer, Irma. *The Joy of Cooking.* St. Louis: A. C. Clayton Printing Co., 1931. Michigan State University Special Collections, East Lansing, Michigan.

Roorbach, G. B. "The World's Food Supply." *World's Food* 74 (November 1917): 1–33.

Rorer, Sarah. "Food." In *Talks upon Practical Subjects*, edited by Marion Harland. 2d ed. New York: Warner Brothers, 1895. Michigan State University Special Collections, East Lansing, Michigan.

Rose, Mary Swartz. *Everyday Foods in War Time.* New York: MacMillan, 1918.

'Round the World Cookery. Reading, Pa.: Culinary Arts Press, 1936.

Sangster, Margaret Elizabeth Munson. *Good Manners for All Occasions: a Practical Manual*. New York: Christian Herald, 1904.

Schapiro, Mary L. "Social Service Dietetics in Relation to Jewish Problems." *Modern Hospital* 14, no. 2 (1920): 147–50.

Sheridan, Carroll Mac, ed. *The Stag Cook Book, Written for Men by Men*. New York: George H. Doran, 1922.

Smiley, Portia. "Courtship Formulas of Southern Negroes." *Journal of American Folklore* 8, no. 29 (June 1895): 155–56.

———. "Folk-Lore from Virginia, South Carolina, Georgia, Alabama, and Florida." *Journal of American Folklore* 32, no. 125 (September 1919): 357–83.

Smith, Esther L. *The Official Cook Book of the Hay System*. Mount Pocono, Pa.: Pocono Haven, 1934. Michigan State University Special Collections, East Lansing, Michigan.

Snyder, Sherwood Percy. *The Practical Hygienic Preparation of Foods: A Treatise on Foods and their Effects upon Health and the Physical and Moral Life*. 10th ed. Dayton, Ohio: Health Publishing, 1913.

Soyer, Nicolas. *Soyer's Paper-Bag Cookery*. New York: Sturgis & Walton, 1911.

Steiner, Edward Alfred. *From Alien to Citizen: The Story of My Life in America*. New York: Fleming H. Revell, 1914.

Stern, Frances, and Gertrude Spitz. *Food for the Worker: The Food Values and Cost of a Series of Menus and Recipes for Seven Weeks*. Boston: Whitcomb & Barrows, 1917.

Stewart, W. Blair. "Some Dietetic Errors and Their Effects." *Journal of the Medical Society of New Jersey* 3 (December 1906): 139–43.

The Suffrage Cook Book. Compiled by Mrs. L. O. Kleber. Pittsburgh: Equal Franchise Federation of Western Pennsylvania, 1915. Division of Rare and Manuscript Collections, Cornell University, Ithaca, New York.

The Sunny Side of Life Book: To Keep Happy, Keep Well—A New Way of Living. Battle Creek, Mich.: Kellogg, 1934.

Surface, Frank M. *American Food in the World War and Reconstruction Period; Operations of the Organizations Under the Direction of Herbert Hoover, 1914 to 1924*. Stanford University, Calif.: Stanford University Press, 1931.

Sylvia of Hollywood. *"No More Alibis!"* Chicago: Photoplay, 1934.

Telford, Emma Paddock. *Good Housekeeper's Cook Book*. New York: Cupples & Leon, 1914.

Thompson, Dr., and Mrs. J. Douglas Thompson. *The Health Recipe Cook Book*. Oakland, Calif.: Thompson Publications, 1927.

Thompson, Henry. *Food and Feeding with an Appendix*. 12th ed. London: F. Warne, 1910.

Thompson, Vance. Preface to *Eat and Grow Thin: The Mahdah Menus*. New York: E. P. Dutton, 1914. Michigan State University Special Collections, East Lansing, Michigan.

Time and Temperature Oven Cooking. St. Louis: American Stove, 1924.

Tucker, Rufus S. "Distribution of Men Physically Unfit for Military Service." *Journal of the American Statistical Association* 18, no. 139 (September 1922): 377–84.

Tyree, Marion Cabell. *Housekeeping in Old Virginia. Containing Contributions from Two Hundred and Fifty Ladies in Virginia and Her Sister States.* Louisville, Ky.: J. P. Morton, 1890.

Ullback, Sylvia. *Pull Yourself Together, Baby!* 1936. New York: Macfadden Book Co., 1939.

Virginia Cookery Book; Traditional Recipes. Richmond, Va.: Virginia League of Women Voters, 1921.

Wallace, Lily Haxworth. *The Rumford Complete Cook Book.* 1908. Cambridge: University Press, 1918.

Ward, Lester F. "Eugenics, Euthenics, and Eudemics." *American Journal of Sociology* 18, no. 6 (May 1913): 737–54.

Washington, Booker T. *Character Building, Being Addresses Delivered on Sunday Evenings to the Students of Tuskegee Institute.* New York: Doubleday, Page, 1903.

Wellman, Mabel Thacher. *Food Planning and Preparation; a Junior Course in Food Study with a Recipe Book for Use at Home and at School.* Philadelphia: Lippincott, 1923.

———. *Food Study; a Textbook in Home Economics for High Schools.* Boston: Little, Brown, 1919.

"Where Cooks Go." *Atlantic Monthly,* September 1912, 430–31.

Wiley, Harvey Washington. *The Lure of the Land: Farming after Fifty.* New York: Century, 1919.

———. *Not by Bread Alone: The Principles of Human Nutrition.* New York: Hearst's International Library, 1915.

Williams, Mrs. Mary E. "Teaching Domestic Science to Different Nationalities." *Journal of Home Economics* 2 (June 1910): 271–73.

Wilson, Mrs. Mary A. *Mrs. Wilson's Cook Book; Numerous New Recipes on Present Economic Conditions.* Philadelphia: J. B. Lippincott, 1920. Division of Rare and Manuscript Collections, Cornell University, Ithaca, New York.

Wood, Bertha M. *Foods of the Foreign-Born in Relation to Health.* Boston: Whitcomb & Barrows, 1922.

Wood, T. B., and F. G. Hopkins, *Food Economy in War Time.* Cambridge: University Press, 1916.

SECONDARY SOURCES

Adams, Katherine, and Michael Keene. *Alice Paul and the American Suffrage Campaign.* Urbana: University of Illinois Press, 2008.

Ahlberg, Kristin. *Transplanting the Great Society: Lyndon Johnson and Food for Peace.* Columbia: University of Missouri Press, 2008.

Allen, Anne Beiser. *An Independent Woman: The Life of Lou Henry Hoover.* Westport, Conn.: Greenwood Press, 2000.

Allen, Judith. *The Feminism of Charlotte Perkins Gilman: Sexualities, Histories, Progressivism.* Chicago: University of Chicago Press, 2009.

Allen, Keith. "Sharing Scarcity: Bread Rationing and the First World War in Berlin, 1914–1923." *Journal of Social History* 32, no. 2 (Winter 1998): 371–93.

Allen, Polly Wynn. *Building Domestic Liberty: Charlotte Perkins Gilman's Architectural Feminism.* Amherst: University of Massachusetts Press, 1988.

Allgor, Catherine. *Parlor Politics: In Which the Ladies of Washington Help Build a City and a Government.* Charlottesville: University Press of Virginia, 2000.

Appadurai, Arjun. "How to Make a National Cuisine: Cookbooks in Contemporary India." *Comparative Studies in Society and History* 30, no. 1 (January 1988): 3–24.

Appleby, Joyce. *Capitalism and a New Social Order: The Republican Vision of the 1790s.* New York: New York University Press, 1984.

Bargielowska, Ina Zweiniger. "The Culture of the Abdomen: Obesity and Reducing in Britain, circa 1900–1939." *Journal of British Studies* 44, no. 2 (April 2005): 239–73.

Barnhart, Robert K., ed. *Barnhart Concise Dictionary of Etymology.* New York: Harper Collins, 1995.

Barthes, Roland. *Mythologies.* New York: Hill and Wang, 1957.

Bayor, Ronald, ed. *Race and Ethnicity in America: A Concise History.* New York: Columbia University Press, 2003.

Beckert, Sven. *The Monied Metropolis: New York City and the Consolidation of the American Bourgeoisie, 1850–1896.* New York: Cambridge University Press, 2001.

Bederman, Gail. *Manliness & Civilization: A Cultural History of Gender and Race in the United States, 1880–1917.* Chicago: University of Chicago Press, 1995.

Belasco, Warren. "Food Matters: Perspectives on an Emerging Field." In *Food Nations: Selling Taste in Consumer Societies,* edited by Warren Belasco and Philip Scranton, 2–23. New York: Routledge, 2002.

———. *Meals to Come: A History of the Future of Food.* Berkeley: University of California Press, 2006.

Belasco, Warren, and Philip Scranton, eds. *Food Nations: Selling Taste in Consumer Societies.* New York: Routledge, 2002.

Bennett, Merrill Kelley. *The World's Food: A Study of the Interrelations of World Populations, National Diets, and Food Potentials.* New York: Harper, 1954.

Bentley, Amy. *Eating for Victory: Food Rationing and the Politics of Domesticity.* Urbana: University of Illinois Press, 1998.

Berlage, Nancy. "The Establishment of an Applied Social Science: Home Economists, Science, and Reform at Cornell University, 1870–1930." In *Gender and American Social Science: The Formative Years,* edited by Helene Silverberg, 185–232. Princeton, N.J.: Princeton University Press, 1998.

Biltekoff, Charlotte. "Hidden Hunger: Eating and Citizenship from Domestic Science to the Fat Epidemic." Ph.D. diss., Brown University, 2006.

———. "The Terror Within: Obesity in Post 9/11 U.S. Life." *American Studies* 48, no. 3 (Fall 2007): 29–48.

Blight, David. *Race and Reunion: The Civil War in American Memory.* Cambridge, Mass.: Belknap Press of Harvard University Press, 2001.

Bobrow-Strain, Aaron. *White Bread: A Social History of the Store-Bought Loaf.* Boston: Beacon Press, 2012.

Bollet, Alfred. *Plagues and Poxes: The Impact of Human History on Epidemic Disease.* 2d ed. New York: Demos Medical Publishing, 2004.

Bonzon, Thierry, and Belinda Davis. "Feeding the Cities." In *Capital Cities at War: Paris, London, Berlin, 1914–1919,* edited by Jay Winter and Jean-Louis Robert, 305–41. New York: Cambridge University Press, 1997.

Bordin, Ruth Birgitta Anderson. *Woman and Temperance: The Quest for Power and Liberty, 1873–1900.* Philadelphia: Temple University Press, 1981.

Boris, Eileen, and Cynthia R. Daniels, eds. *Homework: Historical and Contemporary Perspectives on Paid Labor at Home.* Urbana: University of Illinois Press, 1989.

Boydston, Jeanne. *Home and Work: Housework, Wages, and the Ideology of Labor in the Early Republic.* New York: Oxford University Press, 1990.

———. *The Limits of Sisterhood: The Beecher Sisters on Women's Rights and Woman's Sphere.* Chapel Hill: University of North Carolina Press, 1988.

Brenner, Leslie. *American Appetite: The Coming of Age of a National Cuisine.* New York: Bard, 1999.

Bruce, Robert B. *A Fraternity of Arms: America and France in the Great War.* Lawrence: University Press of Kansas, 2003.

Bruegel, Martin. "How the French Learned to Eat Canned Food." In *Food Nations: Selling Taste in Consumer Societies,* edited by Warren Belasco and Philip Scranton, 113–30. New York: Routledge, 2002.

Brumberg, Joan Jacobs. *Fasting Girls: The History of Anorexia Nervosa.* New York: Vintage Books, 2000.

Budd, Michael Anton. *The Sculpture Machine: Physical Culture and Body Politics in the Age of Empire.* New York: New York University Press, 1997.

Camhi, Jane Jerome. *Women against Women: American Anti-Suffragism, 1880–1920.* Brooklyn, N.Y.: Carlson, 1994.

Capozzola, Christopher. "The Only Badge Needed Is Your Patriotic Fervor: Vigilance, Coercion, and the Law in World War I America." *Journal of American History* 88, no. 4 (March 2002): 1354–82.

———. *Uncle Sam Wants You: World War I and the Making of the Modern American Citizen.* Oxford: Oxford University Press, 2008.

Carney, Judith. *Black Rice: The African Origins of Rice Cultivation in the Americas.* Cambridge, Mass.: Harvard University Press, 2001.

Carroll, Abigail. "Forefathers' Day Dinners and Martha Washington Teas: Commemorative Consumption and the Colonial Revival." *Food, Culture & Society* 12, no. 3 (September 2009): 335–56.

Carter, Susan, et al., eds. Historical Statistics of the United States. Millennial edition online, http://hsus.cambridge.org/HSUSWeb/HSUSEntryServlet.

Carver, Marie Negri. *Home Economics as an Academic Discipline: A Short History.* Tucson: Center for the Study of Higher Education, University of Arizona, 1979.

Chambers, John Whiteclay. *To Raise an Army: The Draft Comes to Modern America.* New York: Free Press, 1987.

Clements, Kendrick. *Hoover, Conservation, and Consumerism: Engineering the Good Life.* Lawrence: University Press of Kansas, 2000.

Coe, Andrew. *Chop Suey: A Cultural History of Chinese Food in the United States.* New York: Oxford University Press, 2009.

Cook, Blanche Wiesen. *Eleanor Roosevelt.* Vol. 1, *1884–1933.* New York: Viking Adult, 1992.

Coppin, Clayton, and Jack High. *The Politics of Purity: Harvey Washington Wiley and the Origins of Federal Food Policy.* Ann Arbor: University of Michigan Press, 1999.

Costigliola, Frank. *Awkward Dominion: American Political, Economic and Cultural Relations with Europe, 1919–1933.* Ithaca, N.Y.: Cornell University Press, 1988.

Counihan, Carole, and Penny Van Esterik, eds. *Food and Culture: A Reader.* New York: Routledge, 1997.

Coveney, John. *Food, Morals and Meaning: The Pleasure and Anxiety of Eating.* London: Routledge, 2000.

Cowan, Ruth Schwartz. *More Work for Mother: The Ironies of Household Technology from the Open Hearth to the Microwave.* New York: Basic Books, 1983.

———. *Sir Francis Galton and the Study of Heredity in the Nineteenth Century.* New York: Garland, 1985.

Craig, Lee A., Barry Goodwin, and Thomas Grennes. "The Effect of Mechanical Refrigeration on Nutrition in the United States." *Social Science History* 28, no. 2 (Summer 2004): 325–36.

Cravens, Hamilton. "Establishing the Science of Nutrition at the USDA: Ellen Swallow Richards and Her Allies." *Agricultural History* 64, no. 2, The United States Department of Agriculture in Historical Perspective (Spring 1990): 122–33.

Cronon, William. *Nature's Metropolis: Chicago and the Great West.* New York: W. W. Norton, 1991.

Crunden, Robert. *Ministers of Reform: The Progressives' Achievement in American Civilization.* New York: Basic Books, 1982.

Cullather, Nick. "The Foreign Policy of the Calorie." *American Historical Review* 112, no. 2 (April 2007): 337–64.

———. *The Hungry World: America's Cold War Battle against Poverty in Asia.* Cambridge, Mass.: Harvard University Press, 2010.

Cummings, Richard Osborn. *The American and His Food: A History of Food Habits in the United States.* Chicago: University of Chicago Press, 1944.

Curry, Lynne. *Modern Mothers in the Heartland: Gender, Health, and Progress in Illinois, 1900–1930.* Columbus: Ohio State University Press, 1999.

Dain, Bruce. *Hideous Monster of the Mind: American Race Theory in the Early Republic.* Cambridge, Mass.: Harvard University Press, 2002.

Davis, Cynthia. *Charlotte Perkins Gilman: A Biography.* Stanford, Calif.: Stanford University Press, 2010.

Davis, Mike. *Late Victorian Holocausts: El Niño Famines and the Making of the Third World.* London: Verso, 2001.

De Grazia, Victoria. *Irresistible Empire: America's Advance through Twentieth-Century Europe.* Cambridge, Mass.: Belknap Press of Harvard University Press, 2005.

Derr, Mark. *A Dog's History of America: How Our Best Friend Explored, Conquered, and Settled a Continent.* New York: North Point Press, 2004.

Deutsch, Sarah. *Women and the City: Gender, Space, and Power in Boston, 1870–1940.* New York: Oxford University Press, 2000.

Deutsch, Tracey. *Building a Housewife's Paradise: Gender, Politics, and American Grocery Stores in the Twentieth Century.* Chapel Hill: University of North Carolina Press, 2010.

Diner, Hasia R. *Hungering for America: Italian, Irish, and Jewish Foodways in the Age of Migration.* Cambridge, Mass.: Harvard University Press, 2001.

Dorr, Gregory Michael. "Fighting Fire with Fire: African Americans and Hereditarian Thinking, 1900–1942." Published online. <www.wfu.edu/~caron/ssrs/Dorr.rtf>. 16 May 2007.

———. *Segregation's Science: Eugenics and Society in Virginia.* Charlottesville: University Press of Virginia, 2008.

Dorsey, Leroy G. *We Are All Americans, Pure and Simple: Theodore Roosevelt and the Myth of Americanism.* Tuscaloosa: University of Alabama Press, 2007.

Dudden, Faye. *Serving Women: Household Service in Nineteenth-Century America.* Middletown, Conn.: Wesleyan University Press, 1983.

Dumas, Alexandre. *Grand Dictionnaire de Cuisine.* 1873 ed. Paris: Éditions Phébus, 2001.

DuPuis, Melanie. *Nature's Perfect Food: How Milk Became America's Drink.* New York: New York University Press, 2002.

Du Vall, Nell. *Domestic Technology: A Chronology of Developments.* Boston: G. K. Hall, 1988.

Dworkin, Shari, and Faye Linda Wachs. *Body Panic: Gender, Health, and the Selling of Fitness.* New York: New York University Press, 2009.

Elias, Megan. *Stir It Up: Home Economics in American Culture.* Philadelphia: University of Pennsylvania Press, 2008.

Enloe, Cynthia. *Bananas, Beaches & Bases: Making Feminist Sense of International Politics.* London: Pandora, 1989.

Fass, Paula. *The Damned and the Beautiful: American Youth in the 1920's.* Oxford: Oxford University Press, 1979.

Faust, Drew Gilpin. *Mothers of Invention: Women of the Slaveholding South in the American Civil War.* Chapel Hill: University of North Carolina Press, 1996.

Fein, Seth. "Culture across Borders in the Americas." *History Compass* 1, no. 1 (2003).

Fernández de la Reguera, Ricard. *España neutral, 1914–1918.* 3d ed. Barcelona: Editorial Planeta, 1969.

Fields, Anne M., and Tschera Harkness. "Classification and the Definition of a Discipline: The Dewey Decimal Classification and Home Economics." *Libraries & Culture* 39, no. 3 (2004): 245–59.

Fitzgerald, Deborah. *Every Farm a Factory: The Industrial Ideal in American Agriculture.* New Haven, Conn.: Yale University Press, 2003.

Flake, Kathleen. *The Politics of American Religious Identity: The Seating of Senator Reed Smoot, Mormon Apostle.* Chapel Hill: University of North Carolina Press, 2004.

Flour, Roderick, Robert Fogel, Bernard Harris, and Sok Chul Hong, eds. *The Changing Body: Health, Nutrition, and Human Development in the Western World since 1700*. New York: Cambridge University Press, 2011.

Floyd, Janet, and Laurel Forster. "The Recipe in Its Cultural Contexts." In *The Recipe Reader: Narratives—Contexts—Traditions*, edited by Janet Floyd and Laurel Forster, 1–14. Aldershot, Hants, England: Ashgate, 2003.

Forth, Christopher E., and Ana Carden-Coyne, eds. *Cultures of the Abdomen: Diet, Digestion, and Fat in the Modern World*. New York: Palgrave Macmillan, 2005.

Fox, Bonnie. "Selling the Mechanized Household: 70 Years of Ads in Ladies Home Journal." *Gender and Society* 4, no. 1 (March 1990): 25–40.

Frank, Dana. "Housewives, Socialists, and the Politics of Food: The 1917 New York Cost-of-Living Protests." *Feminist Studies* 11, no. 2 (Summer 1985): 255–85.

Freiburger, William. "War, Prosperity and Hunger: The New York Food Riots of 1917." *Labor History* 25, no. 2 (Spring 1984): 217–39.

Freidberg, Susanne. *Fresh: A Perishable History*. Cambridge, Mass.: Belknap Press of Harvard University Press, 2009.

Fritschner, Linda Marie. *The Rise and Fall of Home Economics: A Study with Implications for Women, Education, and Change*. Ph.D. diss., University of California, Davis, 1973.

Gabaccia, Donna. *We Are What We Eat: Ethnic Food and the Making of Americans*. Cambridge, Mass.: Harvard University Press, 1998.

Gabaccia, Donna, and Vicki Ruiz, eds. *American Dreaming, Global Realities: Rethinking U.S. Immigration History*. Urbana: University of Illinois Press, 2006.

Gaines, Kevin. *Uplifting the Race: Black Leadership, Politics, and Culture in the Twentieth Century*. Chapel Hill: University of North Carolina Press, 1996.

García, Enric. *¿España neutral?: La marina mercante española durante la primera guerra mundial*. Madrid: Real del Catorce Editores, 2005.

Gerstle, Gary, and John Mollenkopf, eds. *E Pluribus Unum?: Contemporary and Historical Perspectives on Immigrant Political Incorporation*. New York: Russell Sage Foundation, 2001.

Gervais, Michel, Marcel Jollivet, and Yves Tavernier. *La fin de la France paysanne depuis 1914*. Histoire de la France Rurale 4. Paris: Éditions du Seuil, 1977.

Ghaneabassiri, Kamyar. "U.S. Foreign Policy and Persia, 1856–1921." *Iranian Studies* 35, no. 1/3 (Winter-Summer 2002): 145–75.

Giles, Judy. *The Parlour and the Suburb: Domestic Identities, Class, Femininity and Modernity*. Oxford: Berg, 2004.

Gilman, Sander. *Fat: A Cultural History of Obesity*. Cambridge, U.K.: Polit Press, 2008.

Gilmore, Glenda Elizabeth. *Defying Dixie: The Radical Roots of Civil Rights, 1919–1950*. New York: W. W. Norton, 2008.

———. *Gender and Jim Crow: Women and the Politics of White Supremacy in North Carolina, 1896–1920*. Chapel Hill: University of North Carolina Press, 1996.

———, ed. *Who Were the Progressives? Historians at Work*. Boston: Bedford/St. Martin's, 2002.

Glazer-Malbin, Nona. "Housework." *Signs* 1, no. 4 (Summer 1976): 905–22.

Goldin, Claudia. *Understanding the Gender Gap: An Economic History of American Women*. New York: Oxford University Press, 1990.

Goldstein, Carolyn. *Creating Consumers: Home Economists in Twentieth-Century America*. Chapel Hill: University of North Carolina Press, 2012.

———. "From Service to Sales: Home Economics in Light and Power, 1920–1940." *Technology and Culture* 38, no. 1, Gender Analysis and the History of Technology (January 1997): 121–52.

Gordon, Linda. *Pitied but Not Entitled: Single Mothers and the History of Welfare, 1890–1935*. New York: Free Press, 1994.

Grandin, Greg. *Empire's Workshop: Latin America, the United States, and the Rise of the New Imperialism*. New York: Metropolitan Books, 2006.

Gratzer, W. B. *Terrors of the Table: The Curious History of Nutrition*. Oxford: Oxford University Press, 2005.

Grier, Katherine C. *Pets in America: A History*. Chapel Hill: University of North Carolina Press, 2006.

Griffith, R. Marie. *Born Again Bodies: Flesh and Spirit in American Christianity*. Berkeley: University of California Press, 2004.

Grossman, James R. *Land of Hope: Chicago, Black Southerners, and the Great Migration*. Chicago: University of Chicago Press, 1989.

Guterl, Matthew Pratt. *The Color of Race in America, 1900–1940*. Cambridge, Mass.: Harvard University Press, 2001.

Guthman, Julie. "Can't Stomach It: How Michael Pollan et al. Made Me Want to Eat Cheetos." *Gastronomica: The Journal of Food and Culture* 7, no. 3 (Summer 2007): 75–79.

———. *Weighing In: Obesity, Food Justice, and the Limits of Capitalism*. Berkeley: University of California Press, 2011.

Hahamovitch, Cindy. *The Fruits of Their Labor: Atlantic Coast Farmworkers and the Making of Migrant Poverty, 1870–1945*. Chapel Hill: University of North Carolina Press, 1997.

Haley, Andrew. *Turning the Tables: Restaurants and the Rise of the American Middle Class, 1880–1920*. Chapel Hill: University of North Carolina Press, 2011.

Hall, Tom G. "Wilson and the Food Crisis: Agricultural Price Control during World War I." *Agricultural History* 47, no. 1 (January 1973): 25–46.

Hamlin, Kimberly. "Bathing Suits and Backlash: The First Miss America Pageants, 1921–1927." In *There She Is, Miss America: The Politics of Sex, Beauty, and Race in America's Most Famous Pageant*, edited by Elwood Watson and Darcy Martin, 27–52. New York: Palgrave Macmillan, 2004.

Harvey, Paul. *Redeeming the South: Religious Cultures and Racial Identities among Southern Baptists, 1865–1925*. Chapel Hill: University of North Carolina Press, 1997.

Hayden, Dolores. *The Grand Domestic Revolution: A History of Feminist Designs for American Homes, Neighborhoods, and Cities*. Cambridge, Mass.: MIT Press, 1981.

Hays, Sharon. *The Cultural Contradictions of Motherhood*. New Haven: Yale University Press, 1996.

Heldke, Lisa. "Let's Cook Thai: Recipes for Colonialism." *Pilaf, Pozole, and Pad Thai: American Women and Ethnic Food*, edited by Sherrie Inness. Amherst: University of Massachusetts Press, 2001.

Higgs, Robert. "The Boll Weevil, the Cotton Economy, and Black Migration, 1910–1930." *Agricultural History* 50, no. 2 (April 1976): 335–50.

Hochschild, Arlie Russell. *The Commercialization of Intimate Life: Notes from Home and Work*. Berkeley: University of California Press, 2003.

Hoerder, Dirk, and Horst Rossler, eds. *Distant Magnets: Expectations and Realities in the Immigrant Experience, 1840–1930*. New York: Holmes & Meier, 1993.

Hoganson, Kristin. *Consumers' Imperium: The Global Production of American Domesticity, 1865–1920*. Chapel Hill: University of North Carolina Press, 2007.

Holland, Patricia. "Lydia Maria Child as a Nineteenth-Century Professional Author." *Studies in the American Renaissance* (1981): 157–67.

Holt, Marilyn Irvin. *Linoleum, Better Babies, and the Modern Farm Woman, 1890–1930*. Albuquerque: University of New Mexico Press, 1995.

Igo, Sarah Elizabeth. *The Averaged American: Surveys, Citizens, and the Making of a Mass Public*. Cambridge, Mass.: Harvard University Press, 2007.

Inness, Sherrie. "Eating Ethnic." In *Pilaf, Pozole, and Pad Thai: American Women and Ethnic Food*, edited by Sherrie Inness, 1–16. Amherst: University of Massachusetts Press, 2001.

Jackson Lears, T. J. *No Place of Grace: Antimodernism and the Transformation of American Culture, 1880–1920*. New York: Pantheon Books, 1981.

Jacobs, Meg. *Pocketbook Politics: Economic Citizenship in Twentieth-Century America*. Princeton, N.J.: Princeton University Press, 2005.

Jacobson, Matthew Frye. *Whiteness of a Different Color: European Immigrants and the Alchemy of Race*. Cambridge, Mass.: Harvard University Press, 1998.

Johnston, Josée, and Shyon Baumann. *Foodies: Democracy and Distinction in the Gourmet Foodscape*. New York: Routledge, 2010.

Jou, Chin. *Controlling Consumption: The Origins of Modern American Ideas about Food, Eating, and Fat, 1886–1930*. Ph.D. diss., Princeton University, 2009.

Karpinski, Joanne, ed. *Critical Essays on Charlotte Perkins Gilman*. New York: G. K. Hall, 1992.

Kasson, John. *Houdini, Tarzan, and the Perfect Man: The White Male Body and the Challenge of Modernity in America*. New York: Hill and Wang, 2001.

——. *Rudeness and Civility: Manners in Nineteenth-Century Urban America*. New York: Hill and Wang, 1991.

Katzman, David M. *Seven Days a Week: Women and Domestic Service in Industrializing America*. New York: Oxford University Press, 1978.

Kazin, Michael, and Joseph A. McCartin, eds. *Americanism: New Perspectives on the History of an Ideal*. Chapel Hill: University of North Carolina Press, 2006.

Kennedy, David M. *Freedom from Fear: The American People in Depression and War, 1929–1945*. New York: Oxford University Press, 1999.

——. *Over Here: The First World War and American Society*. New York: Oxford University Press, 1980.

Kessler-Harris, Alice. *Gendering Labor History*. Urbana: University of Illinois Press, 2006.

———. *Out to Work: A History of America's Wage-Earning Women in the United States*. New York: Oxford University Press, 1982.

Kevles, Daniel. *In the Name of Eugenics: Genetics and the Uses of Human Heredity*. New York: Knopf, 1985.

Kingsbury, Celia. "In Close Touch with her Government: Women and the Domestic Science Movement in World War One Propaganda." In *The Recipe Reader: Narratives—Contexts—Traditions*, edited by Janet Floyd and Laurel Forster, 88–104. Aldershot, Hants, England: Ashgate, 2003.

Kirby, Ethyn Williams. "Sermons before the Commons, 1640–42." *American Historical Review* 44, no. 3 (April 1939): 528–48.

Kirkland, Anna. "The Environmental Account of Obesity: A Case for Feminist Skepticism." *Signs* 36, no. 2 (Winter 2011): 463–85.

Knobloch, Frieda. *The Culture of Wilderness: Agriculture as Colonization in the American West*. Chapel Hill: University of North Carolina Press, 1996.

Koistinen, Paul. *Mobilizing for Modern War: The Political Economy of American Warfare, 1865–1919*. Lawrence: University Press of Kansas, 1997.

Kolko, Gabriel. *The Triumph of Conservatism: A Re-Interpretation of American History, 1900–1916*. New York: Free Press, 1977.

Komlos, John. *Stature, Living Standards, and Economic Development: Essays in Anthropometric History*. Chicago: University of Chicago Press, 1994.

———, ed. *The Biological Standard of Living on Three Continents: Further Explorations in Anthropometric History*. Boulder, Colo.: Westview Press, 1995.

Komlos, John, and Timothy Cuff, eds. *Classics in Anthropometric History*. St. Katharinen, Germany: Scripta Mercaturae Verlag, 1998.

Laird, Ross. *Brunswick Records: A Discography of Recordings, 1916–1931*. Discographies 87. Westport, Conn.: Greenwood Press, 2001.

Lancaster, Jane. *Making Time: Lillian Moller Gilbreth—A Life Beyond "Cheaper by the Dozen."* Boston: Northeastern University Press, 2004.

Largent, Mark. *Breeding Contempt: The History of Coerced Sterilization in the United States*. New Brunswick, N.J.: Rutgers University Press, 2008.

Leavitt, Sarah Abigail. *From Catharine Beecher to Martha Stewart: A Cultural History of Domestic Advice*. Chapel Hill: University of North Carolina Press, 2002.

L'effort du ravitaillement français, pendant la guerre et pour la paix, 1914–1920. Paris: Librairie Félix Alcan, n.d.

Lentz-Smith, Adriane. *Freedom Struggles: African Americans and World War I*. Cambridge, Mass.: Harvard University Press, 2009.

Levenstein, Harvey. "The American Response to Italian Food, 1880–1930." *Food & Foodways* 1, no. 1 (1985): 1–24.

———. *Paradox of Plenty: A Social History of Eating in Modern America*. Berkeley: University of California Press, 2003.

———. *Revolution at the Table: The Transformation of the American Diet*. Berkeley: University of California Press, 2003.

Lévi-Strauss, Claude. *Totemism*. Translated by Rodney Needham. Boston: Beacon Press, 1963.

Levine, Carol. "The First Ban: How Teddy Roosevelt Saved Saccharin." *Hastings Center Report* 7, no. 6 (December 1977): 6–7.

Link, William A. *The Paradox of Southern Progressivism, 1880–1930*. Chapel Hill: University of North Carolina Press, 1992.

Lowe, Margaret. "From Robust Appetite to Calorie Counting: The Emergence of Dieting among Smith College Students in the 1920s." In *Women and Health in America: Historical Readings*. 2d ed., edited by Judith Walzer Leavitt, 172–90. Madison: University of Wisconsin Press, 1999.

Macleod, David. "Food Prices, Politics, and Policy in the Progressive Era." *Journal of the Gilded Age and Progressive Era* 8, no. 3 (July 2009): 365–406.

Majd, Mohammad Gholi. *The Great Famine and Genocide in Persia, 1917–1919*. Lanham, Md.: University Press of America, 2003.

Margolis, Maxine L. *Mothers and Such: Views of American Women and Why They Changed*. Berkeley: University of California Press, 1984.

Markel, H. "When It Rains It Pours: Endemic Goiter, Iodized Salt, and David Murray Cowie, MD." *American Journal of Public Health* 77, no. 2 (February 1987): 219–29.

Marks, Carole. *Farewell—We're Good and Gone: The Great Black Migration*. Bloomington: Indiana University Press, 1989.

Matthews, Glenna. *"Just a Housewife": The Rise and Fall of Domesticity in America*. New York: Oxford University Press, 1987.

May, Elaine Tyler. *Homeward Bound: American Families in the Cold War Era*. New York: Basic Books, 1988.

McBride, Theresa M. *The Domestic Revolution: The Modernisation of Household Service in England and France, 1820–1920*. London: Croom Helm, 1976.

——. "The Modernization of 'Woman's Work.'" *Journal of Modern History* 49, no. 2 (June 1977): 231–45.

McCusker, John J. *How Much Is That in Real Money? A Historical Commodity Price Index for Use as a Deflator of Money Values in the Economy of the United States*. 2d ed. Worcester, Mass.: American Antiquarian Society, 2001.

McElya, Micki. *Clinging to Mammy: The Faithful Slave in Twentieth-Century America*. Cambridge, Mass.: Harvard University Press, 2007.

McIntosh, E. N. *American Food Habits in Historical Perspective*. Westport, Conn.: Praeger, 1995.

McWilliams, James. *A Revolution in Eating: How the Quest for Food Shaped America*. New York: Columbia University Press, 2005.

Mead, Margaret. "The Changing Significance of Food." In *Food and Culture: A Reader*, edited by Carole Counihan and Penny Van Esterik, 11–19. New York: Routledge, 1997.

Mennell, Stephen. *All Manners of Food: Eating and Taste in England and France from the Middle Ages to the Present*. Oxford: B. Blackwell, 1985.

Merleaux, April. "Sweet Innocence: Child Labor Reform, Mexican Americans, and U.S. Sugar Politics, 1908–1934." Unpublished paper presented at Yale Esquina Latina. February 2005.

Meyer, Stephen. "Adapting the Immigrant to the Line: Americanization in the Ford Factory, 1914–1921." *Journal of Social History* 14, no. 1 (Autumn 1980): 67–82.

Meyerowitz, Joanne. *Women Adrift: Independent Wage Earners in Chicago, 1880–1930*. Chicago: University of Chicago Press, 1988.

Miller, Sally M. *From Prairie to Prison: The Life of Social Activist Kate Richards O'Hare*. Columbia: University of Missouri Press, 1993.

Mintz, Sidney. *Sweetness and Power: The Place of Sugar in Modern History*. New York: Viking, 1985.

Mintz, Steven. *Domestic Revolutions: A Social History of American Family Life*. New York: Free Press, 1988.

Morgan, Ted. *Reds: McCarthyism in Twentieth-Century America*. Vol. 1. New York: Random House, 2003.

Mosse, George L. *The Image of Man: The Creation of Modern Masculinity*. New York: Oxford University Press, 1996.

Motz, Marilyn Ferris, and Pat Browne, eds. *Making the American Home: Middle-Class Women and Domestic Material Culture, 1840–1940*. Bowling Green, Ohio: Bowling Green State University Popular Press, 1988.

Nash, George. *The Life of Herbert Hoover: The Engineer, 1874–1914*. New York: W. W. Norton, 1983.

———. *The Life of Herbert Hoover: The Humanitarian, 1914–1917*. New York: W. W. Norton, 1988.

———. *The Life of Herbert Hoover: Master of Emergencies, 1917–1918*. New York: W. W. Norton, 1996.

Nash, Lee, ed. *Understanding Herbert Hoover: Ten Perspectives*. Stanford: Hoover Institution Press, 1988.

Neuhaus, Jesamyn. *Manly Meals and Mom's Home Cooking: Cookbooks and Gender in Modern America*. Baltimore: Johns Hopkins University Press, 2003.

Nissenbaum, Stephen. *Sex, Diet, and Debility in Jacksonian America: Sylvester Graham and Health Reform*. Westport, Conn.: Greenwood Press, 1980.

Norton, Mary Beth, and Ruth Alexander. "Women Work and Work Culture in Modern America, 1890–1920s." In *Major Problems in American Women's History*, edited by Mary Beth Norton and Ruth Alexander. 4th ed. Boston: Houghton Mifflin, 2007.

Nostrand, Richard, and Lawrence E. Estaville, eds. *Homelands: A Geography of Culture and Place Across America*. Baltimore: Johns Hopkins University Press, 2001.

Nye, David. *Electrifying America: Social Meanings of a New Technology, 1880–1940*. Cambridge, Mass.: MIT Press, 1990.

Offer, Avner. *The First World War: An Agrarian Interpretation*. Oxford: Clarendon Press, 1989.

Ogden, Annegret. *The Great American Housewife: From Helpmate to Wage Earner, 1776–1986*. Westport, Conn.: Greenwood Press, 1986.

Ordish, G. *The Constant Pest: A Short History of Pests and Their Control*. New York: Charles Scribner's Sons, 1976.

Osband, Kent. "The Boll Weevil Versus 'King Cotton.'" *The Journal of Economic History* 45, no. 3 (September 1985): 627–43.

Oxford English Dictionary. Oxford: Oxford University Press, 2006.

Packman, Ana Bégué. *Early California Hospitality: The Cookery Customs of Spanish California.* Glendale, Calif.: Arthur H. Clark, 1938.

Palmer, Phyllis. *Domesticity and Dirt: Housewives and Domestic Servants in the United States, 1920–1945.* Philadelphia: Temple University Press, 1989.

Patenaude, Bertrand M. *The Big Show in Bololand: The American Relief Expedition to Soviet Russia in the Famine of 1921.* Stanford, Calif.: Stanford University Press, 2002.

Paul, Diane B. *The Politics of Heredity: Essays on Eugenics, Biomedicine, and the Nature-Nurture Debate.* Albany: State University of New York Press, 1998.

Pernick, Martin. *The Black Stork: Eugenics and the Death of "Defective" Babies in American Medicine and Motion Pictures since 1915.* New York: Oxford University Press, 1995.

Petrick, Gabriella. "An Ambivalent Diet: The Industrialization of Canning." *OAH Magazine of History,* July 2010.

———. "Feeding the Masses: H. J. Heinz and the Creation of Industrial Food." *Endeavour* 33, no. 1 (March 2009): 29–34.

———. "'Like Ribbons of Green and Gold': Industrializing Lettuce and the Quest for Quality in the Salinas Valley, 1920–1965." *Agricultural History* 80, no. 3 (Summer 2006): 269–95.

Pickus, Noah M. Jedidiah. *True Faith and Allegiance: Immigration and American Civic Nationalism.* Princeton, N.J.: Princeton University Press, 2005.

Pilcher, Jeffrey. *Que Vivan los Tamales! Food and the Making of Mexican Identity.* Albuquerque: University of New Mexico Press, 1998.

Portes, Alejandro. *Immigrant America: A Portrait.* 3d ed. Berkeley: University of California Press, 2006.

Preece, Amelia Grace. *Housework and American Standards of Living, 1920–1980.* Ph.D. diss., University of California, 1990.

Preston, Samuel. *Fatal Years: Child Mortality in Late Nineteenth-Century America.* Princeton, N.J.: Princeton University Press, 1991.

Rabinbach, Anson. *The Human Motor: Energy, Fatigue, and the Origins of Modernity.* New York: Basic Books, 1990.

Rauchway, Eric. "The High Cost of Living in the Progressives' Economy." *Journal of American History* 88, no. 3 (December 2001): 898–924.

Riley, James C. "Height, Nutrition, and Mortality Risk Reconsidered." *Journal of Interdisciplinary History* 24, no. 3 (Winter 1994): 465–92.

———. *Rising Life Expectancy: A Global History.* New York: Cambridge University Press, 2001.

Ritvo, Harriet. *The Platypus and the Mermaid, and Other Figments of the Classifying Imagination.* Cambridge, Mass.: Harvard University Press, 1997.

Rodgers, Daniel. *Atlantic Crossings: Social Politics in a Progressive Age.* Cambridge, Mass.: Belknap Press of Harvard University Press, 1998.

Rossiter, Margaret W. *Women Scientists in America: Before Affirmative Action, 1940–1972*. Baltimore: Johns Hopkins University Press, 1995.

———. *Women Scientists in America: Struggles and Strategies to 1940*. Baltimore: Johns Hopkins University Press, 1982.

Rothbard, Murray. "Hoover's 1919 Food Diplomacy in Retrospect." In *Herbert Hoover—The Great War and Its Aftermath, 1914–1923*, edited by Lawrence Gelfand. Iowa City: University of Iowa Press, 1979.

Rudd, Jill, and Val Gough. *Charlotte Perkins Gilman: Optimist Reformer*. Iowa City: University of Iowa Press, 1999.

Rutherford, Janice Williams. *Selling Mrs. Consumer: Christine Frederick and the Rise of Household Efficiency*. Athens, Ga.: University of Georgia Press, 2003.

Rutkoff, Peter, and Will Scott. *Fly Away: The Great African American Cultural Migrations*. Baltimore: Johns Hopkins University Press, 2010.

Ryan, Barbara. *Love, Wages, Slavery: The Literature of Servitude in the United States*. Urbana: University of Illinois Press, 2006.

Sanders, Elizabeth. *Roots of Reform: Farmers, Workers, and the American State, 1877–1917*. Chicago: University of Chicago Press, 1999.

Schwartz, Hillel. *Never Satisfied: A Cultural History of Diets, Fantasies, and Fat*. New York: Free Press, 1986.

Scott, Anne Firor. *Natural Allies: Women's Associations in American History*. Urbana: University of Illinois Press, 1991.

Scott, Susan, and Christopher J. Duncan. *Demography and Nutrition: Evidence from Historical and Contemporary Populations*. Oxford: Blackwell Science, 2002.

Seashore, Carl E. "Origin of the Term 'Euthenics.'" *Science* 95, no. 2470 (1 May 1942): 455–56.

Seid, Roberta Pollack. *Never Too Thin: Why Women Are at War with Their Bodies*. New York: Prentice Hall Press, 1989.

Selig, Diana. *Americans All: The Cultural Gifts Movement*. Cambridge, Mass.: Harvard University Press, 2008.

Shapiro, Laura. *Perfection Salad: Women and Cooking at the Turn of the Century*. New York: Modern Library, 2001.

Skrabec, Quentin, Jr. *H. J. Heinz: A Biography*. Jefferson, N.C.: McFarland, 2009.

Smith-Rosenberg, Carroll. *Disorderly Conduct: Visions of Gender in Victorian America*. New York: Knopf, 1985.

Sorin, Gerald. *A Time for Building: The Third Migration, 1880–1920*. Baltimore: Johns Hopkins University Press, 1992.

Stage, Sarah, and Virginia Vincenti, eds. *Rethinking Home Economics: Women and the History of a Profession*. Ithaca, N.Y.: Cornell University Press, 1997.

Stavney, Anne. "'Mothers of Tomorrow': The New Negro Renaissance and the Politics of Maternal Representation." *African American Review* 32, no. 4 (Winter 1998): 533–61.

Stearns, Peter. *Fat History: Bodies and Beauty in the Modern West*. New York: New York University Press, 1997.

Stears, Marc. *Progressives, Pluralists, and the Problems of the State: Ideologies of Reform in the United States and Britain, 1909–1926.* Oxford: Oxford University Press, 2002.

Stern, Alexandra Minna. "Making Better Babies: Public Health and Race Betterment in Indiana, 1920–1935." *American Journal of Public Health* 92, no. 5 (May 2002): 742–52.

Stewart, Mary Lynn. *For Health and Beauty: Physical Culture for Frenchwomen, 1880s–1930s.* Baltimore: Johns Hopkins University Press, 2001.

Stigler, George Joseph, and National Bureau of Economic Research. *Domestic Servants in the United States, 1900–1940.* New York: National Bureau of Economic Research, 1946.

Strasser, Susan. *Never Done: A History of American Housework.* New York: Pantheon Books, 1982.

Strickland, Arvarh E. "The Strange Affair of the Boll Weevil: The Pest as Liberator." *Agricultural History* 68, no. 2 (Spring 1994): 157–68.

Stubbs, K. D. *Race to the Front: The Materiel Foundations of Coalition Strategy in the Great War, 1914–1918.* Westport, Conn.: Praeger, 2002.

Sutherland, Daniel. *Americans and Their Servants: Domestic Service in the United States from 1800 to 1920.* Baton Rouge: Louisiana State University Press, 1981.

Swain, Robert. "Ray Lyman Wilbur: 1875–1949." *Science* 111, no. 2883 (31 March 1950): 324–27.

Szymanski, Ann-Marie. *Pathways to Prohibition: Radicals, Moderates, and Social Movement Outcomes.* Durham, N.C.: Duke University Press, 2003.

Taylor, Lynne. "Food Riots Revisited." *Journal of Social History* 30, no. 2 (Winter 1996): 483–96.

Todd, Jan. *Physical Culture and the Body Beautiful: Purposive Exercise in the Lives of American Women, 1800–1870.* Macon, Ga.: Mercer University Press, 1998.

Trotter, Joe William, ed. *The Great Migration in Historical Perspective: New Dimensions of Race, Class, and Gender.* Bloomington: Indiana University Press, 1991.

Tucker, Todd. *The Great Starvation Experiment: The Heroic Men Who Starved So That Millions Could Live.* New York: Free Press, 2006.

Tyrrell, Ian R. *Woman's World/Woman's Empire: The Woman's Christian Temperance Union in International Perspective, 1800–1930.* Chapel Hill: University of North Carolina Press, 1991.

Van Wienen, Mark. "Poetics of the Frugal Housewife: A Modernist Narrative of the Great War and America." *American Literary History* 7, no. 1 (Spring 1995): 55–91.

Verbrugge, Martha. "Gender, Science & Fitness: Perspectives on Women's Exercise in the United States in the 20th Century." *Health and History* 4, no. 1 (2002): 52–72.

Vester, Katharina. "Regime Change: Gender, Class, and the Invention of Dieting in Post-Bellum America." *Journal of Social History* 44, no. 1 (Fall 2010): 39–67.

Vincent, Charles Paul. *The Politics of Hunger: The Allied Blockade of Germany, 1915–1919.* Athens: Ohio University Press, 1985.

Walch, Timothy. *Immigrant America: European Ethnicity in the United States.* New York: Garland, 1994.

Wallerstein, Mitchel. *Food for War—Food for Peace: United States Food Aid in a Global Context*. Cambridge, Mass.: MIT Press, 1980.

Waller-Zuckerman, Mary Ellen. "'Old Homes, in a City of Perpetual Change': Women's Magazines, 1890–1916." *Business History Review* 63, no. 4 (Winter 1989): 715–56.

Weigley, Emma Seifrit. "It Might Have Been Euthenics: The Lake Placid Conferences and the Home Economics Movement." *American Quarterly* 26, no. 1 (March 1974): 79–96.

Weissman, Benjamin. *Herbert Hoover and Famine Relief to Soviet Russia, 1921–1923*. Stanford, Calif.: Hoover Institution Press, 1974.

Welch, David. *Germany, Propaganda and Total War, 1914–1918: The Sins of Omission*. London: Athalone Press, 2000.

White, Barbara Anne. *The Beecher Sisters*. New Haven: Yale University Press, 2003.

Whorton, James C. *Crusaders for Fitness: The History of American Health Reformers*. Princeton, N.J.: Princeton University Press, 1982.

Wiebe, Robert H. *The Search for Order, 1877–1920*. New York: Hill and Wang, 1967.

Wienen, Mark Van. "Poetics of the Frugal Housewife: A Modernist Narrative of the Great War and America." *American Literary History* 7, no. 1 (Spring 1995): 55–91.

Wilkerson, Isabel. *The Warmth of Other Suns: The Epic Story of America's Great Migration*. New York: Random House, 2010.

Williams-Forson, Psyche. *Building Houses out of Chicken Legs: Black Women, Food, and Power*. Chapel Hill: University of North Carolina Press, 2006.

Wilson, Joan Hoff. *Herbert Hoover: Forgotten Progressive*. Boston: Little, Brown, 1975.

Winter, Jay, and Jean-Louis Robert, eds. *Capital Cities at War: Paris, London, Berlin, 1914–1919*. New York: Cambridge University Press, 1997.

Winter, Jay. *The Great War and the British People*. 2d ed. Balsingstoke: Palgrave, 2003.

Wood, David L. "American Indian Farmland and the Great War." *Agricultural History* 55, no. 3 (July 1981): 249–65.

Yellin, Jean Fagan, and Cynthia D. Bond. *The Pen Is Ours: A Listing of Writings by and about African-American Women*. New York: Oxford University Press, 1991.

Young, Nancy Beck. *Lou Henry Hoover: Activist First Lady*. Lawrence: University Press of Kansas, 2004.

Zuckerman, Larry. *The Rape of Belgium: The Untold Story of World War I*. New York: New York University Press, 2004.

INDEX

Italic page numbers refer to illustrations or illustration captions.

production in, 61, 191 (n. 11), 215
(n. 23); wartime food regulations in,
61–62, 215 (n. 28); food riots in, 62;
food shortages in, 63–64; national
cuisine, 67–69, 126–27, 128, 141. *See
also* Foreign foods
Frederick, Christine, 152, 154, 166,
177–78, 182–83
Fruits and vegetables, elevated
importance of, 47–48, 183
Funk, Casimir, 48

Garlic, 143
Germ theory of disease. *See* Hygiene
German Americans, 30, 194 (n. 35)
German occupation of France and
Belgium, 15, 62, 191 (n. 11)
Gilman, Charlotte Perkins, 88–89
Gluttony, 8, 19, 20, 22, 23, 131, 169, 246
(n. 41)
Goldberger, Joseph, 110
Graham, Sylvester, 41

Harding, Warren, 24
Height, as proxy for nutrition levels, 104,
106, 267 (n. 4)
Heinz, Henry, 142
Heinz, Howard, 19
Hoarding, 17, 29, 30, 32, 62, 164, 193–94
(n. 35); comparison to overeating,
163–64
Home economics, 3, 6, 77–100 passim;
dissemination of nutrition science
through, 26, 42, 45, 48, 85; success
of basic reforms, 83; resistance
to, 84; centrality of science to,
84–85; expansion of in response to
World War I, 91–92; relationship
of to suffrage campaign, 96–97;
relationship of to racial sciences, 104
Hoover, Herbert, 5, 12, 17–35 passim,
39, 51, 53–54, 56, 58–74 passim,
92, 111, 164, *165*, 196 (n. 69), 203
(n. 170), 222–23 (n. 126); as head of
Commission for Relief in Belgium,

14–15, 58, 191 (n. 10), 203 (n. 169);
international reputation of, 15, 63;
enthusiasm for strong government,
31–32, 34, 222 (n. 120); cult of
personality around, 33–34, 163
Hoover, Lou Henry, 23, 67, 116
Housewife, 77–100 passim;
modernization of role, 6, 79, 81,
82, 85–88, 90, 93–95, 100, 184,
226 (n. 53); as pivot of world food
system, 66–67; history of, 78–79;
professionalization of role, 79, 85–86,
88, 90, 95, 100, 226 (n. 55); familial
rhetoric surrounding, 79, 90–91, 96;
uniforms for, 85, 86, *87*; resistance to
term "housewife," 95–96
Hull House, 89
Hunger: of European civilians, 12, 72,
182; strategic use of in foreign policy,
71–73. *See also* Fasting
Hygiene, 50, 84, 85, 100, 104, 106, 120,
123, 126, 144; germ theory of disease,
52, 84

Immigrants, 7, 78, 123–27, 132–37,
139, 140, 155, 233 (n. 14); and
race, 126, 135; and beliefs about
body fat, 160, 257 (n. 16). *See also*
Americanization
Immigration Restriction Act of 1924,
125, 155
Imported food, 130–31, 147, 244 (n. 4),
254 (n. 165); in Europe, 14, 15, 214
(n. 18)
Industrialization of food and agriculture,
44, 89, 142, 144, 151–52, 153–54, 183,
184; and relationship of to weight
gain, 161. *See also* Canned food
Intelligence: as basis for modern
housework, 82–83, 88, 100, 224
(n. 25)
Inter-Allied food board, 59
Italian cuisine: pasta, 7, 57, 140–45,
192 (n. 15), 251 (n. 117); garlic, 143;
broccoli, 148

Race: and diet, 3, 7, 102–13 passim, 119, 123, 128–30, 144, 145, 233 (n. 20); and associations with enjoying eating, 30–31; racial degeneration, 50, 107, 118–20, 233 (n. 16); and intelligence, 82–83; and immigrant groups, 126, 135. *See also* Eugenics; Euthenics
Racial sciences. *See* Eugenics; Euthenics
Rationalizing food habits, 3, 4, 5, 8, 37–57 passim, 146, 181, 184
Rationing, 5, 35; desires for, 11–12, 30–31, 202 (n. 148); in Lever Act, 17–18; in Germany, 29; secret support of U.S. food administrators for, 31–32
Refrigeration, 3, 49, 81, 183
Regional cuisines, 152–54, 255–56 (n. 205). *See also* Southern diets
Religiosity in food conservation campaign, 26–29
Religious organizations: in temperance movement, 21; role of in food conservation campaign, 27–29, 199 (n. 120)
Requisitioning of food, 15–16
Restaurants: United States Food Administration rules for, 19, 193–94 (n. 35); foreign, 135, 141, 145, 148, 251 (n. 116)
Rice, 108–9, 235 (nn. 49–50). *See also* Asian cuisines
Richards, Ellen, 137
Rickets, 22, 85
Rombauer, Irma, 147, 167
Roosevelt, Franklin D., 31–32
Rose, Flora, 84

Science. *See* Eugenics; Euthenics; Home economics; Nutrition science; Statistics; Technology
Self-control, 4, 5, 8, 11, 14, 19, 20, 34, 35; political value of, 4, 5, 14, 29, 30–31, 33, 35, 36, 179, 181–82; moral value of, 20, 26, 36, 38, 51, 56, 186–87; racial beliefs about, 30–31, 116; applied to weight loss, 157–58, 159,

160, 166–80 passim, 186–87. *See also* Asceticism; Willpower
Self-denial. *See* Asceticism
Self-discipline. *See* Self-control
Servitude: the servant problem, 3, 80; associations with housework, 6, 77–78, 79, 80–81, 88, 99–100, 184; early history of, 78–79, 80; decline of in twentieth century, 79; and African Americans, 92; and World War I, 92
Seventh-Day Adventists, 27
Sherman, Henry, 26
Slavery, 79, 90; and familial rhetoric, 91. *See also* Mammy figures
Smiley, Portia, 101–2, 121–22
Smith-Hughes Act, 83
Smith-Lever Act, 83
Smoot, Reed, 28
Southern diets, 109–11; nostalgia for Old South cuisine, 101–2, 152–53, 154
Spaghetti. *See* Pasta
Spain, 64
Spices, 129, 130, 131, 143, 147–48. *See also* Foreign foods; Pleasure of eating
Statistics, 155, 159, 194 (n. 39), 256 (n. 211)
Stature. *See* Height, as proxy for nutrition levels
Stedman, Myrtle, 174
Substitute foods: for meat, 5, 43–44, 52–53; for wartime food conservation, 11, 12, 15, 18, 23, 25, 26, 51–52; to optimize nutrition, 45–46, 51. *See also* Nutritional equivalency among foods
Suffrage, woman, 6, 96–99, 129, 230 (n. 111), 231 (n. 118), 231 (n. 125). *See also* Antisuffrage campaign
Sunday, Billy, 27, 60
Sylvia of Hollywood. *See* Ullback, Sylvia

Taft, William, 175
Talley, Marion, 168
Tarbell, Ida, 99
Taste. *See* Pleasure in eating; Spices
Taylor, Alonzo, 23, 63

Made in the USA
Coppell, TX
21 January 2024